APPLETON & LANGE'S

PRACTICE TESTS
for the **USMLE**
Step 2

DR. JOEL S. GOLDBERG
ASSISTANT PROFESSOR OF MEDICINE
DEPARTMENT OF MEDICINE
HAHNEMANN UNIVERSITY SCHOOL OF MEDICINE
PHILADELPHIA, PENNSYLVANIA

APPLETON & LANGE
Stamford, Connecticut

Copyright © 1999 by Appleton & Lange

All rights reserved. This book, or any parts thereof, may not be used or reproduced in any manner without written permission. For information, address Appleton & Lange, Four Stamford Plaza, PO Box 120041, Stamford, Connecticut 06912-0041.

www.appletonlange.com

99 00 01 02 / 10 9 8 7 6 5 4 3 2 1

Prentice Hall International (UK) Limited, *London*
Prentice Hall of Australia Pty. Limited, *Sydney*
Prentice Hall Canada, Inc., *Toronto*
Prentice Hall Hispanoamericana, S.A., *Mexico*
Prentice Hall of India Private Limited, *New Delhi*
Prentice Hall of Japan, Inc., *Tokyo*
Simon & Schuster Asia Pte. Ltd., *Singapore*
Editora Prentice Hall do Brasil Ltda., *Rio de Janeiro*
Prentice Hall, *Upper Saddle River, New Jersey*

ISBN 0–8385–0372–1

Acquisitions Editor: Jessica M. Hirshon
Production Editor: Mary Ellen McCourt
Production Service: Rainbow Graphics, LLC
Cover Designer: Libby Schmitz

PRINTED IN THE UNITED STATES OF AMERICA

ISBN 0-8385-0372-1

90000

9 780838 503720

For Mickey, Daniel, and Kasey

Contributors

Mary S. Applegate, MD, MPH
Medical Director
Bureau of Women's Health
New York State Department of Health
Director
Preventive Medicine Residency Program
University at Albany School of Public Health
Albany, New York

Christina Clay, MD
Department of Medicine
Thomas Jefferson University Hospital
Philadelphia, Pennsylvania
Department of Medicine
Crozer-Chester Medical Center
Upland, Pennsylvania

Edward A. Emmett, MD, MS
Professor and Director
Center for Occupational and Environmental Health
    Policy and Practice
Department of Medicine
Jefferson Medical College of Thomas Jefferson
    University
Philadelphia, Pennsylvania

Joyce C. Frye, DO, MBA
Instructor of Obstetrics/Gynecology
Medical Director, the Women's Group
Jefferson Medical College of Thomas Jefferson
    University
Philadelphia, Pennsylvania

Vivian Gahtan, MD
Assistant Professor of Surgery
Section of Vascular Surgery
Yale University School of Medicine
New Haven, Connecticut

Morris D. Kerstein, MD
Professor and Vice Chair
Department of Surgery
Mt. Sinai Hospital and Medical Center
New York University School of Medicine
New York, New York

Julie A. Peters, MD
Resident, Department of Psychiatry
Yale University School of Medicine
New Haven, Connecticut

Ivan Oransky, MD
Resident, Department of Psychiatry
Yale University School of Medicine
New Haven, Connecticut

R. Douglas Ross, MD
Associate Professor and Vice Chairman
Chief of Obstetrics and Gynecology
Allegheny University of Health Sciences
Hahnemann School of Medicine
Philadelphia, Pennsylvania

Contents

Preface

Appleton & Lange's Practice Tests for the USMLE Step 2 is a new and exciting tool for exam preparation. This is a current book of practice exams designed to mimic actual testing conditions. Keeping with the trend of computer-based testing, a CD-ROM is included to help familiarize the reader with the format and functionality of the electronic exam.

The test questions have been prepared by specialists in each area and were designed after extensive feedback from students who have taken the examination, and in accordance with the guidelines set forth by the National Board of Medical Examiners. We have ensured that the types of questions presented, as well as the material covered, are typical of the most recent administration of the USMLE Step 2. Additionally, the exact proportion of questions in each subject area is comparable to the actual examination.

In summary, this book will provide you, the student, with six practice tests that will better enable you to simulate and prepare for the licensing exam by providing an excellent and comprehensive review for the USMLE Step 2.

Joel S. Goldberg
Philadelphia, Pennsylvania

Acknowledgments

I wish to extend my appreciation to my Editor at Appleton & Lange, Ms. Jessica Hirshon. Jessica has provided guidance and assistance in all phases of development of this exciting new text. With Jessica's assistance this project has easily overcome the usual production hurdles, developing into an up-to-date and comprehensive new study tool.

I would also like to thank the co-authors of this book for their participation. This exceptional group of physicians devoted countless hours in the preparation of their material.

Practice Test 1
Questions

Questions 1 Through 4

You are called to the newborn nursery to examine a 2-day-old newborn who is slightly jaundiced. Examination discloses a normal-appearing full-term infant in no distress, with good color and cry. The infant's chest is clear, and the heart is regular in rate and rhythm without murmurs. You are unable to find any abnormalities during the remainder of your examination. The history is obtained from the nursing staff and the mother, and appears unremarkable except that the baby's mother received virtually no prenatal care. The mother did have a test for syphilis that was negative, she was immune to rubella, and there is no blood group incompatibility. While further questioning the mother, she admits to you that she used intravenous drugs during the pregnancy "once in a while."

1. Which of the following conditions is this infant likely to be at risk for?

   (A) future central nervous system (CNS) malignancy
   (B) cleft palate
   (C) hepatitis B
   (D) Niemann–Pick disease
   (E) neuroblastoma

2. Which of the following is true about hepatitis B?

   (A) The incubation period is 2 to 5 months.
   (B) Breast feeding by mothers with hepatitis B surface antigen (HBsAg) is contraindicated.
   (C) There is an increased risk of abortion or malformations following hepatitis during the first trimester.
   (D) There is a vaccine available for hepatitis B, but it carries a very small risk of acquired immune deficiency syndrome (AIDS).
   (E) Ingestion of contaminated food or water is a common mode of transmission.

3. Differential diagnosis of jaundice in the newborn includes

   (A) Tourette's syndrome
   (B) clavicular fracture
   (C) hyperuricemia
   (D) homocystinuria
   (E) biliary atresia

4. Which of the following is true about the transmission of hepatitis B from pregnant carriers to their infants?

(A) Hepatitis B tends to be more severe in infants and children.

(B) Only about 2.5% of infants born to positive mothers will be positive for HBsAg at birth.

(C) The presence of hepatitis Be antigen (HBeAg) in maternal carriers does not correlate highly with transmission of hepatitis B infection to their offspring.

(D) Newborns are rarely symptomatic, and most of those infected will not go on to be carriers.

(E) The risk of chronic liver disease or hepatocellular carcinoma is not increased in these infants.

5. The most common female genital tract malignancy in the United States is

(A) vulvar cancer
(B) vaginal cancer
(C) cervical cancer
(D) endometrial cancer
(E) ovarian cancer

Questions 6 Through 8

A 28-year-old man presents with chronic diarrhea, arthritis, and a microcytic anemia. He has not traveled outside the continental United States recently and cannot associate the diarrhea with any particular food or medication. His physical examination is unremarkable apart from conjunctival pallor and some joint stiffness when he first begins to move about after sitting in the waiting room for 20 minutes.

6. The MOST likely diagnosis is

(A) lymphoma of the bowel
(B) amyloid infiltration
(C) chronic pancreatitis
(D) ulcerative colitis
(E) tropical sprue

7. Which of the following is true of ulcerative colitis?

(A) rarely involves the rectum
(B) diffuse, continuous inflammation
(C) may mimic peptic ulcer disease (PUD)
(D) usually associated with weight loss
(E) transmural involvement is common

8. Which of the following laboratory test results is MOST likely to occur in this patient?

(A) low serum iron
(B) elevated total iron-binding capacity (TIBC)
(C) low vitamin B_{12} levels
(D) elevated reticulocyte count
(E) low ferritin

9. A 21-year-old college student presented to student health services with complaints of cough and fever for a few days. On physical examination, an erythematous maculopapular rash was seen, and Koplik's spots were present on the oral mucosa. Which of the following is true concerning this illness?

(A) This illness is more common and more severe in children, compared with infants or adults.

(B) In the typical form, the rash appears first on the torso and then spreads to the extremities.

(C) Conjunctivitis, excessive lacrimation, and photophobia are common symptoms.

(D) Prompt administration of immune globulin soon after exposure does not alter the course of the illness.

(E) Antibody protection after infection lasts for only 2 to 3 years.

10. A man returned from a hunting trip in northern California and found a tick clinging to his scalp. He removed the tick. About 4 days later, he presented with the following symptoms: headache, chills, fever, and vomiting. The site of the tick bite was ulcerated, and the

regional lymph nodes were enlarged. No rash was noted. The most likely diagnosis is

(A) Rocky Mountain spotted fever
(B) tularemia
(C) relapsing fever
(D) plague
(E) dengue fever

Questions 11 and 12

A 64-year-old man presents with a 2-cm lesion at the floor of his mouth and two palpable lymph nodes in the left side of the neck. No other evidence of disease exists. Biopsy confirms the diagnosis of squamous cell carcinoma.

11. What is the MOST appropriate therapy?

   (A) comprehensive irradiation to base of the tongue, larynx, and right neck
   (B) excision of the tumor and left radical neck dissection
   (C) bilateral neck irradiation
   (D) comprehensive irradiation of the nasal pharynx and right neck
   (E) multimodal therapy: surgery, irradiation, and cyclic chemotherapy

12. All of the following structures are removed in radical neck dissection EXCEPT the

   (A) sternocleidomastoid muscle
   (B) external carotid artery
   (C) internal jugular vein
   (D) spinal accessory nerve
   (E) submaxillary gland

13. An obese 61-year-old nulliparous woman, last menstrual period (LMP) 4 years ago, presents for a routine examination without complaints. She is a non–insulin-dependent diabetic with hypertension. After the pelvic examination, she informs you that she has been using her friend's estrogen-containing vaginal cream for vaginal dryness and had two episodes of vaginal bleeding. A pelvic exam reveals a slightly enlarged uterus with no palpable adnexal masses. The MOST appropriate management for this patient's complaints is

(A) reassessment in 3 months
(B) Pap smear
(C) transvaginal ultrasound
(D) office endometrial biopsy
(E) dilation and curettage (D&C) and hysteroscopy

14. The pathologist reports that the endometrial tissue is consistent with grade 3 adenocarcinoma of the endometrium. The patient undergoes a total abdominal hysterectomy, bilateral salpingo-oophorectomy, and pelvic and para-aortic lymph node sampling. Surgical pathology documents a grade 3 adenocarcinoma invading the outer half of the myometrium and positive pelvic lymph nodes. Peritoneal cytology is positive for malignancy. Her stage is

(A) stage IA, grade 3
(B) stage IIB, grade 3
(C) stage IIIC, grade 3
(D) stage IVA, grade 3
(E) stage IVB, grade 3

15. What is the MOST appropriate management for this patient?

(A) total abdominal hysterectomy and bilateral salpingo-oophorectomy
(B) external beam irradiation to the whole pelvis followed by total abdominal hysterectomy and bilateral salpingo-oophorectomy
(C) total abdominal hysterectomy, bilateral salpingo-oophorectomy, pelvic and para-aortic lymph node dissection
(D) option C, followed by tailored external beam irradiation
(E) vaginal hysterectomy followed by external beam irradiation

Questions 16 Through 20

A 65-year-old man, whom you have followed for several years, with mild hypertension presents with progressive dyspnea, orthopnea, paroxysmal nocturnal dyspnea, and peripheral edema. You obtain an electrocardiogram (ECG) (see Figure 1.1).

16. The correct interpretation of this ECG is

    (A) anterior septal myocardial infarct
    (B) left bundle branch block (LBBB)
    (C) left ventricular hypertrophy
    (D) right bundle branch block (RBBB)
    (E) trifascicular block

17. Digoxin may be an effective intervention in this patient because he has most likely developed

    (A) heart failure secondary to anemia
    (B) heart failure secondary to an arteriovenous fistula
    (C) low-output heart failure
    (D) cardiac failure secondary to hyperthyroidism
    (E) infection-induced cardiac failure

18. When this patient is started on digoxin, what percentage of the oral dose might be expected to be absorbed?

    (A) 10 to 20%
    (B) 20 to 35%
    (C) 35 to 50%
    (D) 50 to 75%
    (E) over 75%

19. The patient is started on digoxin and hydrochlorothiazide for control of his hypertension and heart failure, with some improvement. However, he continues to have evidence of left-sided heart failure with mild orthopnea, and captopril is started. Within a short time, the patient's orthopnea is resolved; however, he notes at a routine follow-up appointment that his breasts are swollen and tender. This is MOST likely due to

    (A) hydrochlorothiazide
    (B) captopril
    (C) multivitamins
    (D) normal aging
    (E) digoxin

20. The patient decides that the benefits of continuing the digoxin outweigh the discomfort of the gynecomastia, but at his next check-up reports that now he has developed a persistent nonproductive cough that is intolerable. This is MOST likely due to

    (A) hydrochlorothiazide
    (B) captopril
    (C) multivitamins
    (D) normal aging
    (E) digoxin

21. A 62-year-old man presents with bone pain in his legs that worsens on standing. The skin over his tibia is erythematous and warm. Laboratory studies reveal an elevated alkaline phosphatase. An x-ray taken on this patient is shown in Figure 1.2. The MOST likely diagnosis is

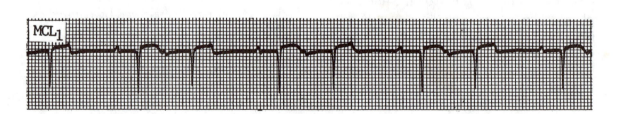

Figure 1.1

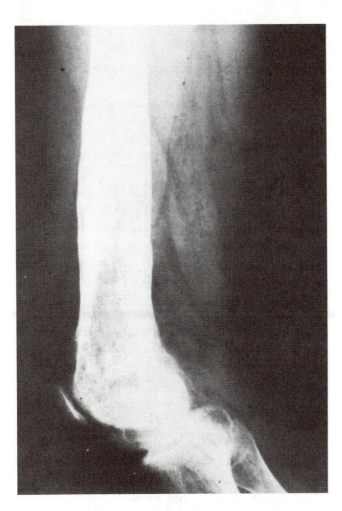

Figure 1.2

(A) osteomalacia
(B) osteoarthritis
(C) calcium pyrophosphate deposition disease
(D) osteomyelitis
(E) Paget's disease

Questions 22 and 23

A 55-year-old man presents with right upper quadrant pain and intermittent referred pain to the right shoulder. Transaminases are moderately elevated.

22. Which study would you obtain next?

    (A) abdominal x-ray series
    (B) colonoscopy
    (C) diagnostic laparoscopy
    (D) upper gastrointestinal (UGI) series
    (E) abdominal ultrasound

23. A lesion is identified in the right lobe of the liver. Needle biopsy is diagnostic for hepatocellular carcinoma. All of the following are true regarding this tumor EXCEPT

    (A) alpha-fetoprotein is markedly elevated
    (B) chronic hepatitis B is a common etiologic factor
    (C) cirrhosis is a common etiologic factor
    (D) the fibrolamellar variant portends a worse prognosis
    (E) aflatoxin B1 has been assoiciated with hepatocellular carcinoma

Questions 24 Through 27

A 19-year-old male presents to your office with a history of a rash for about one week. He reports that he has been camping in Pennsylvania recently during a family vacation. The patient admits to a penicillin allergy but denies taking any medications. He reports that his vaccinations are up to date. No other members of the family have any similar findings or medical complaints. He reports that the rash is not itchy. He admits to consistent lethargy and fatigue with only intermittent headache, fever, and chills. His physical examination is unremarkable except for the rash. On observation, you note that the rash is annular, on his left thigh, and is slightly erythematous. There are distinct margins. The center of the rash is lighter in color than the periphery of the lesion (see Figure 1.3 on page 6).

24. The MOST likely diagnosis is

    (A) atypical measles
    (B) rubella
    (C) tinea corporis
    (D) pityriasis rosea
    (E) Lyme disease

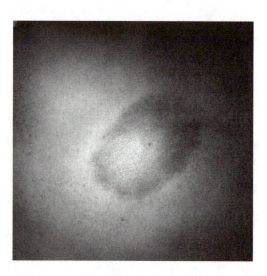

Figure 1.3

25. Which of the following is true regarding Lyme disease?

   (A) Initial signs and symptoms usually resolve without treatment in about 3 months.
   (B) Initial lab data include a elevated immunoglobulin G (IgG) titer.
   (C) The causative agent is the fungus *Borrelia burgdorferi.*
   (D) It is a tick-borne illness *(Ixodes).*
   (E) Intermittent migrating musculoskeletal pains are never present initially.

26. Which of the following has been described in the early phase of this disease?

   (A) abnormal deep tendon reflexes
   (B) tinnitus
   (C) Nikolsky's sign
   (D) rectal prolapse
   (E) testicular swelling

27. The BEST initial treatment steps in the case presented would include

   (A) starting amoxicillin PO for a total course of 4 to 6 weeks, followed by a Lyme titer
   (B) intravenous amoxicillin, 1 g daily for 6 weeks

   (C) doxycycline, 100 mg twice daily for 3 weeks
   (D) intrathecal ceftriaxone, twice daily for 6 weeks
   (E) doxycycline, 100 mg three times daily for 6 weeks

Question 28

A 24-year-old nulliparous patient presents to your office 6 weeks after the first day of her last normal menstrual period. A home pregnancy test is positive. Her physical examination is significant for the presence of a 6-week-size uterus. The beta-subunit of human chorionic gonadotropin (hCG) performed 3 days earlier at her primary care physician's office is positive at 26,000 mIU/mL. A pelvic ultrasound is interpreted as being consistent with a molar gestation. The chest x-ray is normal.

28. Which of the following management options do you recommend to her after evacuation of the hydatidiform mole?

   (A) weekly urine chorionic gonadotropin until four consecutive negative values
   (B) weekly urine chorionic gonadotropin until negative, then monthly for 6 months
   (C) weekly serum beta-subunit hCG until negative, then every 6 months for 1 year
   (D) weekly serum beta-subunit hCG until three consecutive negatives, then monthly for 6 months
   (E) monthly serum beta-hCG determinations until negative, then every 2 months for 1 year

Questions 29 Through 31

A 65-year-old man is diagnosed with a carcinoma of the ascending colon. His preoperative carcinoembryonic antigen (CEA) level was elevated.

29. Which of the following would MOST likely be associated with his condition?

   (A) spiking fevers
   (B) anemia

(C) perirectal abscess

(D) rectal fistula

(E) steatorrhea

30. To which of the following organs is the patient's cancer MOST likely to metastasize?

(A) lung

(B) bone

(C) stomach

(D) skin

(E) liver

31. At surgery, the patient is found to have a tumor invading into the pericolonic fat. Two out of ten lymph nodes have metastatic disease. Which of the following is true about his subsequent care?

(A) No further radiologic studies are needed.

(B) He should be offered adjuvant chemotherapy for his stage IIIB disease.

(C) Follow-up colonoscopy is unnecessary.

(D) Follow-up of his CEA level will prolong his survival.

(E) Follow-up of his CEA level will not help detect recurrence of disease earlier.

Questions 32 Through 34

A 45-year-old alcoholic man on a recent binge arrives at the emergency department with acute onset of hematemesis after several episodes of emesis. He is being fluid resuscitated with normal saline, and blood has been ordered for transfusion. He is heme positive on rectal examination. A nasogastric tube has been passed into the stomach, and blood is being lavaged with normal saline.

32. In your differential diagnosis, the possible reasons for the hemorrhage described include all of the following EXCEPT

(A) gastric ulcer

(B) diverticulosis

(C) bleeding esophageal varices

(D) Mallory–Weiss tear

(E) gastritis

33. The lavage was performed until almost clear. The patient's vital signs stabilized. Upper endoscopy was performed, which shows evidence of a Mallory–Weiss tear without active bleeding. All of the following are true regarding the management of this diagnosis EXCEPT

(A) gastric lavage and decompression are essential

(B) the majority of patients are managed nnoperatively

(C) electrocautery at the time of endoscopy is sometimes necessary

(D) gastrectomy is the treatment of choice

(E) the patient is volume resuscitated as needed from the bleeding event

34. Instead of showing a Mallory–Weiss tear, the endoscopy demonstrates esophageal varices without active hemorrhage. The patient's intravenous fluids are adjusted appropriately to decrease the amount of sodium administered. Four hours later, he has another episode of hematemesis (600 mL). Appropriate management at this point could include

(A) furosemide (Lasix)

(B) sclerotherapy

(C) balloon tamponade

(D) vasopressin

(E) correction of his coagulopathy

Questions 35 and 36

35. Identify the poor prognostic indicator for metastatic gestational trophoblastic neoplasia.

    (A) serum beta-hCG level of < 40,000 mIU/mL
    (B) metastasis to the ovaries
    (C) metastatic gestational trophoblastic neoplasia following an ectopic pregnancy
    (D) brain or liver metastasis
    (E) age less than 18 years at diagnosis

36. Three weeks later, the beta-hCG level has tripled and a CT of the head shows a metastatic lesion to the brain. After discussing treatment options, the patient refuses radiation therapy and chooses chemotherapy. Which of the following options do you recommend for the patient?

    (A) methotrexate
    (B) actinomycin D
    (C) methotrexate and actinomycin D (MAD)
    (D) methotrexate alternating with cyclophosphamide (MaC)
    (E) methotrexate, actinomycin D, and cyclophosphamide (MAC)

Questions 37 and 38

A 47-year-old man presents to your office with a decline in his exercise tolerance over the last month and the new onset of peripheral edema. On physical examination, his liver edge is smooth and palpable 5 cm below the costal margin. He has an increase in jugular venous pressure during inspiration. He gives a history of stage II Hodgkin's disease, treated approximately 20 years previously.

37. What is further evaluation likely to reveal?

    (A) a massively enlarged heart
    (B) a pericardial knock
    (C) atrial fibrillation
    (D) renal failure
    (E) ST elevations

38. Which of the following is the MOST common cause of constrictive pericarditis in the United States?

    (A) trauma
    (B) uremia
    (C) tuberculosis
    (D) idiopathic
    (E) rheumatic fever

39. An observational study examined 649 cases of lung cancer, finding 647 of them to have a history of smoking. Of 649 controls, there were 622 who had a past history of smoking. The incidence (or risk) of lung cancer among smokers may be calculated as follows:

    (A) $647/(647 + 622)$
    (B) $(647 \times 27)/(2 \times 622)$
    (C) $647/649$
    (D) $2/649$
    (E) cannot be calculated using the data given

Questions 40 Through 42

You are asked to evaluate a 46-year-old patient who was admitted to the hospital 2 days ago for pancreatitis. He has become markedly tremulous and begun to experience hallucinations. A clouded state of consciousness is noted.

40. Which of the following is the MOST likely type of psychotic disturbance to be experienced by this patient?

    (A) auditory hallucinations
    (B) visual or tactile hallucinations
    (C) olfactory hallucinations
    (D) delusions
    (E) catatonia

41. Which of the following conditions is MOST likely to occur in patients with this disorder?

    (A) ataxia
    (B) convulsions
    (C) hypothermia
    (D) delusions
    (E) tremulousness

42. Upon being questioned, the patient states that "bugs are crawling all over my body." Which of the following is the correct name for this manifestation?

    (A) formication
    (B) trichotillomania
    (C) akathisia
    (D) confabulation
    (E) koro

Questions 43 Through 45

43. A childless couple presents for discussion, evaluation, and treatment of infertility. They have had unprotected coitus for two years. She is 31 years old, he is 32, and neither has conceived a pregnancy. He is in good health in spite of a "baseball injury." Her history is significant for oligomenorrhea for 3 years. A gynecologic examination, serum prolactin and thyroid-stimulating hormone (TSH), and hysterosalpingogram are normal. The next step for this couple should be

    (A) semen analysis
    (B) intrauterine insemination (IUI)
    (C) sperm penetration assay
    (D) operative laparoscopy
    (E) in vitro fertilization (IVF)

44. Assuming the test you ordered is "normal," what is the MOST likely cause of this couple's infertility?

    (A) ovulation factor
    (B) cervical factor
    (C) uterine factor
    (D) tubal factor
    (E) male factor

45. The MOST common etiology for tubal infertility currently is

    (A) *Chlamydia trachomatis*
    (B) *Neisseria gonorrheae*
    (C) *Mycoplasma hominis*
    (D) *Streptococcus faecalis*
    (E) *Pseudomonas aeruginosa*

Questions 46 Through 49

A 36-year-old woman comes to the emergency department with a 1-day history of abdominal pain. On physical examination, she has marked tenderness in the left upper quadrant. She gives a history of alcohol and drug use but denies recent use of either. Laboratory evaluation reveals an amylase which is elevated; serum glutamic oxaloacetic transaminase (SGOT), serum glutamic pyruvic transaminase (SGPT), and gamma-glutamyl transpeptidase (GGT) are also elevated. Her complete blood count (CBC) shows a white blood cell (WBC) count of 14.2, hemoglobin 10.1 with a mean corpuscular volume of 76, and platelets of 92,000.

46. The MOST common predisposing factor to this condition is

    (A) intravenous drug use
    (B) excessive alcohol use
    (C) biliary duct stones
    (D) pregnancy
    (E) diabetes mellitus

47. Another common laboratory abnormality is

    (A) hypervolemia
    (B) hypercholesterolemia
    (C) hyperglycemia
    (D) hypercalcemia
    (E) hypercarbia

48. Interpretation of the most valuable blood test is confused in the presence of

    (A) diabetes mellitus, type II
    (B) gastric ulcer
    (C) renal failure
    (D) sulfonamide therapy
    (E) gastric carcinoma

49. In AIDS patients, the disorder can be triggered by infection with

    (A) toxoplasmosis
    (B) *Mycobacterium tuberculosis*
    (C) *Mycobacterium avium* complex
    (D) *Pneumocystis carinii*
    (E) herpesvirus

50. The percentage of hemoglobin values that is below minus 2 standard deviations from the mean is

   (A) 1%
   (B) 2%
   (C) 4%
   (D) 8%
   (E) 16%

Questions 51 and 52

An anxious 45-year-old mother brings her 15-year-old daughter in for evaluation because she has not yet menstruated. The mother started menstruating at age 14 and is concerned because menstruation now occurs earlier than when she was developing. The daughter is not concerned, although all of her friends started menstruating at least a year ago. Pubic and axillary hair growth started 2 years ago. The daughter is of average height and weight. Her growth spurt started about 1 year ago. The remainder of your history and physical examination is within normal limits.

51. Your next step should be to

   (A) determine the karyotype of the parents and the patient
   (B) start oral contraceptives as a simple way to induce menstrual flow and confirm patency of the uterus and cervix
   (C) determine the levels of FSH, luteinizing hormone (LH), prolactin, DS, and hCG to start the evaluation
   (D) reassure the mother that her daughter is developing within the normal limits
   (E) perform a progesterone withdrawal test on the daughter

52. The daughter's MOST likely diagnosis is

   (A) Meyer–Rokitansky–Kustner–Hauser (MRKH) syndrome
   (B) precocious puberty
   (C) constitutional delay
   (D) pubertal development within normal limits
   (E) Turner syndrome

Questions 53 and 54

A 55-year-old man from China is known to have chronic liver disease secondary to hepatitis B infection. He has recently felt unwell, and his hemoglobin level has increased from 13 g/dL to 19.5 g/dL.

53. In which of the following is sexual transmission common but requires the presence of another infectious agent before becoming clinically apparent?

   (A) hepatitis A
   (B) hepatitis B
   (C) hepatitis C
   (D) hepatitis D
   (E) hepatitis E

54. The blood test MOST likely to be helpful in the diagnosis of his current problem is

   (A) alkaline phosphatase
   (B) alpha-fetoprotein
   (C) aspartate transaminase (AST)
   (D) AST/alanine transaminase (ALT) ratio
   (E) unconjugated bilirubin

55. A patient is found to be positive for hepatitis B core antibody (anti-HBc) but negative for hepatitis B surface antibody (anti-HBs). Which of the following does NOT apply?

   (A) The patient could be a carrier of hepatitis B.
   (B) The patient's status could be clarified by testing for hepatitis B surface antigen (HBsAg) and IgM hepatitis B core antibody.
   (C) The patient has been exposed to hepatitis B in the past but has recovered and is now immune.
   (D) The patient could be in the "core window" of the recovery phase of an acute hepatitis B infection.
   (E) The patient's anti-HBc could not have been caused by hepatitis B immunization.

Questions 56 Through 58

A 38-year-old white married woman comes to her family physician with a history of vague abdominal pain. She is certain she has cancer. Exhaustive medical examinations and general hospitalizations have failed to reveal any abnormality save for "spastic colitis." However, she continues to believe she has cancer, saying "the doctors just haven't found it yet." She wakes up at about 4 A.M. and has lost at least 15 pounds in the past 6 weeks, which she attributes to cancer. Her speech is monotonous and slow. Tears well up in her eyes as she speaks about her youngest child joining the Navy 7 months ago. Since then, she has felt worthless and has found no pleasure in anything. Although she never feels good, she believes she feels worse in the morning. She had previously been well. She denies any previous history of similar symptoms and has never seen a psychiatrist.

56. Which of the following is the MOST likely axis I diagnosis?

   (A) hypochondriasis
   (B) major depression, single episode
   (C) bipolar disorder
   (D) an undiscovered abdominal tumor
   (E) somatoform disorder

57. Which of the following is the MOST likely axis II diagnosis?

   (A) obsessive–compulsive personality disorder
   (B) borderline personality disorder
   (C) diagnosis deferred
   (D) life stressors
   (E) global assessment of functioning (GAF) of 45

58. This patient

   (A) should not be asked about suicide
   (B) should be asked about suicide
   (C) may be successful in an attempt to commit suicide
   (D) may make a suicidal manipulative gesture
   (E) is most likely to commit suicide by prescription drug overdose

59. A 30-year-old nulliparous woman presents, complaining of light, infrequent menses, flushes, and hot flashes. She had normal menses until 8 months ago. Her pubertal development was normal. She is otherwise in good health. Her vaginal smear shows small intermediate and parabasal cells. A urine pregnancy test is negative. Her serum FSH is 45 mIU/mL. The MOST likely diagnosis is

   (A) Asherman syndrome
   (B) hypothalamic hypogonadotropic amenorrhea
   (C) pituitary gonadotrope-secreting adenoma
   (D) premature ovarian failure
   (E) Sheehan syndrome

Questions 60 and 61

After an occurrence of fever and malaise, a 23-year-old pregnant woman in her first trimester presents with a history of a nonspecific maculopapular rash that lasted 3 days; she also had cervical lymphadenopathy.

60. Her unborn child may be at increased risk for which of the following congenital cardiac abnormalities?

   (A) tetralogy of Fallot
   (B) atrial septal defect
   (C) myocardial necrosis
   (D) aortic stenosis
   (E) arrhythmias

61. The infant is also at increased risk for developing which of the following endocrinopathies?

   (A) diabetes insipidus
   (B) precocious puberty
   (C) gout
   (D) gigantism
   (E) hypothyroidism

Questions 62 Through 65

A 44-year-old woman corners you at a dinner party to complain that she has been taking an over-the-counter (OTC) H_2 blocker off and on for a year. She feels better while she is taking it, but shortly after stopping it, her upper abdominal discomfort returns. You refer her to your partner for evaluation.

62. The first step in evaluation should be

    (A) an upper endoscopy
    (B) a UGI radiograph with barium
    (C) a trial of prescription-strength H_2 blocker
    (D) an antacid preparation four times a day
    (E) a CT scan of the abdomen and pelvis

63. Which of the following is true regarding gastric ulcers?

    (A) pain is usually relieved by food
    (B) caused by gastric hypersecretion
    (C) no chance of malignancy
    (D) often associated with *Helicobacter pylori*
    (E) UGI studies have a 70% false-negative rate

64. On endoscopic evaluation, your partner locates a gastric ulcer. The biopsy shows only acute and chronic inflammatory changes, but culture does grow *H. pylori.* The recommended treatment is

    (A) OTC H_2 blockers for 6 months
    (B) prescription-strength H_2 blockers for 6 weeks
    (C) proton-pump inhibitor
    (D) sucralfate plus a proton-pump inhibitor
    (E) amoxicillin, metronidazole, and bismuth for 2 weeks

65. Which of the following is true regarding *H. pylori*?

    (A) The organism is commonly found in histologically normal stomach tissue.
    (B) It may be the most common human infective agent worldwide.

    (C) The epidemiology of this organism is well known.
    (D) Eradication of the organism results in a 50% cure rate of the associated ulcer.
    (E) It is not often found on biopsies of patients with active antral gastritis.

66. When a screening test for human immunodeficiency virus (HIV) is performed, an enzyme-linked immunosorbent assay (ELISA) test is first done and it is repeated if positive. If the second test is positive, a Western blot test is performed for confirmation. Subsequently, a p24 antigen test may also be performed. This serial interpretation has which of the following effects?

    (A) increases both the sensitivity and the specificity
    (B) increases the predictive value positive and slightly decreases the sensitivity
    (C) increases the predictive value positive and slightly increases the sensitivity
    (D) increases both the specificity and the predictive value negative
    (E) has no effect on the sensitivity or specificity

Questions 67 Through 69

A 35-year-old woman with insulin-dependent diabetes mellitus (IDDM) for 20 years is seen with an erythematous, edematous, nontender right foot. Frank pus is draining from an ulcer on the plantar surface over the third metatarsal head. She has a weak but palpable foot pulse. Her temperature is 102°F; serum glucose level, 400 mg%; and WBC count, 23,000/mm^3.

67. The MOST likely cause of the original ulceration is

    (A) arterial insufficiency
    (B) neuropathy
    (C) infection
    (D) self-mutilation
    (E) spider bite

68. The MOST important intervention for control of the sepsis is

    (A) intravenous antibiotics
    (B) control of hyperglycemia
    (C) surgical debridement
    (D) hydration
    (E) foot x-rays

69. In a patient with a diabetic foot infection, all of the following bacterial organisms are likely to be cultured EXCEPT

    (A) *Staphylococcus*
    (B) *Proteus*
    (C) *Escherichia coli*
    (D) *Bacteroides*
    (E) *Clostridium*

70. The death rate from cancers in U.S women from most to least frequent is

    (A) breast, colon, lung, ovarian
    (B) ovarian, breast, colon, lung
    (C) breast, ovarian, lung, colon
    (D) breast, lung, ovarian, colon
    (E) lung, breast, colon, ovarian

Questions 71 Through 73

In a community of 100,000 persons, there were 1000 existing cases of disease X at the beginning of 1993. During 1993, 100 new cases of this disease were diagnosed, while 500 persons died of disease X during the year. Assume that disease X is a nonrepeating chronic illness.

71. The annual prevalence of disease X for this population during 1993 was

    (A) 75 per 100,000
    (B) 101 per 100,000
    (C) 500 per 100,000
    (D) 1000 per 100,000
    (E) 1100 per 100,000

72. The risk for disease X for this population during 1993 was

    (A) 75 per 100,000
    (B) 101 per 100,000
    (C) 500 per 100,000
    (D) 1000 per 100,000
    (E) 1100 per 100,000

73. The risk of death from disease X this population during 1993 was

    (A) 75 per 100,000
    (B) 101 per 100,000
    (C) 500 per 100,000
    (D) 1000 per 100,000
    (E) 1100 per 100,000

Questions 74 Through 76

74. A 62-year-old woman (P2002) presents for a routine examination. Her history is significant for a weight loss of 25 pounds in the last 6 months and recent increasing abdominal girth. Her last gynecologic exam was 4 or 5 years ago. She has had no gynecological problems or surgery in the past. On physical examination, there is a protuberant abdomen with a fluid wave. Her cervix appears normal. Bimanual examination is difficult, but nodularity in the cul-de-sac was noted on rectovaginal exam. A chest x-ray is negative. An ultrasound examination reveals ascites and ill-defined pelvic masses. The next procedure to be performed is

    (A) ultrasound of the pelvis
    (B) cystoscopy
    (C) exploratory laparotomy
    (D) CT of the chest
    (E) intravenous pyelogram (IVP)

75. At the operation, you find the following: 2 L of ascites, tumor extensively involving the ovaries, tumor replacing most of the omentum, and tumor implants on the diaphragm. The liver parenchyma was uninvolved. The frozen section revealed moderately differentiated papillary serous carcinoma consistent with an ovarian primary tumor. Her stage is

    (A) I
    (B) IIC
    (C) IIIB
    (D) IIIC
    (E) IV

76. In this case, suboptimal debulking was performed. The MOST common adjunctive therapy offered is

    (A) intraperitoneal radioisotope
    (B) multiple-agent chemotherapy to include cisplatin or carboplatin and paclitaxel or cisplatin and cyclophosphamide
    (C) single-agent chemotherapy with melphalan
    (D) whole abdomen external beam irradiation
    (E) whole pelvis external beam irradiation

Questions 77 Through 79

A 61-year-old woman develops exertional angina and has two episodes of syncope. Her last menstrual period was at age 54, but she has had no hormonal replacement. A resting ECG is normal. Her fasting cholesterol is 250 mg/dL. Her diastolic blood pressure is greater than 90 mm Hg on three separate occasions. Her mother and father are both alive, with only mild hypertension.

77. The MOST likely diagnosis is

    (A) mitral stenosis
    (B) mitral insufficiency
    (C) aortic stenosis
    (D) aortic insufficiency
    (E) tricuspid stenosis

78. The patient does not follow recommendations to change her diet and take medication to control her blood pressure. She presents to the emergency department with acute myocardial infarction. She has no symptoms of bradycardia, but temporary pacing may be indicated for

    (A) persistent bradycardia
    (B) Mobitz I block
    (C) first-degree AV block
    (D) new fascicular block
    (E) LBBB

79. The following morning, her bradycardia persists, and, despite optimal medical management, she becomes symptomatic from the hypotension. A temporary pacemaker is placed, which functions when the ventricular rate falls below 60 beats per minute. This type of pacemaker is called

    (A) asynchronous
    (B) atrial synchronous
    (C) ventricular synchronous
    (D) ventricular inhibited
    (E) atrial sequential

80. A 30-year-old woman has a several-year history of multiple somatic complaints for which she has had a thorough medical workup and has been treated by many physicians. However, all their efforts have failed to influence her chronic but fluctuating history of malaise and somatic distress. She now complains of an array of symptoms, including dyspareunia, irregular and painful menses, back pains, chest pains, lightheadedness, nausea, heartburn, painful urination, and "twitching legs," all in a vague but dramatic manner. Examination and laboratory testing again disclose no abnormality. The MOST likely diagnosis is

    (A) Münchhausen syndrome
    (B) factitious disorder
    (C) malingering
    (D) hypochondriasis
    (E) somatization disorder

81. A 50-year-old woman, who was an unrestrained passenger in an automobile accident, is brought into the emergency department by the paramedics. She had direct impact of her face against the windshield. She has significant facial lacerations extending into her oral cavity and obvious facial fractures, with instability of the midface. She is in respiratory distress secondary to secretions and aspiration of blood. Her airway needs to be maintained quickly. What is the safest approach to provide an adequate airway for her?

(A) tracheostomy
(B) nasotracheal intubation
(C) cricothyroidotomy
(D) endotracheal intubation
(E) oxygen (4 L) by the way of nasal cannula

Questions 82 Through 85

A 64-year-old white male is admitted from the emergency department with an acute myocardial infarction.

82. Shortly after transfer to the cardiac care unit (CCU), his blood pressure begins to fall. His color is ashen and extremities cool. The benefit of nitroprusside in this situation is a result of

(A) vasoconstriction
(B) increased ventricular afterload
(C) changes in heart rate
(D) decreased afterload in heart failure
(E) changes in contractility

83. After the administration of thrombolytic therapy, his cardiac function improves and he is moved out of the CCU into a telemetry bed. Four days after admission, he develops chest pain, which gets worse when he takes a deep breath. On physical examination, he has a friction rub. The MOST likely diagnosis is

(A) a new area of myocardial infarction
(B) pneumonia

(C) viral infection
(D) pericarditis secondary to transmural infarction
(E) dissecting aneurysm

84. A number of interventions are of proven benefit in the postinfarction period. Which of the following has been documented to improve survival?

(A) aggressively lowering lipid levels
(B) nitroglycerin
(C) calcium channel blockers
(D) alpha-adrenergic antagonists
(E) nitroprusside

85. Which of the following conditions would make one cautious in the use of beta blockers for this man?

(A) hypertension
(B) tachycardia
(C) fever
(D) resting tremor
(E) congestive heart failure (CHF)

86. A 25-year-old man presents with a known diagnosis of Crohn's disease. All of the following are common findings for these patients EXCEPT

(A) abdominal pain
(B) weight loss
(C) diarrhea
(D) liver disease
(E) palpable mass

Questions 87 and 88

87. The MOST common clinical presentation of early cervical cancer is

(A) asymptomatic
(B) bleeding
(C) foul-smelling vaginal discharge
(D) lower back pain
(E) pelvic pain with leg edema

88. A 19-year-old nulliparous woman has a colposcopy for evaluation of an abnormal Pap smear. The endocervical currettage is positive. A cold-knife conization is performed. Histology reveals microinvasive squamous cell carcinoma (1.5 mm), and the cone margins are free of neoplasia. She is HIV negative. She desires to preserve fertility. Appropriate management for this patient is

(A) radical hysterectomy with lymph node dissection
(B) total abdominal hysterectomy
(C) repeat cold-knife cone biopsy in 6 months
(D) serial Pap smears and colposcopy as necessary
(E) vaginal hysterectomy

Questions 89 Through 91

A 21-year-old college student who recently returned from doing volunteer work in Mexico goes to her physician because her eyes look yellow. She has had a low-grade fever and generalized muscle aches. She also complains of prolonged jet lag. Laboratory studies show elevations of SGOT, SGPT, GGT, and bilirubin. She also has a very mild normocytic anemia.

89. The MOST likely viral etiology for this presentation is

(A) hepatitis A
(B) hepatitis B
(C) hepatitis C
(D) hepatitis D
(E) hepatitis E

90. The jaundice is visible in the eyes but not the skin first because of

(A) the high type II collagen content of scleral tissue
(B) the high elastin content of scleral tissue
(C) the high blood flow to the head with consequent increased bilirubin
(D) secretion via the lacrimal glands
(E) the lighter color of the sclera

91. Which of the following can be prevented by vaccination?

(A) cytomegalovirus (CMV)
(B) Epstein–Barr virus (EBV)
(C) hepatitis A
(D) hepatitis D
(E) hepatitis E

Questions 92 and 93

Three members of a family of eight are admitted to the hospital with similar findings: nausea, vomiting, abdominal cramps, sudden edema of the eyelids, subconjunctival hemorrhages, and photophobia. Each complains of muscle soreness and pain with chills and fever. Two have transient neurologic signs and one develops myocarditis. The family lives on a farm on the outskirts of town. They grow and home-can most of their fruits and vegetables. Their meat supply is obtained from farm hogs, chickens, and hunted wildlife.

92. The MOST likely diagnosis is

(A) dermatomyositis
(B) *Ascaris* infestation
(C) trichinosis
(D) schistosomiasis
(E) salmonellosis

93. The disease could have been prevented by

(A) ensuring that meat and meat products are federally inspected
(B) rodent control
(C) prophylactic active immunization
(D) quarantining the patients
(E) sufficiently cooking ingested meat

94. A 3-year-old child presents with her parents, who are concerned that she continues to wet her bed nightly. While she has mastered toilet training during the daytime for approximately 6 months, she has yet to have a dry night. She has no symptoms of burning or frequency. You should

(A) recommend a thorough urologic evaluation by the child's pediatrician

(B) suggest the use of a bell and pad to behaviorally train the child

(C) question the parents about family stressors

(D) reassure the parents that this is the normal progression of sphincter control

(E) prescribe imipramine

95. Which of the following complications are associated with Crohn's disease?

(A) malnutrition

(B) enteroenteric fistula

(C) toxic megacolon

(D) enterocutaneous fistula

(E) all of the above

Questions 96 Through 99

A 26-year-old man is brought to the psychiatric emergency department by his parents, who are worried about his behavior. In 3 weeks, he has missed 8 days of work and has been witnessed performing bizarre behaviors, including cocking his head to the sky for minutes at a time as if listening to someone speaking to him, and refusing to sit in any chair except one close to the door and backed against a wall. When asked why he has not been reporting to work, he replies, "They're all in on it there." His parents tell you they are concerned because their son was usually outgoing and personable, but he has not left the house except to go to work for a month. On interview, he appears tense and makes little eye contact.

96. The MOST appropriate diagnosis in this patient is

(A) major depressive disorder

(B) paranoid schizophrenia

(C) paranoid personality disorder

(D) schizophreniform disorder

(E) social phobia

97. The MOST appropriate therapy for this patient is

(A) insight-oriented psychotherapy

(B) haloperidol

(C) lorazepam

(D) fluoxetine

(E) behavioral therapy

After being placed on the medication you prescribed, the patient is reported to have a decrease in his bizarre behaviors and returns to work on a regular basis. However, a year later, he stops taking his medications, and relapses into his former behaviors after a week. Although his parents tolerate his relapse for some time, after a month they bring him back to the psychiatric emergency department, saying he refuses to speak to them, will not leave the house or return his friends' phone calls, and "appears suicidal."

98. The MOST appropriate diagnosis in this patient at this time is

(A) major depressive disorder

(B) paranoid schizophrenia

(C) paranoid personality disorder

(D) schizophreniform disorder

(E) social phobia

After a brief hospitalization, the patient once again agrees to take his medication, with a good deal of improvement. For 20 years, he performs well at his job and is promoted several times. One day, however, his coworkers notice him making bizarre movements, including grimacing and lip smacking. His parents, with whom he still lives, report that he often appears as if he is "dancing" without any music being played. Fearing he is again having a relapse, they bring him to the psychiatric emergency department.

99. The MOST appropriate intervention at this time is

(A) addition of propranolol to his medication regimen

(B) an increase in his current medication

(C) addition of benztropine to his medication regimen

(D) discontinuation of his medication and switching to another medication with similar actions but a different side effect profile

(E) addition of lorazepam to his medication regimen

100. A 19-year-old man is diagnosed with a left inguinal hernia on his entrance examination into the military. All of the following statements regarding inguinal hernias are true EXCEPT

(A) a smaller defect is at lower risk for the development of a complication than a larger one

(B) nearly all inguinal hernias in children are indirect and result from a persistent processus vaginalis

(C) some patients have radiation of pain into the scrotum

(D) the groin is the most common location for hernia development

(E) a direct hernia is secondary to a defect in the transversalis fascia

Questions 101 and 102

An 80-year-old, 60-kg, nursing home patient is rescued after smoking in bed and is brought into the burn unit. You determine his burns to be third degree to the anterior chest, abdomen, and right hand and part of the forearm; circumferential second degree to the entire left lower extremity; and first degree to the rest of the right upper extremity, the left upper extremity, and face.

101. What is the approximate total body surface area of the burn?

(A) 15 %

(B) 20%

(C) 60%

(D) 80%

(E) 40%

102. What is the total volume resuscitation this patient should receive within the first 24 hours?

(A) 11,200 mL/24 hours

(B) 9,600 mL/24 hours

(C) 8,000 mL/24 hours

(D) 6,000 mL/24 hours

(E) 15,000 mL/24 hours

103. Which of the following is associated with a functional murmur?

(A) long diastolic murmur at the apex

(B) soft diastolic murmur and clubbing

(C) abnormal ECG

(D) occurs sometime in more than 25% of children

(E) high-pitched diastolic type murmur at the base

104. Which of the following will cause insulin requirements to INCREASE in a child with IDDM?

(A) fever

(B) emotional upset

(C) returning to school after summer camp

(D) addition of corticosteroids

(E) all of the above

Questions 105 and 106

A 23-year-old woman (G1,P0010) calls you at 1 A.M. because she was having intercourse and the condom broke. Her LMP was 12 days earlier and she is extremely upset about the possibility of becoming pregnant.

105. You advise her

(A) to douche immediately

(B) to come to the office in the morning for an intrauterine device (IUD) insertion

(C) that you will phone in a prescription for diethylstilbestrol in the morning

(D) that you will phone in a prescription for an oral contraceptive in the morning with instructions to take three pills at once and another three pills in 24 hours

(E) that she should come to the office in the morning for an examination

106. The next afternoon she calls you again. She has taken the medication and has been feeling extremely nauseated. You ask her to come to the office. On exam, you notice that her uterus is top normal size and slightly softened. On further questioning, you learn that she has had several recent sexual partners, that her last period was actually approximately 1 week early and lighter than normal, and that she has been noticing urinary frequency. You next order

(A) urinalysis
(B) liver function studies
(C) thyroid functions studies
(D) urine hCG
(E) quantitative serum beta-subunit of hCG

Questions 107 and 108

A 21-year-old man with signs of urethritis, conjunctivitis, and arthritis has just received a presumptive diagnosis of an accompanying sexually transmitted disease (STD).

107. What is the MOST likely organism to cause the associated STD?

(A) *Neisseria gonorrhoeae*
(B) *Chlamydia trachomatis*
(C) *Treponema pallidum*
(D) *Gardnerella vaginalis*
(E) *Haemophilus ducreyi*

108. The treatment of choice for this infection is

(A) doxycycline
(B) penicillin
(C) metronidazole
(D) trimethoprim–sulfamethoxazole
(E) gentamicin

Questions 109 and 110

A 24-year-old man comes to the emergency department complaining of severe abdominal pain and saying that he needs emergent surgery. On examination, he is noted to have multiple surgical scars on his abdomen. Despite multiple laboratory tests and x-rays, no evidence of an acute abdomen can be ascertained. A review of previous hospitalizations indicates that, even after multiple abdominal explorations, no pathology has been discovered. Upon being confronted with these facts, the patient signs out against medical advice.

109. The MOST likely diagnosis in this patient is

(A) Munchausen syndrome
(B) a subtle colonic perforation
(C) Ménière syndrome
(D) hypochondriasis
(E) Tourette syndrome

110. The patient is admitted to another hospital, where, after thorough questioning, a psychiatrist determines that the subject is being untruthful during the interview. It is noted that the patient is able to present his medical complaints in considerable detail, in a manner that arouses the interest of the interviewer. Which of the following would BEST describe the patient's presentation of his purported medical history and problems?

(A) logorrhea
(B) perseveration
(C) pseudologia fantastica
(D) dissociation
(E) echolalia

111. A 38-year-old construction worker falls off a scaffold. The report was loss of consciousness at the scene. In the trauma bay, the patient is making strange mumbling sounds, unable to follow commands, unable to elicit eye opening to sternal rub, but withdraws to painful stimuli. What is the Glasgow Coma Scale score for this patient?

(A) 10
(B) 12
(C) 15
(D) 7
(E) 3

Questions 112 and 113

A 42-year-old man presents with flushing. He also notes some right upper quadrant discomfort when leaning over to tie his shoes. He has not lost any weight. A 24-hour urine test for 5-hydroxyindoleacetic (5-HIAA) acid is elevated.

112. The probable diagnosis is

   (A) carcinoid syndrome
   (B) Gaucher's disease
   (C) acute hepatitis
   (D) phenylketonuria
   (E) allergy to monosodium glutamate (MSG)

113. Which of the following signs and symptoms is associated with this diagnosis?

   (A) an enlarged left ventricle
   (B) chronic productive cough
   (C) edema of the head and neck
   (D) constipation
   (E) dysuria

Questions 114 and 115

A 30-year-old man comes into a community clinic with complaints of several lesions at the base of his penis. He is sexually active and has never had anything like this before. He complains that he has had these painful lesions for about 7 days.

114. What is the MOST likely causative organism?

   (A) *Chlamydia trachomatis*
   (B) herpes simplex virus, type 2 (HSV-2)
   (C) *Haemophilus ducreyi*
   (D) *Treponema pallidum*
   (E) *Neisseria gonorrhoeae*

115. What will MOST likely provide the definitive diagnosis for this acute infection?

   (A) serologic assay
   (B) viral isolation from tissue culture
   (C) Tzanck preparation
   (D) darkfield examination of tissue
   (E) routine bacterial culture

116. A 25-year-old steel worker is seen for preoperative evaluation for an elective right inguinal hernia repair. The BEST way to identify the high-risk patient for potential operative bleeding is

   (A) bleeding time
   (B) platelet count
   (C) prothrombin time
   (D) partial thromboplastin time
   (E) history of bleeding problems

Questions 117 Through 121

A 21-month-old child is brought into your office by new foster parents. The child's first 18 months were marked by a lack of medical care. He was known to be a low-birth-weight baby. The child appears malnourished and enters the exam room with a waddling gait. The child's head appears oddly misshapen, and he is noted to have a pot belly and thickening at the wrists and ankles. A strange bumpy appearance is noted at his costochondral junctions, and a fellow physician states that it looks like "rachitic rosary." Plain films reveal several pseudofractures and widened epiphyseal plates (see Figure 1.4).

117. The MOST likely diagnosis is

   (A) vitamin A toxicity
   (B) vitamin D deficiency
   (C) chronic halitosis
   (D) thiamine deficiency
   (E) hypoparathyroidism

118. Which of the following is a clinical sign of rickets?

   (A) craniotabes
   (B) shrinking at the costochondral junctions
   (C) thickening of the knees and pelvis
   (D) rapid growth
   (E) conjunctivitis

119. The daily requirement for vitamin D is

   (A) 100 IU
   (B) 400 IU
   (C) 600 IU

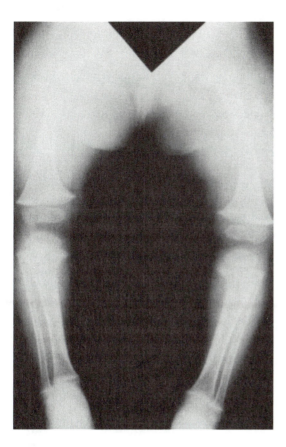

Figure 1.4

(D) 1000 IU

(E) 50 IU

120. In the absence of vitamin D, serum calcium may be maintained by

(A) parathyroid hormone secretion

(B) decreased renal excretion of phosphate

(C) small dietary increases

(D) decreased renal excretion of alkali

(E) increased amounts of vitamin A in the diet

121. Which of the following clinical disorders is NOT associated with an increased incidence of vitamin D deficiency?

(A) cystic fibrosis

(B) hepatic disease

(C) celiac disease

(D) chronic anticonvulsant therapy

(E) obesity

122. A 54-year-old veteran is admitted for a coronary artery bypass grafting (CABG). He receives three units of packed red blood cells intraoperatively. The MOST common complication of red blood cell transfusion is

(A) hepatitis A

(B) febrile transfusion reaction

(C) AIDS

(D) hemolytic reaction

(E) hepatitis B

Questions 123 Through 126

A 55-year-old woman has finally agreed to a routine physical exam at the urging of her daughter. She offers no complaints. Her last visit to a doctor was for her postpartum exam 20 years earlier. Her family history is significant for death of her mother at age 63 from myocardial infarction and death of her father at age 60 from colon cancer. She smokes 1 pack per day. Her height is 5'3" and weight is 146 pounds (66.3 kg). Her blood pressure is 130/88. Dipstick urinalysis is normal except for +1 occult blood.

123. In addition to lung cancer, this woman should be informed that her smoking history puts her at increased risk for

(A) bladder cancer

(B) cervical cancer

(C) myocardial infarction

(D) osteoporosis

(E) all of the above

124. Cardiovascular disease in women

(A) is the second leading cause of death after breast cancer

(B) is 4.5 times more likely to be fatal in the first year after symptomatic myocardial infarction than in men

(C) causes the same symptoms that it does in men, primarily typical angina

(D) can be satisfactorily evaluated with ECG treadmill testing

(E) occurs at the same age as it does in men

125. Microscopic hematuria

    (A) is common in older women not taking estrogen, who have bladder wall thinning due to atrophy, and requires no evaluation
    (B) is probably normal if there are fewer than five red blood cells (RBCs)/hpf
    (C) should always be evaluated with culture, cytology, cystoscopy, and ultrasound or IVP until a cause is found
    (D) is significant in women on anticoagulant therapy only 2% of the time
    (E) is common among smokers and requires no evaluation

126. Ten days after her visit, this woman's Pap smear is returned from the laboratory with a reading of HGSIL. You advise her to have

    (A) colposcopy
    (B) cone biopsy
    (C) LEEP
    (D) LLETZ
    (E) vaginal hysterectomy

Questions 127 Through 129

On careful questioning of a 14-year-old girl who presented to your office complaining of fatigue and is noted on laboratory results to have a hematocrit of 28, you obtain the history that for several years she has been ingesting a substance shown in Figure 1.5, which she refers to as "sour dirt." There is no history of any previous mental or physical disorder.

127. Which of the following terms would BEST describe this practice?

    (A) normal behavior in a 14 year old
    (B) pica
    (C) rumination
    (D) anorexia nervosa
    (E) malingering

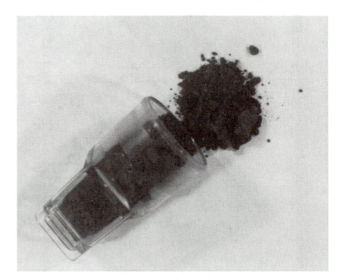

Figure 1.5

128. Which of the following is MOST likely to be observed in an infant who practices such behavior?

    (A) pervasive developmental disorder
    (B) lead poisoning
    (C) morbid obesity
    (D) retinopathy
    (E) moon facies

129. For a diagnosis of this disorder, a substance without nutritive value must be ingested for how long a period of time?

    (A) 1 week
    (B) 2 weeks
    (C) 1 month
    (D) 3 months
    (E) 1 year

130. An 8-year-old otherwise healthy boy presents with a massive lower GI hemorrhage. The MOST likely cause for bleeding is

    (A) midgut volvulus
    (B) anal fissure
    (C) intussusception
    (D) Meckel's diverticulum
    (E) esophageal varices

131. A study in Uganda found a proportional mortality resulting from cancer of 1%. This compares to findings of a proportional mortality from cancer of 6% in the United States. What may be concluded on the basis of the above findings?

(A) Relative risk of dying from cancer in the United States compared to Uganda is 6%.

(B) Uganda has a lower prevalence of cancer than in the United States.

(C) A larger proportion of death in Uganda may be attributed to causes other than cancer.

(D) Uganda has a lower cancer-specific mortality rate than the United States.

(E) More carcinogens are present in the environment in the United States than in Uganda.

132. Treatment of AIDS with measures such as zidovudine (AZT) and trimethoprim–sulfamethoxazole has which of the following direct effects on AIDS in the adult population?

(A) decreased incidence of AIDS

(B) increased incidence of AIDS

(C) decreased prevalence of AIDS

(D) increased prevalence of AIDS

(E) no effect on incidence or prevalence of AIDS

Questions 133 Through 136

An 18-year-old woman is noted on her physical exam for college to have a murmur. She is referred for evaluation, where an echocardiogram reveals mitral valve prolapse.

133. The MOST common physical finding is

(A) a continuous machinery murmur

(B) a pansystolic murmur

(C) a widely split and fixed S2

(D) increased intensity of the pulmonary component of the second heart sound

(E) a late midsystolic murmur

134. Following a dental procedure, the patient develops a fever that lasts 1 week. She notes slender red marks under her nails and raised red lesions in the pads of her fingers and toes. Most of the physical findings associated with this disease process are secondary to

(A) direct bacterial invasion

(B) bacterial toxins

(C) vascular phenomena

(D) valvular damage

(E) preexisting cardiac dysfunction

135. Appropriate prophylaxis before a dental procedure in this woman could include which of the following?

(A) amoxicillin, 2 g PO 1 hour before a procedure

(B) amoxicillin, 500 mg PO four times a day for a week following a procedure

(C) clindamycin, 2 g PO 1 hour before a procedure

(D) gentamicin, 1.5 mg/kg IV 30 minutes before a procedure

(E) gentamicin, 500 mg PO 1 hour before a procedure

136. The MOST likely organism to cause this disease process is

(A) *Streptococcus viridans*

(B) *Staphylococcus aureus*

(C) *Streptococcus pneumoniae*

(D) *Actinobacillus*

(E) *Eikenella corrodens*

137. Assume that surveillance for a specific disease has been implemented and that an appropriate screening test is being sought. Which of the following is MOST important for an effective surveillance system screening test?

(A) high complexity

(B) high specificity

(C) high predictive value positive

(D) low predictive value negative

(E) low flexibility

DIRECTIONS (Questions 138 through 150): Each group of items in this section consists of lettered headings followed by a set of numbered words or phrases. For each numbered word or phrase, select the ONE lettered heading that is most closely associated with it. Each lettered heading may be selected once, more than once, or not at all.

Questions 138 Through 142

(A) Goodpasture syndrome
(B) Pasture syndrome
(C) hemolytic–uremic syndrome
(D) systemic lupus erythematosus (SLE)
(E) acute poststreptococcal glomerulonephritis
(F) polyarteritis nodosa
(G) cortical necrosis
(H) renal cyst
(I) fatal acetaminophen overdose
(J) pyelonephritis
(K) renal calculi

138. The majority of patients have no permanent impairment of renal function in what disorder in addition to (E), (H), and (J)?

139. Associated with nephritis and pulmonary hemorrhage

140. The female/male ratio for this type of nephritis is 4:1

141. Thought to be a hypersensitivity reaction involving medium-sized vessels in its chronic form

142. Usually preceded by a gastroenteritis syndrome

Questions 143 Through 147

Match the laboratory findings with the diseases that feature purpura.

(A) normal platelet count, normal megakaryocytes
(B) decreased platelet count, decreased megakaryocytes
(C) decreased platelet count, increased megakaryocytes
(D) decreased platelet count, normal megakaryocytes
(E) normal platelet count, decreased factor VIII
(F) decreased platelet count, decreased factor VI
(G) normal platelet count, decreased factor X
(H) platelet clumping, elevated glucose
(I) elevated prostate-specific antigen (PSA), elevated platelet count

143. Idiopathic thrombocytopenic purpura (ITP)

144. Aplastic anemia

145. Acute lymphocytic leukemia

146. von Willebrand disease

147. Anaphylactoid purpura

Questions 148 Through 150

(A) pica
(B) bulimia nervosa
(C) anorexia nervosa
(D) amphetamine dependence
(E) central diabetes insipidus
(F) Wilson's disease
(G) dysphagia

148. A 27-year-old patient with schizophrenia is brought to the hospital for acute mental status changes. He is noted to have a sodium level of 109.

149. A 15-year-old girl who has lost 30 pounds in the last 6 months is noted by her dentist to have poor dentition.

150. A 16-year-old girl who has lost 30 pounds over the last 6 months denies food when it is offered to her.

Answers and Explanations

1–4. (1-C, 2-A, 3-E, 4-B) Use of drugs during pregnancy continues to be a national problem. Nothing in the history suggests increased risk of CNS malignancy. Rather, the focus of this discussion is on a mother who, through intravenous drug use, is a carrier of hepatitis B surface antigen. The Centers for Disease Control and Prevention (CDC), American Academy of Pediatrics, and American College of Obstetricians and Gynecologists have all recommended universal screening of pregnant women. A, B, C, and D in question 3 are incorrect because they do not result in jaundice. Mothers who are HBeAg positive are at greatest risk of transmission to their offspring. Transmission probably occurs at the time of delivery, and only 2.5% of infants are antigen positive at birth. Management of the infant includes administration of hepatitis B immune globulin (HBIG) and the first three doses of vaccine at birth. If the infant is antigenemic at 9 months, he or she is considered a vaccine failure and is managed as a carrier. Breast feeding is not contraindicated.

5. (D) In American women, breast cancer is the most common, followed by cancer of the colon, rectum, lung, and endometrium. Approximately 31,000 cases of endometrial cancer are diagnosed annually. Ovarian cancer is the second most common gynecologic malignancy, with approximately 19,000 new cases diagnosed annually. It is the leading cause of death of all gynecologic malignancies. Worldwide, cervical cancer is the most frequently diagnosed gynecologic cancer; however, in the United States, there has been a 70% decline in mortality since the introduction of Papanicolaou (Pap) smear screening in the late 1940s.

6. (D) Joint involvement in inflammatory bowel disease may involve sacroiliitis or specific large-joint peripheral arthritis. The latter type of arthritis parallels the course of the bowel disease. The sacroiliitis (spondylitic variety) follows an independent course. Lymphoma, amyloid, pancreatitis, and tropical sprue are not as common and are not commonly associated with arthritis.

7. (B) Ulcerative colitis almost always involves the rectum (some experts would say always) and is a diffuse, continuous process unlikely to have skip areas. It is Crohn's disease that can mimic PUD, is associated with weight loss, and often has transmural and lymph node involvement.

8. (A) With a microcytic anemia, the patient is most likely to have an iron-deficiency anemia associated with some chronic blood loss from his inflammatory bowel disease. This would typically result in a low serum iron, elevated TIBC, and low ferritin. However, inflammatory processes are often associated with elevations of ferritin and suppression of the TIBC—findings more typical of an anemia of chronic disease. Therefore, although an elevated TIBC and low ferritin are possible, the most likely to occur is a low serum iron. B_{12} deficiency can be seen in chronic bowel processes because of malabsorption; however, this would give a macrocytic anemia. In iron-deficiency and inflammatory processes, the reticulocyte count is low secondary to decreased production. It is elevated in hemolytic states in which adequate stores exist to mount a brisk response and in the recovery phase after replacement of iron (or correction of any other deficiency).

9. **(C)** Measles is more common in children but not more severe. The risk of complications are highest among the very young or the very old. The incubation period for measles is 10 to 12 days. Usually, the first symptoms are fever and malaise, followed by cough, coryza, and conjunctivitis. Prompt administration of immune globulin to exposed individuals can alter clinical disease.

10. **(B)** Tularemia is a fatal bacteremia of rabbits and certain rodents, and secondarily an accidental infection of domestic animals and humans. The common characteristics are a sudden and dramatic onset of chills, fever, headache, and vomiting. The primary lesion usually ulcerates.

11. **(B)** The proper treatment is excision of the tumor and radical neck dissection in the presence of clinically palpable nodal disease.

12. **(B)** In performing a radical neck dissection, the carotid artery and its branches are not removed. However, for the complete removal of lymph nodes and draining areas, it is essential to remove the sternocleidomastoid muscle, internal jugular vein, submaxillary gland, and spinal accessory nerve.

13. **(D)** Endometrial carcinoma needs to be excluded in virtually all women who admit to any degree of postmenopausal bleeding. Four fifths of endometrial cancers develop after menopause. For most, postmenopausal bleeding is the only symptom. An endometrial biopsy performed in the office is the initial step in evaluation. A Papanicolaou (Pap) smear will infrequently suggest endometrial cancer. A transvaginal sonogram will identify the thickness of the endometrial stripe and identify intrauterine pathology, but it cannot make or refute the diagnosis of endometrial cancer. A D&C and hysteroscopy is of value in assessing the patient with a nondiagnostic endometrial biopsy. This patient has multiple risk factors for endometrial cancer; obesity (causes conversion of Δ_4-androstenedione to estrone) increases 3 to 10×, nulliparity's anovulatory cycles with unopposed estrogen increase the risk 2.5×, diabetes mellitus increases the risk 3×, and atypical hyperplasia increases the risk 8 to 29×.

14. **(C)** Surgical staging for endometrial cancer includes total abdominal hysterectomy, bilateral salpingo-oophorectomy, peritoneal washings for cytology, and pelvic and para-aortic lymph node sampling in conjunction with physical examination, chest x-ray, cystoscopy, and proctosigmoidoscopy. International Federation of Gynecology and Obstetrics (FIGO) IA is limited to the endometrium. IIB has invasion of the cervical stroma. This patient is staged as IIIC, grade 3 because of the pelvic lymph metastases. IVA has invasion to the bladder and/or bowel mucosa. IVB has distant metastases including lungs, vagina, abdomen, bone, intra-abdominal, and/or inguinal lymph nodes.

15. **(D)** Surgery is the principal means for the diagnosis, staging, and treatment of endometrial cancer. Staging endometrial cancer includes total abdominal hysterectomy, bilateral salpingo-oophorectomy, peritoneal washings for cytology, and pelvic and para-aortic lymph node sampling. Surgical pathologic findings and assessment of potential metastatic sites documents the degree of tumor spread into the myometrium and the degree of extrauterine spread to the adnexa, peritoneal cavity, and retroperitoneum. The decision to recommend postoperative radiation therapy is based on these surgical pathologic findings. Primary radiotherapy is used when contraindications to surgery are present. Chemotherapy palliates but does not cure.

16. **(B)** The ECG demonstates prolongation of the QRS interval, an RS complex in lead V1, and absent septal Q waves in leads V1 and V6 consistent with a diagnosis of LBBB. An anterior septal myocardial infarct would show ST elevations in the anterior chest leads. Enlargement of the left ventricle causes large T waves, especially in the lateral chest leads. RBBB causes a left axis deviation.

17. **(C)** Digoxin is most effective in the treatment of low-output cardiac failure while the other options are examples of high-output failure. The patient scenario is most suggestive of hypertensive heart disease, which typically results in low-output failure. Other diseases that can give this pattern of failure include ischemic cardiomyopathy, valvular disease, some types of congenital heart disease, and dilated cardiomyopathies.

18. **(D)** The bioavailability of digoxin in the standard tablet formulation is 50 to 75%. A preparation in which digoxin is dissolved in an encapsulated gel gives higher bioavailability, requiring a slight adjustment in the standard maintenance dose. Previously marketed preparations with poor bioavailability are no longer available in the United States.

19. **(E)** The estrogenic activity of various medicines, including digoxin, cimetidine, diazepam, ketaconazole, and spironolactone, can cause gynecomastia.

20. **(B)** Angiotensin-converting enzyme (ACE) inhibitors can all cause a nonproductive cough, especially within the first one or two months of therapy. These symptoms respond to decreasing the dose of discontinuing the medication.

21. **(E)** The major biological change in Paget's disease is an elevated alkaline phosphatase. Because studies have shown that as many as 90% of patients with Paget's disease are asymptomatic, diagnostic chance findings of abnormalities on radiologic examination or blood chemistry screening are invaluable in diagnosing this condition.

22. **(E)** Abdominal ultrasound should provide an accurate noninvasive means of assessing for pathologic disease involving the hepatobiliary system. Diagnostic laparoscopy is invasive and may miss intraparenchymal lesions. An abdominal x-ray series would not likely provide definitive information. The UGI series may demonstrate whether ulcer disease is present but would not provide information regarding the hepatobiliary system. A colonoscopy would not provide information regarding pathologic findings of the right upper quadrant unless a lesion involving the hepatic flexure of the colon is present.

23. **(D)** The fibrolamellar variant of hepatocellular carcinoma has a distinctly better prognosis. All of the other statements are true.

24–27. **(24-E, 25-D, 26-E, 27-E)** Measles and rubella are incorrect choices because they do not cause a single localized lesion. Pityriasis rosea likewise would result in multiple lesions, including a "herald patch" and Christmas tree distribution. Tinea corporis is a possibility, but in the face of a recent camping trip and malaise, Lyme disease would be the primary consideration.

   Lyme disease is a tick-borne, spirochetal (not fungal) disease caused by *Borrelia burgdorferi*. It is characterized by a distinctive skin lesion known as erythema chronicum migrans. Initial signs and symptoms often resolve within 3 to 4 weeks, regardless of treatment, though the rash may recur. There is then a latent period of weeks to months, after which time neurologic, cardiac, or musculoskeletal manifestations may appear. The classic neurologic triad is meningitis, cranial neuropathy (including Bell's palsy), and peripheral radiculoneuropathy. Cardiac involvement may include atrioventricular (AV) block, pericarditis, or cardiomegaly. Migratory arthralgias and arthritis involving large joints, especially the knee, are the most common latent manifestation. Treatment of choice is amoxicillin in younger children and doxycycline or minocycline in older individuals. Duration of treatment should include at least one 4-week generation cycle, so 6 weeks is advised. Tetracycline does not penetrate the CNS very well, so it is not advised. Plain erythromycin does not work at all.

28. **(D)** Approximately 20% of women with a hydatidiform mole develop bilateral theca lutein cysts. They are the result of ovarian hyperstimulation by the very high levels of hCG that are frequently seen in women with hydatidiform moles. The theca lutein cysts will regress spontaneously after evacuation of the mole, but it may take up to 12 weeks before the ovaries are back to their normal size. Close follow-up with the very sensitive serum beta-hCG assay allows early identification of those hydatidiform moles that will behave in a maligant fashion. A rise in serum beta-hCG level or a plateau in the level identified over three weekly determinations results in a diagnosis of malignant hydatidiform mole. A woman with malignant hydatidiform mole requires a thorough evaluation for metastases and chemotherapy. A complete mole is most common, arises from fertilization of a blighted ovum, and has a 46,XX karyotype. A partial mole is 69,XXY.

29. **(B)** The major symptoms of colorectal cancer are rectal bleeding, pain, and change in bowel habits. Fortunately, many colorectal cancers are being detected by screening tests before these signs of advanced disease develop. By the use of stool tests for occult blood, sigmoidoscopy, and colonoscopy, many are being found at early and asymptomatic stages. The clinical presentation in an individual patient is related to the size and location of the tumor. Bleeding and the development of iron-deficiency anemia are classic signs of carcinomas of the ascending colon.

30. **(E)** An abdominal mass or symptoms and signs of liver metastasis may be the earliest clinical manifestation of an underlying colorectal cancer. Distant spread to the lungs and bone may be silent until very advanced.

31. **(B)** If not done preoperatively, staging with computed tomography (CT) of the abdomen

and at many centers the chest, is recommended in patients with positive nodes. Adjuvant chemotherapy with 5-fluorouracil (5-FU) and leucovorin or levamisole has been shown to increase disease-free survival and overall survival in patients with IIIA and IIIB disease. Stage IIB patients probably benefit as well, but the advantage is less striking. Routine colonoscopy is recommended because of the likelihood of second colonic primaries. Routine follow-up of the CEA level is done. It has never been shown to affect overall survival or disease-free interval. In patients with nromal preoperative levels, there is no indication for repeated study. Following the CEA level in patients whose levels were elevated preoperatively does appear to allow the detection of recurrence at an earlier point and make resection of isolated recurrences more likely. The resection of isolated primaries has been associated with prolonged disease-free periods.

32. **(B)** Hematemesis is indicative of a bleeding source proximal to the ligament of Treitz. Diverticulosis would be more likely to be associated with hematochezia. All the other diagnoses listed could explain hematemesis in this patient.

33. **(D)** A Mallory–Weiss tear is a longitudinal tear of the gastric mucosa near the esophagogastric junction. This lesion usually occurs after vomiting and forceful retching. Most of the patients are alcoholics. The vast majority are self-limited events that do not require surgical intervention. If surgery is required for persistent hemorrhage, the management is to oversew the tear, not gastrectomy.

34. **(A)** Diuretics are not appropriate in a patient who requires continuing resuscitation. All of the other options are directed at stopping the hemorrhage.

35. **(D)** A widely used clinical classification of metastatic gestational trophoblastic neoplasia (known as the Duke, Hammond, or NCI classification) categorizes patients who have metastatic gestational trophoblastic neoplasia

into a high-risk and a low-risk group based on the following criteria:

Poor prognosis—any single high-risk factor:

1. Prechemotherapy serum beta-hCG level of > 40,000 mIU/mL
2. Duration of disease of > 4 months
3. Brain and/or liver metastasis
4. Failed prior chemotherapy
5. Antecedent term pregnancy

Good prognosis—absence of high-risk factors.

36. **(E)** Whole-brain irradiation can be used alone or in combination with chemotherapy. Patients with poor-prognosis metastatic gestational trophoblastic neoplasia require multiagent chemotherapy. The most common regimen gives methotrexate, actinomycin D, and cyclophosphamide (MAC) every 3 weeks. An alternative regimen used for patients with very high-risk disease is known as EMA-CO (etoposide, methotrexate, and actinomycin D alternating with cyclophosphamide and oncovin).

37. **(B)** In patients with constrictive pericarditis, ventricular filling is suddenly checked at the end of the early diastolic pressure dip, and therefore a loud third heart sound (pericardial knock) is frequently heard. Atrial fibrillation is common in long-standing cases, but this patient has relatively new symptoms. The heart size is often normal or only mildly enlarged. Renal failure is more often associated with pericardial effusions. ST elevations are suggestive of myocardial strain or infarct.

38. **(D)** In the United States and Western Europe, constrictive pericarditis is most often idiopathic. Other causes include radiation, neoplasm, trauma, and connective tissue disorders. Tuberculosis and bacterial infections are unusual in the United States.

39. **(E)** This is a case-control study that does not include the size of the populations at risk. Therefore, incidence cannot be calculated. The measure that would be useful here would be the odds ratio (which is [647 ×

27]/[2 × 622]). The odds ratio is an approximation of the relative risk, which may be obtained in cohort studies. The relative risk is the ratio of the incidence in the exposed cohort to the incidence in the unexposed cohort. Calculation of incidence requires knowledge of both the number of cases occurring in a specific population for the numerator and the size of that population for the denominator. The case-control study does not have population size.

40. **(B)** This patient, who likely has pancreatitis secondary to chronic alcoholism, is suffering from alcohol withdrawal, manifested by delirium tremens. Although auditory halucinations, delusions, and even olfactory hallucinations can occur in patients suffering from the delirium tremens, visual and tactile hallucinations are most common.

41. **(E)** As its name implies, delirium tremens most often presents with tremors, usually continuous, with an amplitude of more than 8 Hz, after 6 to 8 hours of no ingestion of alcohol. Any of the other symptoms can occur with progression of the condition.

42. **(A)** Formication, a prickling sensation that bugs are crawling on one's body, is a common manifestation of delirium tremens. Trichotillomania refers to pulling out of one's hair. Akathisia, a common side effect of antipsychotic medications, means restlessness. Confabulation is common in Korsakoff's syndrome, which affects alcoholic patients, and is the fictionalization of events, usually in an attempt to disguise difficulties with memory. Koro is a state of extreme anxiety sometimes seen in Southeast Asian men who fear their penises are shrinking into their bodies.

43. **(A)** The work-up is significant for the absence of the semen analysis. Approximately 40% of infertility is related to the male factor; therefore, the semen analysis is a mandatory part of the infertily evaluation. A varicocele is present in 25% of infertile men. The sperm penetration assay is of dubious value in evaluation of infertility. Laparoscopy is limited to

patients with histories or findings of endometriosis, pelvic infection, or an abnormal hysterosalpingogram. IUI and IVF are treatments of specific conditions. The incidence of infertility is approximately 10 to 15% of all reproductive-age couples. Infertility increases as follicle-stimulating hormone (FSH) levels increase and is directly associated with normal menstrual function.

44. **(A)** Anovulation is a common cause of infertility. This woman's history is highly indicative of ovulatory dysfunction. Information about cervical factors such as thick mucus or infection was not given. The hysterosalpingogram should eliminate most tubal and uterine causes. Clomiphene citrate is the first-line ovulation-inducing agent. A normal reproductive tract and male partner and an intact hypothalamic–pituitary–ovarian axis should be demonstrated prior to ovulation induction. Human menopausal gonadotropins may be used in clomiphine failures. Supraovulation and ovarian hyperstimulation are risks. IVF is only a last resort in a patient such as this.

45. **(A)** *Chlamydia trachomatis* is the leading cause of tubal infertility in the United States. It is frequently subclinical. Up to 75% of infertile patients with tubal factor and previous *Chlamydia* exposure (by serology) report no history of pelvic infection. The incidence of infertility increases from 15 to 30 to 50% after the first, second, and third episodes of pelvic inflammatory disease, respectively.

46. **(B)** In the United States, excessive alcohol use is most commonly associated with acute pancreatitis. Intravenous drug use, stones, and diabetes are also predisposing factors. Pregnancy alone is not an associated process. Alcohol is also the most common cause of chronic pancreatitis.

47. **(C)** Hyperglycemia is very common in pancreatitis secondary to a combination of factors, including decreased insulin release, increased glucagon release, and elevated adrenal glucocorticoids and catecholamines.

Patients are usually intravascularly volume depleted. Hypocalcemia is a poor prognostic sign.

48. **(C)** Amylase accumulates in the setting of renal failure and thus becomes a less valuable diagnostic test. Numerous other conditions involving the pancreas, the gut, and the salivary glands can raise amylase levels. Sulfonamides cause pancreatitis; therefore, an elevated amylase is not confusing, but rather a useful test for pancreatitis. Morphine can elevate amylase levels in the absence of pancreatitis.

49. **(C)** Pancreatitis in AIDS can be caused by cytomegalovirus and *Cryptosporidium* as well as *Mycobacterium avium* complex. Drugs are another cause of AIDS-related pancreatitis.

50. **(B)** Approximately 2% of the sample is below minus 2 standard deviations from the mean. Approximately 16% of the sample would be below minus 1 standard deviation from the mean.

51–52. **(51-D, 52-D)** The daughter is developing within normal limits. The normal sequence of pubertal development is directed by the maturation of the hypothalamic ovarian axis. FSH and then LH secretion cause the ovary to secrete estradiol, which leads to thelarche (median 9.8 years), adrenarche (median 10.5 years), and the growth spurt. Menarche should occur within 2 to 3 years of thelarche (median 12.8 years) and before the age of 16. A limited evaluation is appropriate only if reassurance of the mother and daughter is not satisfactory. McCune–Albright syndrome and isosexual precocious puberty are associated with precocious puberty, whereas Turner syndrome and constitutional delay are associated with delayed onset of puberty. MRKH is a congenital absence of the vagina, uterus, and tubes caused by müllerian agenesis. Precocious puberty is secondary sexual change before age 8. Approximately 75% of precocious puberty in females is idiopathic. 21-Hydroxylase deficiency congenital adrenal hyperplasia is the most common cause of excessive hormone secretion.

53. **(D)** Hepatitis B and D are most commonly transmitted sexually in the United States. Hepatitis D infection does not become symptomatic without coinfection by hepatitis B. Hepatitis B is endemic in many areas of Asia.

54. **(B)** Hepatoma is the most likely diagnosis in this man. In China, it is estimated that the lifetime risk of hepatoma in people with chronic hepatitis B is close to 40%. Alpha-fetoprotein elevations over 500 to 1000 μg/L in the absence of a colonic tumor, germ cell tumor, or pregnancy suggest hepatoma. Paraneoplastic syndromes are not common but include erythrocytosis, hypercalcemia, and secondary porphyria.

55. **(C)** If this patient were immune, the hepatitis B surface antibody (anti-HBs) would be positive. Anti-HBc develops in all hepatitis B virus (HBV) infections and persists indefinitely. It can indicate current or past HBV infection. HbsAg can be identified in serum 30 to 60 days after exposure to HBV and persists for a variable period; persistence for over 6 months is indicative of a carrier state. Anti-HBs develops after a resolved infection and is thought to be responsible for a long-term immunity. The IgM core antibody develops early and persists for at least 6 months; therefore, it is helpful in identifying a recent infection. If the HbsAg is positive and IgM anti-HBc is negative, a carrier state is likely. The hepatitis B vaccine induces anti-HBs, not anti-HBc, because the antigen used in the vaccine is the surface (not core) antigen.

56. **(B)** This patient, with melancholia, early morning awakening, loss of appetite, weight loss, and psychomotor retardation for a period of greater than 6 months after an identifiable stressor, meets DSM-IV (Diagnostic and Statistical Manual, 4th edition) criteria for a major depressive episode. Disorders such as hypochondriasis and somatoform disorder can be diagnosed only if a major axis I disorder is not present. The patient has no evidence of manic episodes.

57. **(C)** In the presence of an axis I diagnosis, it is not possible to make an axis II diagnosis. Life stressors are axis IV, and the GAF is axis V.

58. **(B)** Patients for whom psychiatrists have any index of suspicion for suicidal ideation or plans should always be asked about suicide. It has been demonstrated that discussing suicide with patients does not increase their risk of suicide attempts. Unfortunately, there has yet to be discovered a good prognostic indicator for the relative success of suicide attempts among depressed patients or a way to predict how they might commit suicide.

59. **(D)** The patient has the signs and symptoms of menopause. Menopause before the age of 40 is premature ovarian failure. An FSH level greater than 40 mIU/mL is confirmatory. Asherman syndrome is intrauterine scarring resulting in amenorrhea. Hypothalamic hypogonadotropic amenorrhea is not an acceptable choice because of the elevated FSH. A pituitary adenoma with FSH hypersecretion is very rare. Sheehan syndrome is pituitary necrosis with a lack of gonadotropin production and is a rare phenomenon most commonly occurring after a hypovolemic episode (eg, postpartum hemorrhage).

60. **(C)** The "3-day measles" or rubella is characterized by a relatively mild maculopapular rash that lasts 3 days or less. The rash begins on the face and spreads downward. Contraction of rubella during the first trimester is particularly dangerous and may result in numerous congenital abnormalities of the fetus. Possible cardiac manifestations included are patent ductus arteriosus, pulmonary stenosis, and myocardial necrosis.

61. **(B)** Precocious puberty has been associated with congenital rubella infection, as have diabetes mellitus, growth retardation, and growth hormone deficiency.

62. **(A)** If a patient presented for the first time with complaints typical of PUD, it would not be unreasonable to try an H₂ blocker (or

antacids if the symptoms were mild). Although the OTC preparations are not as strong, a one-year trial has already occurred, and evaluation should proceed to the next level. UGI is less expensive, but it is less sensitive and less specific; therefore, peptic ulcer disease is best defined by endoscopy.

63. **(D)** Gastric and duodenal ulcers can often be distinguished clinically. Gastric ulcer pain is frequently worsened by oral intake, and some weight loss is common. Gastric ulcers are caused by decreased mucosal protection from gastric acid by *H. pylori* infection, nonsteroidal anti-inflammatory drugs (NSAIDs), and intestinal metaplasia. Gastric hypersecretion is more often the cause of duodenal ulcers. There is in fact a risk of gastric ulcers becoming malignant, whereas duodenal ulcers are rarely anything but benign. Both types of ulcers are associated with infection by *H. pylori*. UGI studies have an approximately 30% false-negative rate.

64. **(E)** *H. pylori* is not effectively treated by any single-drug regimen. A combination of agents is required because of the organism's ability to develop antibiotic resistance. Fortunately, the course of treatment required is short because about 20% of patients develop side effects severe enough to limit their compliance.

65. **(B)** *H. pylori*, a gram-negative micro-aerophilic organism, may be the most common infection worldwide. No reservoir other than the human stomach has been identified, and the epidemiology is unknown. The organism is fastidious but can be cultured with careful technique. It is found in nearly all biopsies showing active antral gastritis with polymorphonuclear cell infiltration, whereas the organism is unusual in the histologically normal stomach. Eradication of the organism results in an 85 to 90% cure rate.

66. **(B)** The ELISA test is repeated because of the high number of false positives (ie, low specificity). Repeating the test greatly increases the predictive value positive. However, there

is a slight chance that the test may be falsely negative, and this chance is increased by the serial testing. Thus, it slightly decreases the sensitivity. The initial screening by ELISA is very sensitive, but not so specific. The subsequent tests are both very sensitive and very specific. They are performed later because they are more expensive. Cost is controlled by screening using the ELISA test.

67. **(D)** The location of the ulcer on the plantar surface over a metatarsal head is classic for a neuropathic ulcer, also known as a mal perforans ulcer. This ulcer has become secondarily infected. The fact that this patient also has an inflamed foot without pain indicates the presence of significant neuropathy. It is unlikely that arterial insufficiency is significant for this wound because the patient had a palpable foot pulse. Self-mutilation and spider bite would be extremely unlikely.

68. **(C)** The most important intervention for controlling a pyogenic infection is adequate debridement and drainage of the infected tissue. Intravenous antibiotics, control of hyperglycemia, and adequate hydration are also essential to the management of this patient. Foot x-rays are helpful in determining gas in the tissues and evidence of more advanced osteomyelitis.

69. **(E)** Diabetic foot infections are usually caused by mixed flora consisting of gram-positive, gram-negative, and anaerobic organisms. All of the organisms listed are common except for *Clostridium*.

70. **(E)** Lung cancer resulted in 52,000 deaths in 1995. Most cases are related to smoking. Breast cancer accounted for 43,600 deaths in 1995. A woman's lifetime risk is 11%. Colon cancer ended the lives of 29,000 women in 1995. Ovarian cancer caused 13,200 deaths in 1995.

71–73. **(71-E, 72-B, 73-C)** The annual prevalence of X is computed using the number of existing cases of disease during 1993 (old and new cases = 1100) as the numerator and the entire population at the beginning of the year as the denominator. The risk of disease X is the annual incidence of disease X during 1993 and is equal to the number of new cases of disease X (100 divided by the population at risk at the beginning of the year; 100,000 minus the 1000 existing cases), so it is 100 divided by 99,000, or 101. Risk of death, or mortality proportion, is deaths from a specific cause divided by the population at risk of death from that cause at the begining of the time period.

74. **(C)** This patient's clinical presentation is highly suggestive of ovarian carcinoma, the fifth most common malignancy. Weight loss, increased abdominal girth, ascites, adnexal masses, and cul-de-sac nodularity are very suggestive of ovarian malignancy. Imaging studies such as sonography or CT may be helpful. CT does a better job of imaging retroperitoneal structures. Chest x-ray is used to rule out metastatic disease. Barium enema is performed if there is a suspicion of colon involvement. Exploratory laparotomy is required to make the diagnosis (including stage) and initiate therapy. If the disease appears to be confined to the pelvic organs, retroperitoneal exploration and upper abdominal exploration and biopsies are necessary. The goal is to remove (debulk) as much tumor as possible.

75. **(D)** Only about 30% of patients have stage I or II disease. Stage I is limited to the ovaries. Stage II includes pelvic extension. Stage III has disease outside the true pelvis or positive inguinal or retroperitoneal nodes. Stage IIIC has positive nodes or implants greater than 2 cm. Stage IV has distant metastatic disease, pleural effusion with positive cytology, or liver parenchymal metastases. Debulking (cytoreductive surgery) is performed to shift the residual cells into the growth fraction where they are more susceptible to chemotherapy. Also, debulking may help relieve ascites formation and prevent potential bowel obstruction.

76. **(B)** The value relative to the risks of chemotherapy (adjunctive therapy) is clear except in low-grade tumors confined to the ovary (stage IA, IB). Therefore, most patients receive adjuvant chemotherapy. Melphalan, an alkylating agent, is the most commonly used agent. When used more than 12 cycles, it is associated with acute nonlymphocytic leukemia. Cisplatin, carboplatin, or paclitaxel is used alone or in combination. Radiocolloids or whole abdomen irradiation is also used. In stage II to IV patients, combination chemotherapy followed by a second-look laparotomy is the norm.

77. **(C)** Aortic stenosis is most likely to be associated with angina pectoris and syncope. Increased oxygen requirement, myocardial hypertrophy, low diastolic pressure, and shortening of diastole are contributory factors to the syncope.

78. **(E)** There is a possible indication (but not an obligation) to insert a temporary pacemaker if a new LBBB occurs. If LBBB and a Mobitz II AV block occur, there is general agreement on the usefulness of pacing. A temporary pacemaker is not required for first-degree block. For second-degree block of the Wenckebach type, pacing is required only if symptoms of bradycardia and hypotension cannot be controlled medically. The necessity for temporary pacing during an acute myocardial infarction does not necessarily indicate that permanent pacing will be required.

79. **(D)** The ventricular inhibited pacemaker functions when the heart rate falls below a preset interval. If a QRS is detected, the pacemaker is inhibited. If a QRS is not sensed, the pacing stimulus is not inhibited and the ventricle is stimulated.

80. **(E)** Somatization disorder usually begins in the twenties and runs a fluctuating course, although the patient is rarely free of symptoms. These patients do not have symptoms of melancholia. Although they may include conversion phenomena in their list of com-

plaints, the diagnosis of conversion disorder should be reserved for those in whom conversion symptoms are primary. Hypochondriasis is characterized by unrealistic interpretations of actual physical signs and symptoms and by an obsessive fear that one is ill. The diagnosis of malingering should be reserved for those patients with an identifiable secondary gain from hospitalization or medical attention.

81. **(C)** Cricothyroidotomy is the safest way to obtain an airway in an emergency department setting. Tracheostomy can be more time consuming and more prone to complications, especially by less experienced persons. Nasotracheal and endotracheal intubation are not appropriate in this setting and can lead to significant iatrogenic complications. Oxygen by way of nasal cannula would be inadequate for oxygenation and would not address protection of her airway.

82. **(D)** With the impaired cardiac function of cardiogenic shock, stroke output is increased by nitroprusside as left ventircular end-diastolic pressure falls. Nitroprusside is an arterial vasodilator. It has no direct effect on heart rate or contractility.

83. **(D)** Pericarditis secondary to transmural infarction is very common, and most cases appear within 4 days. The most common manifestation of pericarditis is a friction rub along the left sternal border. Signs and symptoms last only a few days. The pain is pleuritic, worsened by inspiration, swallowing, coughing, or lying down. It is frequently associated with a low-grade fever. While all five options are possible and must be evaluated with chest x-ray and repeat ECG, postinfarct pericarditis is the most common.

84. **(A)** Beta blockers, antiplatelet agents, warfarin, and lowered lipid levels have all been shown to improve the prognosis of patients after myocardial infarction. While control of lipids, beta blockers, and antiplatelet agents are useful in the longer run, warfarin does not seem to add much after 6 months. Calcium channel blockers, alpha-adrenergic antagonists, and nitroprusside have roles in the management of hypertension, coronary artery disease, and myocardial infarction, but they do not improve prognosis in the postinfarction period.

85. **(E)** Relative contraindications to the use of beta blockers include CHF, heart block, diabetes mellitus (masks symptoms of hypoglycemia), and bradycardia. Beta blockers are useful drugs in the treatment of hypertension and tremors. Tachycardia and fever require investigation but do not pose specific problems to the use of beta blockers.

86. **(D)** Liver disease is relatively uncommon (< 5%). The other four choices are relatively common, with diarrhea and abdominal pain being the most common complaints.

87. **(A)** The key is "early." Early disease is not associated with symptoms. As the tumor grows and invades, tissue necrosis causes bleeding and/or foul-smelling discharge. Bleeding is the most common symptom of cervical carcinoma. The symptoms of advanced local disease include lower back pain, sciatic pain, uremia, and lower extremity edema. Distant disease is usually metastasic to the liver or lung. Most cases are diagnosed between ages 45 and 50. Risk factors include early intercourse, multiple sex partners, cigarette smoking, human papillomavirus (HPV), and HIV.

88. **(D)** Microinvasive carcinoma of the cervix in some circumstances is amenable to less radical therapy. Patients with microinvasion have a very small risk of pelvic lymph node metastasis; therefore, less radical therapy may acheive the same outcome. Patients should have clear margins and absence of lymphovascular space involvement. Positive margins are associated with a higher incidence of residual cancer. Cigarette smoking, HPV, HIV, multiple partners, and early intercourse are recognized risk factors.

89. (A) The viral hepatitis most commonly acquired on short-term trips of this nature is hepatitis A. Like hepatitis E, the most likely route of spread is fecal–oral. Fortunately, the mortality rate with hepatitis A is low, and fulminant hepatitis A is rare. Chronic hepatitis does not occur. There is no carrier state.

90. (B) The sclera are high in elastin content, which has an affinity for bilirubin. Unconjugated hyperbilirubinemia is caused by overproduction, decreased uptake, or decreased conjugation.

91. (C) Effective vaccines are available for hepatitis A and B. Because hepatitis D is always seen in association with hepatitis B, vaccination for hepatitis B almost eliminates the likelihood of symptomatic hepatitis D infection, but does not prevent it specifically. No vaccine is yet available for CMV, EBV, or hepatitis E or C.

92. (C) The first sign of trichinosis is a sudden appearance of edema of the upper eyelids. Shortly thereafter, muscle soreness and pain, skin lesions, thirst, profuse sweating, chills, weakness, prostration, and eosinopilia appear. Respiratory and neurologic symptoms may develop 3 to 6 weeks after onset.

93. (E) The main source of transmission is eating food that contains raw or insufficiently cooked pork; therefore, prevention would be to properly cook pork. Heating to a temperature of 65.5°C (150°F) or cooling to –25°C (–13°F) for 10 days will destroy the cysts, which are not visible to a meat inspector.

94. (D) Control of daytime urination usually occurs by age 2 or 3, while lack of nighttime control is not a major concern until age 4. A physical exam may be helpful if physical symptoms are present or the patient is unable to master daytime sphincter control. Questioning about family stressors may be indicated if the child fails to progress with nighttime sphincter control. More extensive behavioral or pharmacologic treatments may

be considered at that time. In the meantime, encouragement, avoiding fluids after supper and before bedtime, and simple rewards for dry nights will likely be successful.

95. (E) All of the options are complications associated with Crohn's disease.

96. (D) This patient is exhibiting classic positive and negative symptoms, and age of onset, of paranoid schizophrenia: bizarre behaviors, likely auditory hallucinations, paranoid delusions, and decline in daily function. The presence of psychosis (auditory hallucinations, a delusional system) rules out a personality disorder or a social phobia. Similarly, the absence of feelings of worthlessness, trouble sleeping, or frank suicidal ideation makes major depressive disorder a less fitting diagnosis. However, DSM-IV requires a persistence of symptoms of at least 6 months for the diagnosis of schizophrenia, so the most appropriate diagnosis at this time is schizophreniform disorder.

97. (B) The patient will most benefit from administration of an antipsychotic such as haloperidol. In the presence of psychosis, especially paranoid delusions, insight-oriented and behavioral therapy would be counterproductive. Lorazepam, a benzodiazepine, might sedate the patient and calm him down but would do nothing to control his psychotic symptoms. Fluoxetine, a member of the serotonin-specific reuptake inhibitor (SSRI) family of antidepressants, would also be of little or no help in a psychotic patient.

98. (B) The patient is experiencing a relapse of his symptoms, and because their duration now exceeds 6 months, he can be diagnosed with paranoid schizophrenia.

99. (D) While at first glance his behavior may appear bizarre, and thus perhaps a relapse of his psychotic symptoms, the patient is in reality suffering from tardive dyskinesia, one of the long-term side effects of administering traditional antipsychotics. Thus, increasing his haloperidol dosage will only make things worse. Unfortunately, tardive dyskinesia is irreversible, but there is some evidence that switching to a newer class of antipsychotics with a different side effect profile, such as clozapine, can prevent worsening of dyskinetic symptoms. Benztropine, an anticholinergic agent, has been shown to be effective as a prophylactic measure against tardive dyskinesia when given in conjunction with traditional antipsychotics but is of little use once tardive sets in. While benzodiazepines such as lorazepam and beta blockers such as propranolol may be effective in managing the movement disorders characteristic of tardive dyskinesia, the most important step in managing the condition is discontinuation of the offending agent.

100. **(A)** A smaller defect is worrisome secondary to an increased risk of incarceration and possible strangulation of the hernia contents. All of the other statements are correct.

101. **(E)** The head, each arm, and one side of each lower extremity is 9%. The anterior chest and abdomen is 18%. The entire back is 18%. The perineum is 1%. First-degree burns are not included in this calculation.

102. **(B)** The total volume resuscitation this patient should receive is 4 mL/kg/percent area burn ($4 \times 60 \times 40$). Half the total volume should be administered in the first 8 hours and the other half over the subsequent 16 hours. First-degree burns are not included in this calculation.

103. **(D)** Murmurs not associated with significant hemodynamic abnormalities are referred to as functional or innocent murmurs. Functional murmurs are noted on routine examination in over 30% of children. The most common is a medium-pitched, vibratory, systolic ejection murmur. Others include innocent pulmonic murmurs that are high-pitched and early systolic, and venous hums caused by turbulence of blood in the jugular system. A normal ECG is associated with an innocent murmur. Diastolic murmurs are not

considered to be innocent murmurs. They are found in a number of cardiac lesions. Examples include pulmonary valve insufficiency (associated with a high-pitched blowing diastolic murmur along the left sternal border), mitral stenosis (long diastolic rumbling murmur at the apex), and mitral insufficiency (rumbling mid-diastolic murmur at the apex).

104. **(E)** Stress from these conditions will require additional insulin doses. Infections are short-term stresses, which will raise blood sugar levels. Because physical activity will decrease the insulin requirements, returning to school where there is more sedentary time will require additional insulin doses.

105. **(E)** Douching is of limited value in preventing pregnancy due to the rapid transit of sperm through the genital tract. Postcoital contraception or "morning after" contraception can be accomplished with good effectiveness in several ways. Five-day therapy started within 72 hours of the event with diethystilbestrol (DES) 25 to 50 mg/day, ethinyl estradiol 5 mg/day, or conjugated estrogen 30 mg/day have all been used with subsequent pregnancy rates of 0.6 to 1.6% compared to an estimated midcycle clinical pregnancy rate of 7%. Side effects of severe nausea, vomiting, breast tenderness, and menstrual irregularity limit compliance with 5-day therapy. More recently, four tablets of a combination oral contraceptive with 0.05 mg of ethinyl estradiol and 0.5 mg/dL of levonorgestrol (Ovral) in doses of two tablets 12 hours apart have become the treatment of choice, with equal effectiveness and shorter duration of side effects. Pharmacies generally dispense the entire package of pills rather than the small dose needed; thus, instructions to the patient must be very specific. Insertion of a copper IUD is also very effective but has the risk of introducing bacteria into the upper genital tract.

106. **(D)** It is generally preferable to examine the patient prior to prescription, unless a thorough history can be obtained from a well-

known patient. Previous similar accidents may have already resulted in a pregnancy. "Implantation bleeding" may be confused with menses. A urine hCG should detect a pregnancy within 14 days after conception. Urinary frequency is a common early symptom in pregnancy.

107. **(B)** *Chlamydia trachomatis* is the most likely STD associated with the triad of urethritis, conjunctivitis, and arthritis. This syndrome is called Reiter syndrome.

108. **(A)** The treatment of choice for *Chlamydia trachomatis* is doxycycline. Tetracycline is also an alternative. Metronidazole is the treatment of choice for *Gardnerella vaginalis*. Penicillin is still the treatment for syphilis. Cephalosporins are becoming significant therapy for gonococcal infections.

109. **(A)** Münchhausen syndrome is a condition characterized by continued and habitual presentation for surgery and/or hospitalization for an imagined acute illness. The patient gives a meticulous history, all of which is false, but insists on medical attention. This syndrome is a chronic, factitious disorder with physical symptoms. It differs from hypochondriasis in that patients suffering from hypochondriasis usually have an actual physical complaint that they interpret as signifying a terrible disorder (eg, "I have this terrible headache which means I must have a brain tumor"). Tourette syndrome is a disorder usually diagnosed in children, which is characterized by facial tics and inappropriate swearing. Ménière syndrome is a disease that affects the inner ear, involving deafness associated with tinnitus and vertigo.

110. **(C)** The patient displays uncontrollable lying in which he voluntarily presents involved and elaborate fantasies. This form of habitual, pathological lying may not just involve the patient's medical problems, but often involves other areas of his life. Logorrhea refers to rapid speech, often illogical, which is often seen in manias. Perseveration is the insistence on performing a task or repeating a phrase. Dissociation, which may be a main factor in fugue and other states, refers to the ability to hold two conflicting ideas in concert. Echolalia is the pathological repetition of words spoken by another person.

111. **(D)** The Glasgow coma scoring is calculated as follows: (1) Eye: 4—spontaneously opens, 3—opens to command, 2—opens to pain, 1—no response; (2) Verbal: 5—spontaneous speech, 4—disoriented, 3—incomprehensible words, 2—incomprehensible sounds, 1—no response; (3) Motor: 6—spontaneous movement, 5—localizes pain, 4—withdraws to pain, 3—decorticate posturing (flexor), 2—decerebrate (extensor), 1—no response. A patient receives a score from each of these three areas and then the total is determined. In this case, the patient's total score is 7 (Eye—1, Verbal—2, Motor—4).

112. **(A)** The carcinoid syndrome is characterized by elevated levels of 5-HIAA in the urine. Symptoms most commonly occur when the disease has metastasized to the liver. Appendiceal carcinoids can sometimes be found incidentally. These cancers are relatively slow growing and therefore the 5-year survival rates are over 90%. Treatment is resection when possible and management of symptoms when resection is impossible. Gaucher's and hepatitis will produce an enlarged liver, but flushing and 5-HIAA are not present. Allergy to MSG causes flushing but is not associated with 5-HIAA or hepatomegaly.

113. **(C)** The carcinoid syndrome is associated with right heart lesions (tricuspid or pulmonary stenosis or regurgitation), whose murmurs are made worse by inspiration. An enlarged left ventricle would be more suggestive of mitral or aortic dysfunction. Edema of the head and neck is not uncommonly seen in bronchial carcinoids. Bronchospasm can be seen with any site of origin but is not associated with a chronic infectious process. Abdominal pain and diarrhea are additional common manifestations. Neither constipation nor dysuria are associated with the carcinoid syndrome.

114. (B) The cause of initial onset of multiple painful genital lesions of a sexually transmitted origin is most likely herpes simplex, type 2.

115. (B) Viral isolation of HSV-2 from tissue culture is the definitive method for identification of this viral infection. The yield is further increased if this is a primary infection and when the lesions are vesicular (as opposed to ulcerative). Presumptive diagnosis can be made from the Tzanck preparation in the office setting. Darkfield examination technique establishes the definitive diagnosis of *Treponema pallidum* infection. Fluorescent monoclonal antibody stain helps establish the diagnosis of *Chlamydia trachomatis*.

116. (E) The best way to identify the high-risk patient for operative bleeding is through obtaining a detailed history.

117–121.   (117-B, 118-A, 119-B, 120-A, 121-E) Hypervitaminosis A results in nausea, drowsiness, papilledema, and hyperostosis of the long bones. Thiamine deficiency results in depression, drowsiness, peripheral neuritis, and tachycardia (beriberi). Hypoparathyroidism results in dry skin, abdominal pain, muscle pain and cramps, and positive Chvostek and Trousseau signs. The signs listed are typical of vitamin D deficiency, a key vitamin in bone metabolism. All of the choices listed are early signs of rickets except conjunctivitis. Symptoms may be present after several months of vitamin D deficiency. Four hundred IU of vitamin D is present in about 32 ounces of whole milk and recommended for individuals between 6 months and 24 years of age. Two hundred IU is suggested as the recommended daily allowance (RDA) for those above 24 years of age. Parathyroid hormone will mobilize calcium from bone. Obesity itself has not been linked with an increased incidence of vitamin D deficiency. Anticonvulsants can interfere with metabolism of vitamin D, leading to a deficiency when combined with poor sun exposure.

122. (B) A febrile transfusion reaction is the most common. Hepatitis B and AIDS have decreased since the 1980s. Cytomegalovirus is the most commonly transmitted infectious agent. Hepatitis A is transmitted by way of an enteral route of transfusion.

123. (E) Cigarette smoking increases the risk for bladder and cervical cancer, cardiovascular disease, and for bone loss, which leads to osteoporosis.

124. (B) Cardiovascular disease is the leading cause of death and is more likely to present with atypical angina. Onset of disease is typically one decade later than in men. Evaluation is best initiated with thallium treadmill or stress echocardiography.

125. (B) Evaluation of hematuria tailored to the clinical situation should be carried out even when benign explanations such as atrophy are present. Twenty percent of women with microscopic hematuria on anticoagulants have significant disease.

126. (A) Evaluation of the abnormal Pap smear should begin with colposcopy.

127. (B) Pica, which refers to the ingestion of nonnutritive substances, including paint, plaster, string, hair, cloth, or dirt, can start in infancy. It is not a normal behavior. Rumination, which in cows refers to redigestion of food, is characteristic of depressive and obsessive disorders and refers to the inability to discard a particular thought. While it is possible that this patient also suffers from anorexia nervosa, the most appropriate diagnosis is pica. Finally, it is unlikely that a patient with a hematocrit of 28 is malingering.

128. (B) Although pica may be comorbid with any number of mental disorders, lead poisoning is the most common and most concerning disorder that presents concomitantly with pica. Patients who suffer from pica are more likely to be underweight than morbidly obese. Moon facies is a common manifestation of Cushing syndrome, a disorder resulting from high serum levels of corticosteroids.

129. **(C)** DSM-IV requires a period of a month or more for the diagnosis of pica.

130. **(D)** The most common cause for lower GI hemorrhage in children is from a Meckel's diverticulum. In infancy, anal fissures are the leading cause of rectal bleeding. Intussusception is most common in children 8 to 12 months of age. Although they may pass bloody mucus ("currant jelly stool"), it is not usually associated with massive hemorrhage. Significant UGI hemorrhage in infants and children is most often due to esophageal varices from prehepatic occlusion of the portal vein.

131. **(C)** Proportional mortality studies do not measure risk of dying, since the denominator is deaths from all causes rather than the living population. The findings given merely show that a larger proportion of deaths in Uganda may be attributed to causes other than cancer. This could be due to either a protective effect against dying from cancer or an increased risk of dying from some other cause. The data given do not allow differentiation between these possibilities. There are also no data on the prevalence of cancer or the cancer-specific mortality rate.

132. **(D)** When a chronic, incurable disease that may be fatal is so treated that life is lengthened, the net effect from treatment alone is an increase in the prevalence of AIDS, above what it otherwise would be. Thus, an increase in prevalence may not be a bad thing when it is due to longer survival, as it is here. Incidence will not be affected among adults, although it may go down as a result of less maternal transmission to infants. To decrease the incidence of disease, and subsequently the prevalence, measures to prevent AIDS would be needed.

133. **(E)** In mitral valve prolapse, the first heart sound is usually preserved, followed by a systolic click and mid to late systolic mur-

mur. Mitral regurgitation may occur. A continuous machinery murmur is heard below the left clavicle in association with a persistent ductus arteriosus. Pansystolic murmurs are heard in ventricular septal defects, and the intensity of the murmur is no indication of the size. Atrial septal defects result in a right ventricular lift and a fixed, split S2. Pulmonary hypertension causes increased intensity of the second heart sound, particularly the pulmonary component.

134. **(C)** Common findings in endocarditis include splinter hemorrhages and petechiae (which are not specific). Osler's nodes, Roth's spots, Janeway lesons, and stroke. Many of these complications are thought to be embolic, but may include vasculitis. Osler's nodes, splinter hemorrhages, and petechiae result from the deposition of immune complexes and can continue to appear for several days after the initiation of antibiotics. Roth's spots are retinal hemorrhages. Janeway lesions are emboli to the palms and soles.

135. **(A)** The 1997 recommendations of the American Heart Association for dental prophylaxis give several options, including amoxicillin, 2 g PO as a single dose. The PO dose of clindamycin is 600 mg. Gentamicin is recommended for patients undergoing GI or genitourinary (GU) procedures.

136. **(A)** *S. viridans* and *S. bovis* are the most common organisms seen in native valve endocarditis. *S. aureus* is also frequently seen. *S. pneumoniae*, *Actinobacillus*, and *Eikenella* are unusual.

137. **(C)** For a screening test to be effective, the most important single factor to consider is that it have a high predictive value positive. This will be related to both the sensitivity and the specificity of the test and also to the incidence of the disease in the population being tested. If a disease is very rare in the screened population, the predictive value of a positive test may be low, even with both very high sensitivity and specificity. Thus,

part of a surveillance system can entail selection of population at higher risk and targeting them for screening. Some other important attributes for an effective surveillance program are simplicity, acceptability, and flexibility.

138. (K)

139. (A)

140. (D)

141. (F)

142. (C) The ratio of females to males with SLE is 4:1. Goodpasture syndrome is associated with nephritis and pulmonary alveolar hemorrhage, usually affecting young adult males and children. This disorder may follow an acute illness or drug exposure and has been associated with the flu. Hemolytic–uremic syndrome is most common in children under the age of 4, and there is usually a prodrome of gastroenteritis. The pathology of chronic polyarteritis nodosa involves a hypersensitivity reaction of the medium-sized vessel. The majority of patients with acute poststreptococcal glomerulonephritis recover without permanent renal damage as do individuals with renal stones and infections.

143. (C)

144. (B)

145. (B)

146. (E)

147. (A) With idiopathic thrombocytopenic purpura, the platelets are coated with increased amounts of IgG or IgM, resulting in rapid destruction of platelets. The bone marrow responds to this low platelet count with in-

creased young megakaryocytes. ITP follows viral infections in 80% of the cases. Bone marrow suppression may occur after radiation ad cytotoxic drugs, as well as following exposure to insecticides (DDT or Lindane), solvents such as benzene, and other drugs, such as chloramphenicol and sulfonamides. In patients with acute lymphocytic leukemia (ALL), the bone marrow becomes infiltrated with leukemic cells, decreasing the megakaryocytes and peripheral platelets. In von Willebrand disease, there is often mild to moderate bleeding. The platelets are normal, but there is a defect in the adhesion to exposed vascular collagen. Decreased factor VIII is secondary to decreased amount of von Willebrand factor, which transports the factor VIII. The most common symptoms of this autosomal dominant disease are nosebleeds and easy bruising. Anaphylactoid purpura is a vasculitis with leaking of the red cells into the tissue rather than a problem with platelets or clotting factors. The bone marrow and platelet count will be normal. The purpura typically occurs on the buttocks and flexor surfaces of the legs. Renal and intestinal lesions are common.

148. (E) Patients with schizophrenia are often observed drinking very large amounts of water, on the order of gallons per day, and their kidneys can become overwhelmed and not retain sufficient sodium. This manifestation of the disorder is reversible.

149. (B) Bulimia nervosa refers to repeated episodes of binge eating, followed by self-induced vomiting, which can destroy tooth enamel. Patients exhibit marked weight changes.

150. (C) Anorexia nervosa presents with all the physiologic findings of self-induced starvation. It is more common in adolescent girls than boys.

Practice Test 2
Questions

DIRECTIONS (Questions 1 through 38): Each group of items in this section consists of lettered headings followed by a set of numbered words or phrases. For each numbered word or phrase, select the ONE lettered heading that is most closely associated with it. Each lettered heading may be selected once, more than once, or not at all.

Questions 1 Through 5

Match the following diagnostic tests with the numbered statements. Each is a diagnostic test used in the evaluation of a trauma patient.

(A) computed tomography (CT) scan of the chest
(B) diagnostic peritoneal lavage (DPL)
(C) abdominal x-ray series
(D) CT scan of the abdomen
(E) arteriography
(F) chest x-ray
(G) none of the above

1. A 46-year-old man is status post a motor vehicle accident. He was an unrestrained passenger. He has a significant closed head injury and is hemodynamically unstable. What would be the test of choice to assess the patient for a significant intra-abdominal injury?

2. A 25-year-old man, status post a motorcycle accident, presents as alert and awake, with fractures involving his right wrist and an open fracture of his right leg. His abdomen is soft and nontender. He is initially tachycardic and hypotensive, but stabilizes after fluid resuscitation in the emergency department. The orthopedic surgeon wants to take the patient to the operating room as soon as possible for definitive management of the fractures. His medical history discloses several previous abdominal surgical procedures secondary to a stab wound 2 years prior. How will you assess this patient for an intra-abdominal injury?

3. A 37-year-old woman, who was a restrained driver, is status post a motor vehicle accident. You are told by the paramedics that the steering wheel sustained considerable damage. A chest x-ray demonstrates a widened mediastinum. You are concerned that she has a traumatic aortic disruption. What is the definitive study for this life-threatening diagnosis?

4. This diagnostic study is always reliable for diagnosis of ruptured diaphragm.

5. Use of this diagnostic study may result in operation for intra-abdominal injury not requiring operative repair.

Questions 6 Through 8

    (A) a 36-year-old man with paranasal sinus pain, purulent nasal discharge, and lower respiratiory tract symptoms

    (B) a 36-year-old woman with hemoptysis, dyspnea, and hematuria

    (C) a 42-year-old man with chronic active hepatitis B

    (D) a 22-year-old woman with arthralgias of the fingers, wrists, knees, and ankles, and Raynaud syndrome

6. Goodpasture syndrome

7. Wegener's granulomatosis

8. Periarteritis nodosa

Questions 9 Through 14

Match the case presentations with the disorders listed.

    (A) toxoplasmosis
    (B) rubella
    (C) rubeola
    (D) cytomegalovirus
    (E) varicella
    (F) erythema bullosum
    (G) staphylococcal scalded skin syndrome
    (H) roseola
    (I) Fifth disease

9. A 1-year-old child who had a fever as high as 103°F for 3 days, without an identifiable source of infection, presents with a "slapped-cheek" appearance.

10. A 1-year-old child with high fevers for 4 days presents with no fever and feeling well. You note a rash on the trunk, slightly red pharynx, and cervical adenopathy.

11. A baby is found to have patent ductus arteriosus (PDA), cataracts, deafness, and delayed development.

12. A 9-year-old girl presents with a generalized vesicular eruption, with lesions in different stages including crusted macules and vesicles. She was exposed to another child with same rash 2 weeks earlier. (See Figure 2.1.)

13. A 5-year-old unvaccinated child presents with coryza, cough, and conjunctivitis, followed by Koplik's spots.

14. A 3-month-old baby presents with hydrocephalus, chrorioretinitis, and intracranial calcifications.

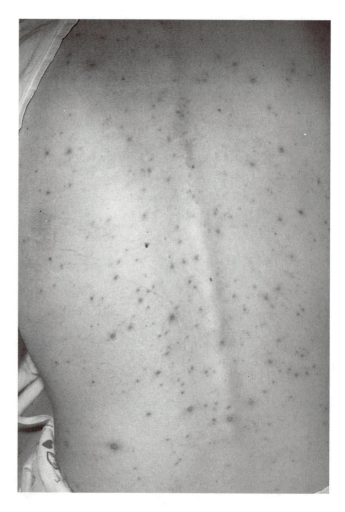

Figure 2.1

Questions 15 Through 17

Match the following diagnoses with the appropriate descriptions.

    (A) Lyme disease

    (B) juvenile rheumatoid arthritis

    (C) serum sickness

    (D) degenerative arthritis

    (E) acute rheumatic fever

    (F) gouty arthritis

    (G) transient synovitis

    (H) fibromyalgia

15. Usually affects children between the ages of 3 and 6, and is associated with a limp and pain. The hip, anterior thigh, or knee is usually involved, and the temperature is normal or slightly elevated. An upper respiratory infection, limited internal rotation, or reduced extension and abduction may be found.

16. Starts with a headache, stiff neck, myalgia, fatigue, lethargy, and lymphadenopathy. May progress to arthritis of the large joints, especially the knee.

17. Fever, myalgia, lymphadenopathy, arthralgias, and arthritis following exposure to blood products, drugs, or infectious agents.

Questions 18 and 19

Match the following diagnoses with the clinical descriptions.

    (A) *Listeria* monocytes

    (B) rotavirus infection

    (C) atypical mycobacteria

    (D) *Salmonella*

    (E) *Shigella*

    (F) adenovirus infection

    (G) *Streptococcus pneumoniae* infection

    (H) Kawasaki disease

    (I) tuberculosis (TB)

    (J) staphylococcal infection

18. A 9-month-old child with a 2-day history of fever and diarrhea, fair urine output, intake of solid foods poor, but good intake of fluids; green stool with more liquid than solid matter

19. A 9-year-old child with a 2 × 3-cm lymph node in the left anterior cervical area that is mobile and tender; weakly positive purified protein derivative (PPD) (5-mm induration)

Questions 20 Through 24

Match the following choices of abdominal pain patterns with the case scenarios.

    (A) pain pattern suggestive of early acute appendicitis

    (B) pain pattern suggestive of urolithiasis

    (C) pain pattern suggestive of perforated viscus

    (D) pain pattern suggestive of cholecystitis

    (E) pain pattern suggestive of pancreatitis

    (F) pain pattern suggestive of early diverticulitis

20. A 50-year-old man presents with acute onset of severe flank pain radiating to the groin, crescendo in nature; he cannot seem to be still during examination; pain is not increased by anterior abdominal palpation.

21. A 70-year-old man describes acute onset of sharp pain in the left lower quadrant spreading to the entire infraumbilical area over 1 to 2 hours; the abdomen is rigid to examination and bowel sounds are absent, with rebound tenderness over the left lower quadrant.

22. A 36-year-old man presents with several hours of vague, poorly localized epigastric pain and anorexia, which recently became well-localized right lower quadrant pain and tenderness to palpation.

23. A 40-year-old man with a history of alcohol abuse and a recent binge presents with epigastric pain radiating through to the midback; the pain is made better with a seated position, leaning slightly forward.

24. A 36-year-old woman is admitted with a chief complaint of abdominal pain that awakens her at night. The pain is described as a steady pain or pressure sensation boring through her back in the right upper quadrant. It lasts several hours, gradually disappears, and is frequently accompanied by nausea.

Questions 25 Through 27

Match the diagnosis with the clinical description.

(A) trisomy 15
(B) Neimann–Pick disease
(C) Lesch–Nyhan syndrome

(D) Down syndrome
(E) autism
(F) attention deficit hyperactivity disorder (ADHD)
(G) post-Lyme disease deficit

25. Poor attention span, distractibility, normal intelligence, poor school performance

26. Repetitive movements, poor communication skills, low intelligence quotient (IQ), poor interpersonal relationships

27. Mental retardation, self-destructive behavior, biting

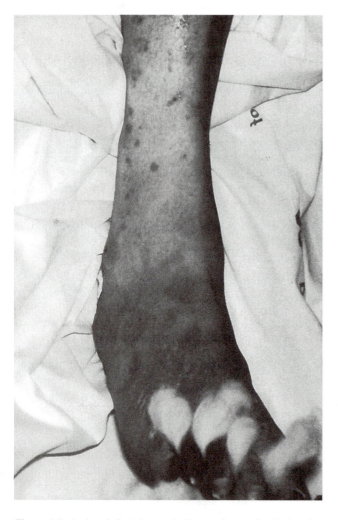

Figure 2.2. Ischemic foot demonstrating a ruborous forefoot and dry gangrene of the digits.

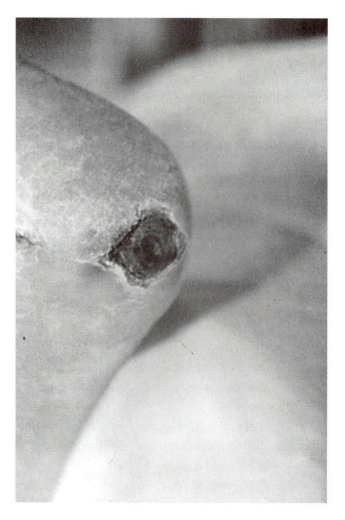

Figure 2.3. Heel decubitus ulcer.

Questions 28 Through 34

Match the following with the numbered statements relating to them.

(A) Figure 2.2

(B) Figure 2.3

(C) Figure 2.4

(D) Figure 2.5

(E) a puncture wound from a nail in the right foot

(F) none of the above

28. May develop as a consequence of deep venous thrombosis (DVT)

29. Cured by antibiotic therapy alone

30. Will require revascularization for limb salvage

31. Usually induced by immobilization and prolonged pressure in areas of decreased sensation

32. Requires tetanus immunization to be up to date

33. Recurrent lymphangitis and cellulitis

34. Compression therapy is the mainstay of therapy in what condition other than venous stasis?

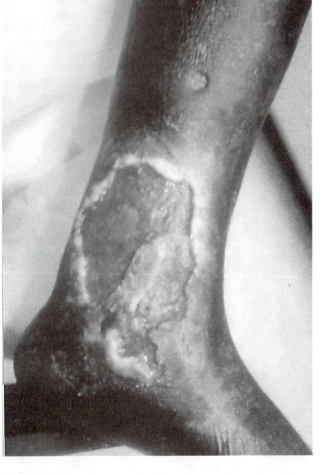

Figure 2.4. Classic venous stasis leg ulcer over the region of the medial malleolus.

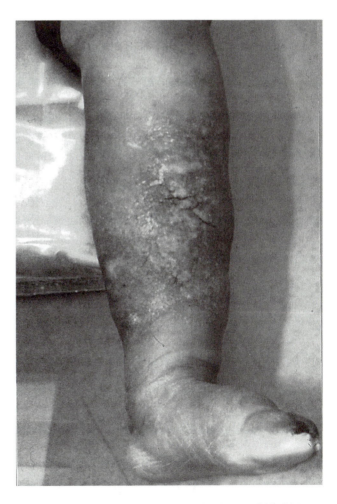

Figure 2.5. Chronic lymphedema with skin changes (skin thickened and hyperkeratotic).

Questions 35 Through 38

Match the diagnosis with the clinical description.

- (A) basal ganglia hemorrhage
- (B) cerebellar hemorrhage
- (C) pontine hemorrhage
- (D) lobar intracerebral hemorrhage
- (E) cocaine-related hemorrhage
- (F) subarachnoid hemorrhage
- (G) arteriovenous malformation (AVM)
- (H) hypertensive encephalopathy
- (I) primary intraventricular hemorrhage

35. A 67-year-old man develops coma over a few minutes. He has ataxic respirations and pinpoint, reactive pupils. Oculocephalic reflexes are absent.

36. A 74-year-old woman develops occipital headache, vomiting, and ataxia. Over the next few hours, she develops a decline in her level of consciousness.

37. In addition to basal ganglia and pontine hemorrhage, his syndrome is almost always associated with chronic hypertension.

38. A 24-year-old man has a history of recurrent, throbbing headaches. He suddenly develops mild right-sided weakness. His blood pressure in the past has been normal but now is slightly elevated.

DIRECTIONS (Questions 39 Through 150): Each of the numbered items or incomplete statements in this section is followed by answers or by completions of the statement. Select the ONE lettered answer or completion that is BEST in each case.

39. When evaluating any of the patients in questions 35 through 38, the physician often has a choice between CT and magnetic resonance imaging (MRI). In which circumstance is CT of the brain superior to MRI?

    (A) demonstrating AVMs
    (B) staging for metastatic malignancy

    (C) imaging small infarcts
    (D) evaluating possible multiple sclerosis
    (E) diagnosing an acute hemorrhage

40. A 10-year-old boy is brought into the office by his anxious parents. His complaint is hair loss. He denies taking any medication and has had no medical problems. There was an attempted break-in at his home 3 months earlier, which was upsetting, but the child sustained no injury. Exam discloses a mild diffuse thinning of the hair without additional abnormalities. Laboratory studies reveal normal thyroid functioning, slight anemia, and a normal chemistry screen. A test for tuberculosis performed 1 year earlier was reported as negative. The child is up to date on vaccines. The child has several pets at home, including a mynah bird, two turtles, and a garden snake. The scalp appears as in Figures 2.6 and 2.7. The MOST likely diagnosis is

    (A) alopecia areata
    (B) tinea capitis
    (C) telogen effluvium
    (D) traction alopecia
    (E) trichotillomania

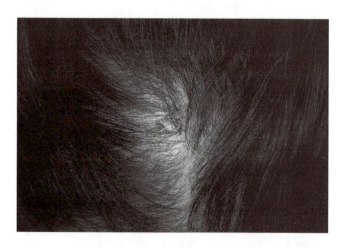

Figure 2.6

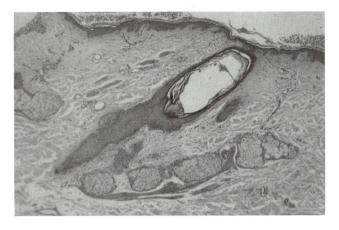

Figure 2.7

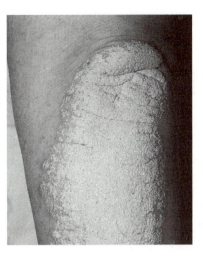

Figure 2.8

41. Which of the following risk factors are associated with rectal cancer?

    (A) diets rich in animal products
    (B) nitrosamine-preserved foods
    (C) hepatitis B virus
    (D) chemical irritants
    (E) Epstein–Barr virus

42. A 23-year-old nulliparous woman presents, complaining of no menses for the last 6 months and irregular menses for the preceding 14 months. Her puberty was normal. Even in college, she never missed more than two menses per year. She has become a committed competitive bicyclist. She recently had a total body fat of 19%. The MOST likely significant laboratory finding explaining the diagnosis is

    (A) elevated endorphins
    (B) suppressed thyroid hormones except rT_3
    (C) elevated thyroid hormones except rT_3
    (D) suppressed gonadotropin-releasing hormone (GnRH)
    (E) elevated GnRH

Questions 43 and 44

A 22-year-old man develops the skin lesion shown in Figure 2.8. He has just started a new job in a chemical plant.

43. Which of the following statements is true of this type of lesion?

    (A) It is an occupational disorder.
    (B) It is an unusual skin disorder.
    (C) Plaque formation is an unusual presentation.
    (D) It is exacerbated by exposure to the sun.
    (E) It is associated with pitting of the nails.

44. There are many options in treating psoriasis, which are chosen depending on the extent and severity of the disease. The BEST choice for this patient whose lesions are limited to the elbows is

    (A) oral corticosteroids
    (B) PUVA (psoralen plus ultraviolet A)
    (C) high-potency steroid ointment
    (D) etretinate
    (E) cyclosporine

45. Students in a junior high school became ill, with symptoms of headache, chills, nausea, and vomiting. Investigation showed that the illness was confined to students who attended the 9:30 to 11:15 home economics classes on that day, where fruit punch and cookies prepared the previous evening were served. The incubation period ranged from 5 minutes to 2 hours. The punch was stored overnight in three 5-gallon water containers with galvanized metal linings. The punch was transferred to plastic pitchers immediately before it was served. Which of the following statements is correct?

(A) The short incubation period suggests staphylococcal food poisoning.

(B) Food poisoning is unlikely here because of the absence of diarrhea and the foods involved in this case (punch and cookies).

(C) The incubation period and the storage of the punch suggests *Clostridium perfringens* as the etiologic agent.

(D) The short incubation period and the storage of the punch suggest chemical food poisoning.

(E) Culture of the remaining punch would probably help in the diagnosis.

46. Earlobe dermatitis and hand eczema in a teenager girl is likely to be an allergy to

(A) copper
(B) nickel
(C) brass
(D) silver
(E) magnesium

Questions 47 and 48

A 38-year-old woman comes to the emergency department with her husband. She is agitated, diaphoretic, and tremulous. She cries out in fear of visual hallucinations, saying, "Police are around that corner, and they're trying to shoot me!" She has a history of one myocarial infarction and 20 years of insulin-dependent diabetes mellitus (IDDM).

47. The MOST important diagnostic test to order immediately for this patient is

(A) a serum glucose level
(B) serum thyroid-stimulating hormone (TSH)
(C) CT scan of the head
(D) electrocardiogram (ECG)
(E) electroencephalogram (EEG)

48. The MOST appropriate intervention in this patient would include

(A) lorazepam (IM)
(B) glucose (PO or IV)
(C) haloperidol (IM)
(D) amoxapine (PO)
(E) fluoxetine (PO)

49. A newborn infant is noted to have low birth weight, narrow palpebral fissures, microcephaly, and flattened nasolabial facies. Which of the following is the MOST likely substance the mother was exposed to prenatally?

(A) lead
(B) mercury
(C) alcohol
(D) benzene
(E) carbon monoxide

50. An obese 24-year-old nulliparous female presents with a long history of irregular bleeding. She does not desire fertility, but is sexually active. She comes to you for management. The FIRST step in the work-up should be

(A) a pelvic ultrasound
(B) an endometrial biopsy
(C) a CT or MRI of the pituitary
(D) a progesterone "withdrawal" test
(E) a pregnancy test

Questions 51 Through 53

A 40-year-old man comes to the emergency department with the inability to adduct or abduct the fingers on his right hand this morning. He is a chronic alcohol user, and he fell asleep last night leaning over the back of a kitchen chair. He is noted to have trouble walking, recent memory deficits, and a tendency to tell elaborate stories that are clearly untrue.

51. The abnormality MOST likely to be the cause of the problem in his hand is

   (A) thiamine deficiency
   (B) alcohol intoxication
   (C) brachial plexus damage
   (D) B_{12} deficiency
   (E) ulnar nerve damage

52. The memory loss, ataxia, and confabulation are likely secondary to

   (A) thiamine deficiency
   (B) B_{12} deficiency
   (C) alcohol intoxication
   (D) alcohol withdrawal
   (E) folate deficiency

53. Acute treatment for this man might include

   (A) prophylactic phenytoin administration
   (B) prophylactic librium administration
   (C) prophylactic carbamazepine administration
   (D) calcium administration
   (E) steroid administration

Questions 54 Through 56

A 14-year-old boy presents to your office with fever and painful joints for the past week. He also complains of a nonproductive cough and sore throat for the past week.

54. Appropriate initial steps for this patient should include

   (A) throat culture for group A streptococcus
   (B) throat culture for *Haemophilus influenzae*

   (C) roentgenograms of involved joints
   (D) attempt at aspiration of joints
   (E) erythrocyte sedimentation rate (ESR)

55. The treatment of choice is

   (A) doxycycline
   (B) clindamycin
   (C) Rocephin (ceftriaxone sodium)
   (D) penicillin
   (E) Augmentin (amoxicillin and clavulanate potassium)

56. Possible complications include

   (A) anemia, thrombocytopenia
   (B) dermatomyositis, polymyositis
   (C) hematuria, proteinuria, red blood cell (RBC) casts
   (D) macrocytosis or target cell formation
   (E) polyuria, polydipsia

Question 57

A 28-year-old woman (G1P1) with regular 28-day cycles presents with menses 1 week late. Her husband has been using condoms for contraception. On bimanual exam, you palpate a 5-cm left adnexal cyst. Her urine pregnancy test is negative. You order a pelvic ultrasound, which is done the next day and reveals a simple cyst with some debris but no septations.

57. The most frequent cystic tumors of the ovary in women of any age group are

   (A) theca lutein cysts
   (B) corpus luteum cysts
   (C) follicular cysts
   (D) benign cystic teratomas
   (E) dysgerminomas

Questions 58 Through 60

A 34-year-old man presents with a history of human immunodeficiency virus (HIV) infection for 6 years. He has a CD4 count of 310 and has had no acquired immune deficiency syndrome (AIDS)-defining illnesses. He presents with a new rash. (See Figure 2.9.)

58. Although you feel confident of the diagnosis, you order a biopsy, which shows

    (A) bacillary angiomatosis
    (B) Kaposi's sarcoma
    (C) melanoma
    (D) mycosis fungoides
    (E) infected excoriations

59. Which of the following statements is true of Kaposi's sarcoma?

    (A) It is associated with parvovirus B-19.
    (B) The incidence was unchanged after homosexuals began practicing safe sex.
    (C) It is associated with human T-lymphotropic virus-I (HTLV-I).
    (D) It is an aggressive disease in older Mediterranean men.
    (E) It can spread beyond the skin.

60. Because he is otherwise well and there are only a few lesions, the patient elects no treatment at this time. He does keep regular appointments for follow-up. Approximately 1 year later, his CD4 count is 100 and the lesions have become confluent, with the addition of many more. They still do not bother him. What would be a reasonable first step?

    (A) Institute therapy with adriamycin.
    (B) Consult a plastic surgeon for resection with grafting.
    (C) Consult radiation oncology.
    (D) Schedule a return visit in 6 months.
    (E) Order a CT scan and start antiretroviral agents.

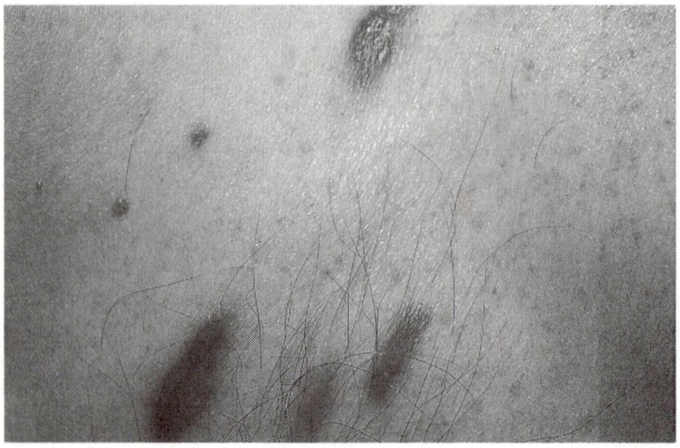

61. A traveler returning from Central Africa is suspected of having malaria despite taking appropriate chemosuppressive medication. Which of the following would NOT constitute an effective treatment option?

    (A) quinidine gluconate
    (B) chloroquine phosphate
    (C) pyrimethamine–sulfadoxine
    (D) proguanil
    (E) quinine

Questions 62 Through 64

A 70-year-old retired construction worker has an asymptomatic, palpable, pulsatile abdominal mass noted during an annual routine physical examination. An abdominal aortic aneurysm (AAA) is suspected.

62. The test you would order to confirm the diagnosis of AAA is

    (A) abdominal aortogram
    (B) abdominal ultrasound
    (C) CT scan
    (D) Doppler pressure index
    (E) MRI

63. Which of the following are complications of infrarenal AAA repair?

    (A) sigmoid colon infarction
    (B) postoperative myocardial infarction
    (C) graft-enteric fistula formation

Figure 2.9

(D) pulmonary embolus and distal embolization

(E) all of the above

64. What is the expected mortality rate of patients undergoing elective AAA repair?

(A) < 5%

(B) 15%

(C) 30%

(D) 50%

(E) 65%

Questions 65 and 66

A 15-year-old girl is brought to the clinic by her mother because of heavy, irregular menses. The mother explains that her daughter's period had been occurring 1 week late every month and lasting 4 days. In the last year, however, menses have been lasting 6 to 7 days. This time, menses did not start for 2 months, were very heavy and crampy, and lasted for 10 days. Her mother states that there has been no sexual activity.

65. The normal menstrual cycle length, duration of flow, and blood loss and their corresponding ranges are

(A) length, 28 ± 7 days; duration, 4 ± 2 days; blood loss, 40 ± 20 mL

(B) length, 21 ± 7 days; duration, 4 ± 2 days; blood loss, 40 ± 20 mL

(C) length, 28 ± 7 days; duration, 7 ± 2 days; blood loss, 40 ± 20 mL

(D) length, 28 ± 7 days; duration, 4 ± 2 days; blood loss, 100 ± 20 mL

(E) length, 32 ± 7 days; duration, 7 ± 2 days; blood loss, 200 ± 20 mL

66. Upon hearing this history, which of the following is the BEST list of your differential diagnoses?

(A) chlamydia infection, ovarian cyst, endometrial carcinoma

(B) anovulation, pregnancy with spontaneous abortion, ovarian cyst, chlamydia infection

(C) chlamydia infection, ovarian cyst, endometrial carcinoma

(D) anovulation, polycystic ovary (PCO) syndrome, chlamydia infection, ovarian cyst, endometrial carcinoma

(E) pregnancy with spontaneous abortion, chlamydia infection, ovarian cyst, endometrial carcinoma

Questions 67 Through 69

A 26-year-old woman has just delivered her third child. She was found to have an iron-deficiency anemia during her prenatal evaluations but had trouble with the iron supplementation because of constipation. The morning after delivery, she tries to ambulate but becomes very dizzy and short of breath. A complete blood count (CBC) shows a hemoglobin of 4.2 g/dL, down from 8 g/dL at her last check-up. You recommend a transfusion of one unit of packed RBCs.

67. Which of the following statements is true about blood transfusions?

(A) A special consent form is required for all blood transfusions.

(B) Directed-donor blood is safer than standard units.

(C) Packed RBCs are preferred over whole blood.

(D) Patients must be rescreened every 48 to 72 hours.

(E) If a patients needs blood, at least two units should be given.

68. The patient wants to know the exact risk of contracting hepatitis from a transfusion. You tell her that it is

(A) 1/500

(B) 1/5000

(C) 1/50,000

(D) 1/500,000

(E) 1/1,000,000

69. During the transfusion, she develops a fever of 101.2°F and one shaking chill before the nurse discontinues the transfusion. Blood bank protocol is followed and blood and urine checked. There is no evidence of hemolysis. Which of the following statements is true about this reaction?

    (A) It could be prevented in the future with acetaminophen or a white blood cell (WBC) filter.
    (B) It is a reaction to RBC antigens.
    (C) It could be prevented by administering irradiated blood.
    (D) The unit was probably contaminated, and the patient should receive antibiotics.
    (E) The use of directed-donor blood decreases the risk of this complication.

70. A 21-year-old man comes to your office with painful, tender, enlarged, draining left inguinal nodes of 2 days' duration. He also complains of chills, fever, malaise, nausea, and pains in the limbs and back. He has just returned from a trip to Vietnam. The MOST likely diagnosis is

    (A) lymphadenopathy of cat scratch fever
    (B) bubonic plague
    (C) tularemia
    (D) lymphogranuloma venereum
    (E) suppurative gonorrhea

71. A patient with known sickle cell disease (Hb SS) presents to labor and delivery 2 weeks after her most recent transfusion (discharge hematocrit, 33%, and hemoglobin A, 55%) complaining of a fever, cough with purulent sputum, shortness of breath, and right-sided chest pain. The MOST likely diagnosis is

    (A) pulmonary embolization
    (B) vaso-occlusive crisis
    (C) placental abruption
    (D) pyelonephritis
    (E) pneumonia

Questions 72 and 73

You are asked to examine a patient with the following symptoms: fever, chills, cough, and pleural pain. The patient tells you that he spent 2 days on a fossil hunt in the Bakersfield area of the Central Valley of California about 2 weeks before the onset of symptoms.

72. The MOST likely diagnosis is

    (A) coccidioidomycosis
    (B) influenza
    (C) tick fever
    (D) pneumonia
    (E) tularemia

73. The MOST likely mode of transmission is

    (A) infection through an open wound
    (B) contact with another person
    (C) inhalation of spores in dust or soil, or from dry vegetation
    (D) contact with an animal
    (E) insect bites

Questions 74 and 75

A 45-year-old woman presents for a gynecologic exam. She has noticed increased vulvar pruritus in the last 2 weeks. Six months ago she resumed sexual activity with a new partner after a 3-year hiatus which began when she underwent total abdominal hysterectomy and bilateral salpingo-oophorectomy for microinvasive cervical carcinoma. She has not used hormone replacement therapy. On exam, you see white coalescent plaques of the labia bilaterally. Vaginal exam reveals a thin, frothy leukorrhea that, on wet mount, reveals motile, flagellated organisms.

74. The MOST likely cause of her vulvar lesions is

    (A) condyloma lata
    (B) condyloma lata and *Trichomonas labialis*
    (C) lichen sclerosis and condyloma acuminata

(D) vulvar intraepithelial neoplasia (VIN)

(E) *Trichomonas labialis* and hyperplastic dystrophy

75. You decide to

(A) treat her with metronidazole, 0.75% gel, and ask her to return in 2 weeks for vulvar biopsy

(B) treat her with metronidazole, 250 mg PO tid for 7 days, and order a rapid plasma reagin (RPR)

(C) treat her with Betadine douche for 5 days

(D) do an immediate vulvar biopsy

(E) order blood tests, including RPR, HIV, hepatitis B antigen; prescribe metronidazole, 2 g PO, and ask her to return in 1 week for vulvar biopsy

Questions 76 and 77

A 68-year-old woman presents to her attending physician feeling unwell and having lost 10 pounds. Physical examination reveals left axillary lymphadenopathy. Biopsy reveals well-differentiated adenocarcinoma. Liver scan and bone scan suggest widespread metastases.

76. Which of the following statements concerning her further management is correct?

(A) The response rate for metastatic, well-differentiated adenocarcinoma of unknown primary site is so poor that no investigation or treatment is indicated.

(B) The pancreas is a common site of origin of this tumor.

(C) Extensive work-up, including colonoscopy, abdominal CT scan, and mammography, will define subsets that benefit from treatment.

(D) Special studies of the excised lymph node are not useful in determining the site of origin.

(E) Metastatic breast cancer is the most common cause of adenocarcinoma of unknown primary site in women.

77. Which of the following markers is likely to be elevated if the patient's primary site is in the breast?

(A) prostate-specific antigen (PSA)

(B) CA 125

(C) alpha-fetoprotein

(D) CA 27.29

(E) CA 19-9

Questions 78 Through 80

A 19-year-old woman develops axillary lymphadenopathy. Biopsy reveals Hodgkin's disease, nodular sclerosing variant.

78. Which of the following statements about staging is correct?

(A) Only one quarter of patients have advanced disease after all staging procedures.

(B) The presence of pruritus indicates stage B Hodgkin's.

(C) If B symptoms are present, chemotherapy, with or without radiation therapy, is a mandatory part of treatment.

(D) Nodular sclerosing forms of Hodgkin's are more commonly diagnosed at advanced stages than the lymphocyte-depleted type.

(E) The increasing use of effective chemotherapy has meant that staging laparotomy is less commonly performed.

79. Which of the following statements comparing Hodgkin's disease and lymphocytic lymphoma is correct?

(A) Lymphocytic lymphoma is more likely to be localized than Hodgkin's at the time of diagnosis.

(B) Involvement of Waldeyer's ring and epitrochlear nodes is similar in both conditions.

(C) The spleen is more frequently involved in Hodgkin's.

(D) Both spread by hematogenous and non-contiguous nodal spread.

(E) Marrow involvement is common in both diseases.

80. In discussing treatment options with the patient, you note that the following is a side effect of the chemotherapeutic agents in CHOP (cyclophosphamide, adriamycin, vincristine, and prednisone).

   (A) hypoglycemia
   (B) papillary necrosis
   (C) congestive heart failure (CHF)
   (D) hypertension
   (E) diarrhea

Questions 81 and 82

You are called to evaluate an infant with constipation. Upon examination, you note that the child has a dry mouth. Further examination reveals generalized weakness, decreased sucking, and decreased gag reflexes.

81. In your opinion, this infant MOST likely has

   (A) polio
   (B) Werdnig–Hoffman syndrome
   (C) Guillain–Barré syndrome
   (D) botulism
   (E) none of the above

82. Immediate treatment steps would include

   (A) intravenous antibiotics
   (B) intensive care unit (ICU) admission for supportive treatment
   (C) botulinum antitoxin
   (D) hyperbaric therapy
   (E) herbal supplements

Questions 83 Through 85

An 80-year-old woman presents with the lesion shown in Figure 2.10 on her right cheek. She notes that she also has some scaly plaques on her forehead. She is an avid sailor.

83. Which of the following is considered a risk factor for this type of skin lesion?

   (A) being native to an equatorial region
   (B) the amount and intensity of exposure to ultraviolet light

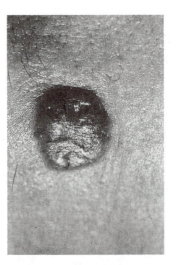

Figure 2.10

   (C) having blue or gray eyes
   (D) living near a high density of electric power lines
   (E) hepatocellular dysfunction (cirrhosis)

84. Which of the following is a true statement about the behavior of this particular type of skin lesion?

   (A) It does not metastasize beyond the skin.
   (B) It may develop in long-standing scars.
   (C) It cannot be treated with x-ray therapy.
   (D) It can be caused by caustic material.
   (E) It never requires surgery.

85. Basal cell carcinomas can often be seen concurrently with squamous cell carcinomas because they share many of the same risk factors. Which of the following is true of squamous cell carcinomas?

   (A) They rarely metastasize if left untreated.
   (B) They may develop in long-standing scars.
   (C) They are resistant to x-ray therapy.
   (D) They require a 5-cm resection margin for adequate surgical treatment.
   (E) They are adequately treated with cryotherapy only.

Questions 86 Through 88

A 50-year-old woman comes to your office complaining of pelvic pressure when standing that is relieved by lying down. She has had six children, all born vaginally, with the largest weighing 4,000 g (10.7 lb). She also complains of leaking a small amount of urine with coughing or sneezing. On exam, you find that she has a large cystocele.

86. The next step in the management of this patient would include

(A) anterior repair

(B) transvaginal hysterectomy and anterior repair

(C) inspection of the remaining endopelvic fascial support to identify any other weaknesses

(D) total abdominal hysterectomy and Burch retropubic urethropexy

(E) a pessary

87. The reason women with genuine urinary stress incontinence leak urine with coughing and/or sneezing can BEST be described as

(A) the pressure of an uninhibited bladder contraction associated with coughing

(B) the presence of a large cystocele with loss of bladder support

(C) the descent of the distal urethra with decreased closure pressure in the distal third of the urethra

(D) the augmentation of pressure transmission through the bladder to the proximal urethra

(E) the descent of the proximal urethra with a loss of pressure transmission (with coughing and sneezing) to the proximal urethra

88. The purpose of a cystometrogram in evaluation of urinary incontinence can BEST be described as

(A) to detect the presence of any uninhibited detrusor contraction

(B) to determine whether the surgery should be performed vaginally or abdominally

(C) to rule out all other causes of incontinence

(D) requiring extensive training and expensive equipment

(E) to determine the Greene's classification

Questions 89 Through 92

A 50-year-old woman presents with a 3-week history of fatigue and pallor. She has noticed some yellowing of her eyes, but has not noticed her urine being darker. Physical examination reveals slight jaundice. Laboratory evaluation reveals a hemoglobin of 6 g/dL with normal white blood cells (WBCs) and platelets. The smear shows polychromatophilia with some spherocytes. The total bilirubin is 2 mg/dL, and direct is .3 mg/dL; haptoglobin, 10 mg/dL, lactic dehydrogenase (LDH), 200 IU/L; and urine bilirubin, negative. The Coombs' test is positive on direct but negative on indirect evaluation.

89. The diagnosis in this woman is MOST likely

(A) iron deficiency

(B) congenital spherocytosis

(C) liver failure and hemolysis

(D) splenomegaly

(E) autoimmune hemolytic anemia (AIHA)

90. The MOST likely cause of this woman's anemia is

(A) external blood loss

(B) decreased red cell production

(C) ineffective erythropoiesis

(D) intravascular hemolysis

(E) extravascular hemolysis

91. Which of the following statements is true about her condition?

(A) It is a result of pyridoxine deficiency.

(B) It is a result of iron deficiency.

(C) There is decreased red cell survival.

(D) There will be a low number of reticulocytes.

(E) RBC transfusion is contraindicated.

92. Which of the following is associated with schistocytes?

    (A) hemoglobin E
    (B) unstable hemoglobins
    (C) immune thrombocytopenic purpura (ITP)
    (D) beta-thalassemia
    (E) prosthetic valves

Questions 93 and 94

A 27-year-old female patient has had IDDM since age 7. During her routine office visit, she has the following vital signs: heart rate, 72; respiratory rate, 13; blood pressure, 140/90. Her glycosylated hemoglobin (HbA1C) is 8.9.

93. The patient's PRIMARY risk for mortality from IDDM is

    (A) renal disease
    (B) ketoacidosis
    (C) cardiovascular disease
    (D) hypoglycemic coma
    (E) stroke

94. The MOST common complication you would expect her to have is

    (A) frequent urinary tract infections
    (B) frequent yeast infections
    (C) background retinopathy
    (D) peripheral neuropathy
    (E) angina

95. A 13-year-old boy is brought into the emergency department by his mother. She reports that the child has recently experienced staring spells and interrupted speech. These episodes last several seconds, after which the child returns to his normal activity. Laboratory studies reveal a glucose of 84, sedimentation rate of 9, and a normal CBC. The child is on no medication, and a recent chest x-ray is reported to have been normal. What will the EEG look like in this patient?

    (A) hypsarrhythmia
    (B) 3/sec spike and dome

    (C) disorganized pattern from the temporal lobe area
    (D) seizure spikes from the optic chiasm
    (E) none of the above

Questions 96 Through 98

A 54-year-old woman had been on hormone replacement therapy for approximately 1 year when a 2-mm cluster of microcalcifications was found in the left upper outer quadrant on routine mammography. She has no family history of breast cancer and had three children by the age of 28, all of whom were breast fed.

96. Upon receiving the mammogram report, you advise the patient to return for an exam. You find no evidence of a mass or of lymphatic enlargement. You then recommend

    (A) breast ultrasound
    (B) a 6-month follow-up mammogram of the left breast
    (C) an office fine-needle aspiration (FNA) biopsy
    (D) an excisional biopsy
    (E) an excisional biopsy with immediate mastectomy and node dissection if the frozen section is positive for malignancy

97. The risk for breast cancer is increased by

    (A) multiparity
    (B) breast feeding
    (C) irregular menses
    (D) postmenopausal breast cancer in a first-degree relative
    (E) late menopause

98. Assuming a theoretic 100-day doubling time for growth of breast cancer, a 2-mm mass detected on mammography has been growing for approximately

    (A) 7 weeks
    (B) 7 months
    (C) 700 days
    (D) 7 years
    (E) 1600 days

99. A 1-year-old girl is evaluated in the office for a rash. The rash is ntoed to be in the inguinal creases and buttocks. These areas are "beefy red" and macerated with satellite pustules and tiny papules. The child appears uncomfortable. The MOST likely cause for this condition is

(A) ringworm

(B) *Candida albicans* diaper rash

(C) contact dermatitis

(D) bullous impetigo

(E) irritant diaper rash

Questions 100 and 101

100. A 38-year-old woman is referred to you for evaluation of an abnormal Papanicolaou (Pap) smear showing necrosis and possibly HGSIL. She complains of a foul-smelling vaginal discharge and occasional postcoital bleeding during the last year. The cervix has a 2 × 1-cm ulcerative lesion replacing the anterior left lateral cervical lip. Appropriate management is a

(A) repeat Pap smear

(B) colposcopy and cervical biopsy

(C) cold-knife cervical conization

(D) cryotherapy

(E) laser vaporization

101. The patient is diagnosed with squamous cell carcinoma of the cervix. There is palpable tumor extension to the left vaginal fornix and left parametrial thickening. Chest x-ray, cystoscopy, and proctoscopy are normal. Intravenous pyelography (IVP) shows left hydronephrosis. CT of the abdomen shows scattered nodules in the liver parenchyma consistent with metastatic disease. The stage is

(A) IB

(B) IIB

(C) IIIB

(D) IVA

(E) IVB

Questions 102 and 103

A 77-year-old woman with a history of atherosclerotic cardiovascular disease and mild, compensated CHF, for which she is taking digoxin, complains of occasional "skipped heartbeats." Cardiac auscultation and an initial ECG revealed no ectopic beats. The physician decided to monitor the patient's rhythm for 24 hours. Figure 2.11 was obtained while the patient was sleeping.

102. The monitor strip in this patient shows

(A) Wenckebach phenomenon

(B) Mobitz type II atrioventricular (AV) block

(C) complete heart block

(D) parasystole

(E) multifocal atrial tachycardia (MAT)

103. Which of the following would be the next step in treating the patient described?

(A) starting propranolol

(B) obtaining a digoxin level

(C) starting amiodarone

(D) implanting a temporary pacemaker

(E) implanting a permanent pacemaker

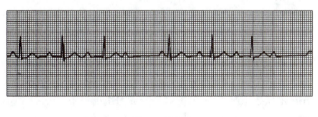

Figure 2.11

Questions 104 and 105

104. A 2-year-old child is being seen for a well-child checkup. Which of the following is a leading potential cause of death for this child for which a preventive measure is available and which should be discussed with the parents?

   (A) lead toxicity
   (B) motor vehicle accident
   (C) tuberculosis
   (D) pneumonia
   (E) influenza

105. Treatment of a person with AIDS using zidovudine (AZT) is

   (A) primary prevention
   (B) secondary prevention
   (C) tertiary prevention
   (D) all of the above
   (E) none of the above

Questions 106 and 107

Since she was 8 years old, a 28-year-old woman has had difficulties talking in class, participating in group discussions, and giving speeches. Despite this, she has risen to middle management at an accounting firm and is known as a good worker. She has no symptoms of anxiety outside the above situations. There is no history of prior psychological assessment or therapy. She denies a history of alcohol or drug abuse. There is no history of medical illness, and she takes no medications. She has a close circle of steady friends. Her father is described as shy and anxious.

   Her main complaint is that she finds herself avoiding meetings that could help with job advancement because "I can't sleep or think if I have to go to one." When she does attend, she states that her voice wavers, her hands tremble, and she feels her heart racing.

106. Which of the following diagnoses is MOST likely in this case?

   (A) panic attacks
   (B) social phobia

   (C) specific phobia
   (D) panic attacks with agoraphobia
   (E) schizoid personality disorder

107. The lifetime prevalence of this disorder from epidemiologic and community-based studies has a range of

   (A) 0.5% to 1%
   (B) 1% to 3%
   (C) 3% to 13%
   (D) 10% to 20%
   (E) 20% to 30%

108. Screening for gestational diabetes is typically performed between 24 and 28 weeks because most patients will have sufficient glucose intolerance caused by a placental hormone. The peripheral tissue resistance to insulin in the pregnant woman is mediated by

   (A) hCG
   (B) human placental lactogen (hPL)
   (C) GH
   (D) luteinizing hormone (LH)
   (E) follicle-stimulating hormone (FSH)

109. An 18-month-old Native American boy is brought to you because his mother is concerned about his carious teeth. You should advise her to

   (A) see a dentist
   (B) stop giving him a bottle
   (C) stop giving him a pacifier
   (D) brush his teeth
   (E) wait until his permanent teeth emerge

Questions 110 and 111

A 25-year-old woman presents to the emergency department after slightly cutting her arms with a razor blade during an argument with her boyfriend. She has a history of intense relationships, many of which have been short-lived, and a history of similar attempts at self-abuse at times of trouble in these relationships.

110. The MOST important question to ask this patient at her initial evaluation in the emergency department is

(A) is there any history of sexual abuse of the patient
(B) is the patient suicidal or homicidal
(C) does the patient possess a cherished "transitional object," such as a teddy bear
(D) is the patient concerned about her sexual orientation
(E) has the patient been engaging in unsafe sexual practices

111. Which of the following is the MOST likely long-term prognosis for this patient with borderline personality disorder?

(A) a progression to schizophrenia
(B) deterioration of relationships and vocational functioning in her 30s and 40s
(C) little risk of episodes of major depressive disorder
(D) increasing stability in relationships and vocational functioning during midlife
(E) little risk of self-harm

112. The leading cause of years of potential life lost for people under age 65 in the United States for 1987 was

(A) heart disease
(B) cancer
(C) stroke
(D) unintentional injuries
(E) pulmonary disease

113. A 26-year-old man has recently been hospitalized for an episode of mania. After he is discharged from the hospital, the optimal serum concentration of lithium for the long-term treatment of this patient's bipolar disorder is

(A) 0 to 0.3 mEq/L
(B) 0.4 to 0.7 mEq/L
(C) 0.8 to 1.2 mEq/L
(D) 1.3 to 1.6 mEq/L
(E) 1.7 to 2.0 mEq/L

114. A 25-year-old man has a 6-month history of believing that "people" are trying to put "bad thoughts" into his head and make him do "bad things." He finds special messages from them in TV news reports and in the newspaper. He is agitated, pacing constantly. His affect is inappropriate, and he laughs as he tells of his persecution. Physical examination is within normal limits. Drug screen is negative. The pharmacologic treatment of choice is

(A) clorazepate
(B) lorazepam
(C) haloperidol
(D) amitriptyline
(E) imipramine

115. A patient reports symptoms of tremors, emotional lability, neurasthesias, and psychomotor disturbances. Which of the following toxic substances might cause this condition?

(A) lead
(B) arsenic
(C) mercury
(D) aromatic solvents
(E) malathion

Questions 116 and 117

A 30-year-old stockbroker comes to your office speaking rapidly and reporting that he has not been sleeping for the last week but feels very energetic. He states that he has learned the ultimate secret to ensure making a killing on the stock market.

116. Medication that is likely to give some relief of symptoms in this patient in a matter of hours rather than days includes

(A) lithium
(B) valproic acid
(C) haloperidol
(D) carbamazepine
(E) amitriptyline

117. Two weeks after starting on lithium, this patient has achieved control of his manic episode. In what range does his serum lithium level likely lie?

    (A) 0.1 to 0.3 mEq/L
    (B) 0.4 to 0.6 mEq/L
    (C) 1.0 to 1.5 mEq/L
    (D) 1.6 to 2.0 mEq/L
    (E) 3.0 to 5.0 mEq/L

Questions 118 Through 120

A 32-year-old woman (G3,P2012) presents to the emergency department because of persistent intermittent spotting for 2 weeks, which began 3 weeks after her last menstrual period (LMP). She had a tubal ligation with the birth of her last child by cesarean 6 years ago. Menses have been regular until now. She has not had routine gynecologic care since her divorce 4 years ago. She began a new sexual relationship 4 months ago. You perform a pelvic exam, taking specimens for additional studies. A wet mount of the vaginal secretions reveals clue cells.

118. The next test you order is a

    (A) rapid *Chlamydia* screen
    (B) rapid group B beta-hemolytic streptococcal assay
    (C) urine hCG
    (D) CBC
    (E) pelvic ultrasound

119. Following surgical tubal ligation

    (A) 80% of pregnancies that occur are ectopic
    (B) the incidence of ovarian cancer is increased
    (C) symptoms of pelvic inflammatory disease (PID) are the same as in nonsterilized women
    (D) the failure rate is highest with Pomeroy-type tubal ligation done at the time of cesarean
    (E) the incidence of ectopic pregnancy increases with length of time since the surgery was performed

120. Bacterial vaginosis

    (A) may be treated with oral or vaginal metronidazole, or oral or vaginal clindamycin, according to the Centers for Disease Control and Prevention (CDC)
    (B) is associated with a combination of aerobic bacteria including *Bacteroides*, *Peptococcus*, and *Mobiluncus* species
    (C) is diagnosed by the presence of "clue cells," a pH < 4.5, and a positive "whiff test"
    (D) is a sexually transmitted disease (STD)
    (E) should be treated only in women who are symptomatic

121. A 42-year-old married woman presents with dysuria and increased urinary frequency. She also complains of frequent headaches, for which she takes Excedrin. The urine dipstick is positive for protein. Which of the following would MOST likely contribute to her dipstick results?

    (A) urinary tract infection (UTI)
    (B) analgesic use
    (C) dietary intake
    (D) pregnancy
    (E) dehydration

Questions 122 and 123

A 22-year-old single man presents to the psychiatric emergency room because he "doesn't know what else to do." He relates that about 1 year ago, he began to hear voices talking to him, which no one else could hear, telling him things about people around him. At other times, he is able to hear people around him talking about him, even though he knows that they are too far away for him to actually be hearing them.

He is presently in his third year of a 5-year plumbing apprenticeship. He is having difficulty at work, and his supervisor has noticed his difficulties concentrating and frequent mistakes. He became particularly concerned after camping outdoors 2 nights ago and experiencing auditory and visual hallucinations, accompanied by the strong feeling that someone was going to sneak up and kill him. He sheepishly admits that he had been drinking quite a few beers and had smoked marijuana. He says that this is only the second time he has ever used marijuana.

122. To meet the criteria for major depression with psychotic features, which of the following must be true?

(A) The delusions and hallucinations involve typical depressive themes such as personal inadequacy, guilt, death, and punishment.

(B) The patient has experienced either depressed mood or anhedonia.

(C) Symptoms of depression began at least 2 weeks before the onset of hallucinations.

(D) The patient has experienced recurrent suicidal ideation.

(E) none of the above

123. Symptoms reported by the patient include

(A) loose association

(B) depersonalization

(C) cannabis abuse

(D) auditory hallucinations

(E) derailment

124. A 5-year-old previously well child has a fever, headache, irritability, and stiff neck. The remainder of his examination is found to be normal. A lumbar puncture reveals clear spinal fluid with 150 WBCs (45 polys, 55 lymphs), protein 40 mg/dL, glucose 55 mg/dL, and serum glucose 80 mg/dL. No bacteria are seen on the Gram stain. A diagnosis of viral meningitis is made. Which of the following statements is true about the diagnosis?

(A) The data is consistent with the diagnosis.

(B) The percentage of polys is too high.

(C) The percentage of lymphs is too low.

(D) The glucose should be lower.

(E) The protein should be higher.

125. AIDS has been recognized in infants as a result of transmission of HIV from infected mothers before, at, or shortly after birth. Estimates of the rate of HIV transmission to such infants (from their infected mothers) in the absence of AZT prophylaxis range from approximately

(A) 1 to 4%

(B) 5 to 14%

(C) 15 to 19%

(D) 20 to 40%

(E) more than 40%

126. A 25-year-old woman comes to your office for a routine physical examination prior to starting graduate school. Your findings on physical examination include hypotension, bradycardia, dependent edema, and lanugo hair. You are MOST concerned about

(A) T-cell lymphoma

(B) CHF

(C) anorexia nervosa

(D) an ovarian tumor

(E) hyperthyroidism

127. During a routine physical exam, a healthy 15-year-old girl tells you that she has been getting in trouble in school for being late to classes during the past year. She says she knows that it is because she washes her hands so many times after going to the bathroom, but she says she cannot stop herself no matter how hard she tries. The MOST likely diagnosis is

(A) Tourette's disorder

(B) Asberger's disorder

(C) obsessive–compulsive personality disorder

(D) obsessive–compulsive disorder

(E) anal-retentive personality disorder

128. A 12-year-old boy has just been cut on the arm by a small piece of glass in his bedroom. The wound is clean upon evaluation in your office. Your initial approach includes irrigating the wound with saline. The child had full basic immunizations and a tetanus booster 3 years ago at the time of a prior injury. The child's father asks when his son needs another tetanus booster. You reply

(A) now
(B) in 2 years
(C) in 3 years
(D) in 5 years
(E) in 7 years

129. A 19-year-old woman comes to your office for a physical examination prior to joining the field hockey team in college. The women is friendly and talkative and says that she is enjoying college. During the physical examination, you notice erosion of tooth enamel and abrasions on the dorsum of her right hand. In this woman, you are most concerned about

(A) caffeine dependence
(B) bulimia nervosa
(C) pica
(D) sports injury
(E) multiple sclerosis

130. During a routine medical follow-up, you find that a 71-year-old woman with a history of hypertension and atrial fibrillation has been feeling depressed and sleeping much of the day. Her husband tells you that she has become forgetful as well. These complaints are new since you saw her 6 months earlier, and you are concerned that they may be related to her medications. You obtain a TSH level, which is elevated. Which of the following medications is MOST likely to be responsible for this woman's symptoms?

(A) fosinopril
(B) lisinopril
(C) hydrochlorothiazide
(D) furosemide
(E) amiodarone

131. A 14-year-old girl with acute abdominal pain is evaluated in the emergency department. A plain film of her abdomen is performed, revealing a normal gas pattern, but a calcification in her left lower quadrant appears. The calcification resembles a tooth. The MOST likely explanation for this finding is

(A) she swallowed the tooth
(B) artifact
(C) a fecalith that looks like a tooth
(D) a dermoid cyst
(E) diverticulum

132. A 9-year-old boy presents to your office on referral by his pediatrician because of a history of inattentiveness, impulsivity, hyperactivity, and aggressiveness, both at home and at school. His parents request that you do "a test" to determine if he has ADHD. You should

(A) order an EEG
(B) order a positron-emission tomography (PET) scan
(C) check endogenous stimulant levels
(D) collect additional history
(E) perform a Wechsler Intelligence Scale for Children

133. A 10-year-old boy presents with his parents, who describe significant difficulties with peer relationships in school and the neighborhood. They state that he likes to be alone, rarely seeking out even his parents for contact. He seems very interested in carefully aligning blocks while waving his arms in an unusual way or running the vacuum cleaner. What developmental line would be MOST helpful to ask about at this point?

(A) gender identity
(B) moral reasoning
(C) language development
(D) ability to understand cause-and-effect relationships
(E) sleep history

134. Which of the following is the MOST frequent epithelial tumor?

(A) choriocarcinoma

(B) clear cell

(C) mucinous

(D) papillary serous

(E) Sertoli–Leydig cell

Questions 135 Through 137

A 72-year-old woman comes to you for advice about her neck. For the past 3 years she has had some bumps, and now as she is preparing for her granddaughter's wedding, she finds all her dresses uncomfortably tight around the neck. She denies any other problems. On physical examination, you find multiple, nontender, enlarged lymph nodes, the greatest being 2 cm in diameter.

135. You recommend

(A) antibiotics

(B) chest x-ray

(C) CT scan and referral to a surgeon for biopsy

(D) thyroid scan

(E) referral to radiation oncology

136. The CT demonstrates diffuse adenopathy throughout the chest and abdomen. The biopsy is positive for a diffuse follicle center lymphoma. She returns to your office to discuss the next step. You tell her that

(A) no treatment is available

(B) treatment is available and she will very likely be cured

(C) treatment is available but is very toxic and at her age not recommended

(D) treatment is available if needed for symptoms

(E) aggressive treatment will prolong her life

137. She responds to monthly pulses of chlorambucil and prednisone and achieves a clinical remission, as documented on physical exam and by CT scan. Two years later, she returns to your office complaining of the develop-

ment of a mass in her right axilla. On examination, her adenopathy is no longer present apart from one large node, which measures 5 cm, and which she assures you has developed in just the past few weeks. The MOST likely explanation for this is

(A) recurrence of her indolent lymphoma

(B) an infection in her arm with reactive nodal enlargement

(C) development of an aggressive lymphoma

(D) metastatic breast cancer to the nodes

(E) a side effect of the chlorambucil

138. A 10-year-old boy is evaluated in the office. The child's parents report that he is the shortest child in his class. He has had a normal childhood, without any serious illnesses or problems. He has had a good appetite and by history consumes a well-balanced diet. He does not take any supplemental vitamins. Both of the child's parents are of normal height. The child is found to be perfectly normal on physical examination. He is at the third percentile for height and weight. His parents are very anxious about the situation. What is the next best step in your evaluation?

(A) growth hormone levels

(B) CBC

(C) somatomedin level

(D) bone age

(E) give growth hormone

139. A 6-week-old infant is evaluated in the office. He is brought in because of a prolonged, barky cough. The child is without fever. He is noted to be without cyanosis. Examination of the infant's chest does not demonstrate any rales, and good air entry is noted. Which of the following is the MOST likely diagnosis?

(A) tracheoesophageal fistula

(B) croup

(C) pulmonary sequestration

(D) bronchiolitis

(E) vascular ring

Questions 140 Through 143

A 19-year-old woman presents for a routine gynecologic exam with a request for oral contraceptives. Her LMP was 24 days earlier. Menses have been regular, with mild discomfort that is relieved by ibuprofen and has not worsened in the last 3 years. On exam, you find a 6-cm left adnexal mass lying anteriorly in the pelvis. You decide to order an ultrasound.

140. The patient is found to have a complex cystic and solid mass. Based on her age, symptoms, and the appearance of the tumor, the MOST likely diagnosis is

    (A) dermoid
    (B) dysgerminoma
    (C) endometrioma
    (D) serous cystadenoma
    (E) serous cystadenocarcinoma

141. The MOST common malignant tumor of the ovary in all age groups is

    (A) Brenner tumor of the ovary
    (B) dysgerminoma
    (C) immature teratoma
    (D) mucinous cystadenocarcinoma
    (E) serous cystadenocarcinoma

142. Which of the following is true of mature cystic teratomas?

    (A) They are rarely bilateral.
    (B) They have a 46,XXX karyotype.
    (C) They can occur from infancy through the postmenopausal years.
    (D) They arise from the epidermal germ cell layer and contain thick liquid sebaceous material in the cyst cavity.
    (E) They are most frequently complicated by rupture into the peritoneal cavity.

143. Which of the following is true of endometriomas?

    (A) Most patients with endometriomas are asymptomatic.
    (B) They are considered neoplasms of the ovary.

    (C) Rupture is most likely to occur in the late luteal phase.
    (D) In the classification of endometriosis, presence of any size endometrioma indicates a classification of "severe."
    (E) Endometriomas can be readily distinguished from other pelvic conditions on MRI.

144. A 6-month-old child is evaluated in the office. The child is noted to have poor growth, hepatomegaly, lymphadenopathy, oral candidiasis, diarrhea, eczema, and low-grade fevers. The MOST likely diagnosis is

    (A) histiocytosis X
    (B) Gaucher's disease
    (C) immunoglobulin G (IgG) deficiency
    (D) toxoplasmosis
    (E) HIV infection

Questions 145 and 146

A 40-year-old woman complains of episodes of severe unilateral facial pain of a stabbing quality that is intermittent for several hours, then disappears for several days. Physical examination is entirely normal.

145. The MOST likely diagnosis is

    (A) trigeminal neuralgia
    (B) herpes zoster
    (C) acoustic neuroma
    (D) Bell's palsy
    (E) diabetic neuropathy

146. The MOST effective therapy for the condition described is
    (A) morphine
    (B) indomethacin
    (C) cimetidine
    (D) carbamazepine
    (E) lidocaine (Xylocaine) gel

Questions 147 and 148

A 27-year-old man comes to your office seeking help for his compulsive masturbation. He relates that on a daily basis he feels the overwhelming urge to masturbate into a high-heeled shoe that he kept as a memento of a previous relationship. He says that this has been going on for the past 3 years and is causing difficulties in his current relationship. In the past 4 months, the strife in his current relationship has caused him to feel sad most days, with some increased sleep latency and lack of interest in normally pleasurable activities. He denies any other depressive or anxious symptomatology.

147. His sexual disorder is BEST described as

   (A) dyspareunia
   (B) pedophilia
   (C) frotteurism
   (D) fetishism
   (E) exhibitionism

148. His mood symptomatology is BEST characterized diagnostically as

   (A) major depression, single episode
   (B) dysthymic disorder
   (C) depressive order due to sexual dysfunction
   (D) adjustment order with depressed mood
   (E) cyclothymic disorder

Questions 149 and 150

A 32-year-old woman presents with a loss of vision, which she describes as like looking through plastic wrap. Fundoscopic examination is normal, without retinal hemorrhage. Over the next few days, her vision gradually returns. She remains well until approximately 1 year later when she presents to the emergency department with acute onset of diplopia. On examination, the patient is asked to look to the right but the left eye does not move past midline. Again, after 10 days, the diplopia resolves.

149. Which of the following signs and symptoms is a common presentation of this disease?

   (A) pain in one or more extremities
   (B) unilateral vision loss
   (C) urinary incontinence
   (D) hearing loss
   (E) changes in intellectual function

150. Which of the following statements concerning this disease is true?

   (A) This disease is most common in equatorial areas.
   (B) The average age of onset is the mid-60s.
   (C) The lesions consist of scattered areas of CNS myelin dissolution combined with destruction of the axon.
   (D) The incidence of cases rises sharply close to the equator.
   (E) Epidemiologic studies are suggestive of an infectious etiology.

Answers and Explanations

1. **(B)** DPL is rapid, easy to perform, and does not require moving a hemodynamically unstable patient to other areas of the hospital. In addition, the sensitivity for detecting an intraperitoneal source of hemorrhage makes DPL the test of choice in evaluating unstable trauma patients for the possibility of intraperitoneal hemorrhage.

2. **(D)** This patient cannot be followed with serial clinical examinations and should have a definitive diagnostic study to assess for intra-abdominal injuries because he is going to the operating room for a number of hours. A CT scan is the optimal choice because he has had prior abdominal surgery. The CT scan provides information regarding the intraperitoneal and retroperitoneal organs. Retroperitoneal injuries would not be readily determined by DPL; therefore, DPL is generally limited to the detection of intraperitoneal injuries. CT scanning is also helpful for evaluating injured solid organs, providing an estimate of the extent of injury and indicating the likelihood of success of nonoperative management.

3. **(E)** While CT scanning of the chest is developing some favor in excluding traumatic aortic disruption, arteriography remains the definitive test. Patients with a deceleration mechanism of injury and a wide or indistinct mediastinum, as seen on chest x-ray, should be evaluated for traumatic aortic disruption.

4. **(G)** While a chest radiograph, DPL, or CT scan may suggest a traumatic diaphragm injury, none has a high degree of accuracy. Exploratory laparotomy or laparoscopy may be necessary.

5. **(B)** DPL confirms the presence of intraperitoneal hemorrhage. This is a nonspecific finding that may require laparotomy. At operation, a liver laceration that is no longer bleeding, or a similar problem not requiring operative repair, may be found as the source of the small amount of blood (20 to 30 mL) necessary to produce a positive DPL.

6. **(B)** Goodpasture syndrome is a condition characterized by antiglomerular and antialveolar basement membrane antibodies that produces interstitial lung disease with pulmonary hemorrhages, as well as glomerulonephritis with hematuria and renal failure. Unlike Wegener's, upper respiratory tract involvement is not seen.

7. **(A)** Wegener's granulomatosis is a necrotizing granulomatous process most commonly presenting with evidence of chronic sinusitis and nasal passage and pulmonary involvement. As in Goodpasture syndrome, renal disease is also common.

8. **(C)** Periarteritis nodosa is a neutrophilic inflammatory disorder of small and medium-sized arteries that has a frequent association with hepatitis B antigenemia with circulating immune complexes. Commonly affected organs are the skin, kidneys, and gastrointestinal (GI) tract.

9–14. **(9-I, 10-H, 11-B, 12-E, 13-C, 14-A)** Erythema infectiosum, or Fifth disease, is caused by a parvovirus. The rash may spread to the trunk and be pruritic. The other answers are incorrect as only Fifth disease typically produces the "slapped cheek" rash without other significant symptoms or findings.

Roseola infantum, a result of human herpesvirus-6, presents with the noted typical pattern of fever followed by a rash. This classic presentation is not noted in any of the other choices.

Rubella infection in pregnancy produces a spectrum of defects resulting in either stillbirths, abortions, or live births with various problems, including red-purple macular "blueberry muffin" lesions, hepatitis, hemolytic anemia, PDA, hearing loss, cataracts, glaucoma, retinopathy, and encephalitis. In childhood, diabetes may develop. Varicella, or chickenpox, presents with the rash as indicated. The rash usually begins on the trunk and spreads to the extremities. It is contagious from a day or so prior to the onset of the rash until all lesions are crusted and drying. The pattern of lesions in various stages of development and resolution is classic for chickenpox and unlike any of the other choices listed.

The typical symptoms and findings of measles are noted.

Most toxoplasmosis infections are asymptomatic at birth. Findings in toxoplasmosis infection, in addition to those noted, include seizures, increased intracranial pressure, and nystagmus. The staphylococcal scalded skin syndrome presents with spreading erythema and tenderness in infants.

15–17. **(15-G, 16-A, 17-C)** Transient synovitis is a nonspecific, self-limited inflammation of the hip joint of unknown etiology. It is usually associated with an upper respiratory infection. There is a normal temperature or low-grade fever. Laboratory tests are normal. The other choices are incorrect as they fall outside of the given age group. If persistent, Legg–Calvé–Perthes disease (aseptic necrosis of the femoral head) needs to be ruled out.

Lyme disease is a multiple-system disease, with symptoms including headache, stiff neck, myalgia, arthralgias, malaise, fa-

tigue, lethargy, and lymphadenopathy. The other choices are incorrect, as those conditions do not present with headaches and lymphadenopathy. Ten percent have cardiac manifestations, including myocarditis, pancarditis, and conduction disturbances. One third of patients will remember having a tick bite. The organism responsible is *Borrelia burgdorferi.*

Serum sickness follows drug reactions (eg, penicillin), insect bites, and transplantation. In the past, injections of antisera made from horses were the major culprits. It is a delayed type of immediate hypersensitivity. The illness may last 7 to 10 days. In the late stages, eosinophilia is present. Degenerative arthritis, gouty arthritis, and fibromyalgia would usually be found in adults. The other choices are incorrect as they do not follow exposure to blood products.

18–19. **(18-B, 19-C)** Rotavirus is the most important cause of acute gastroenteritis in infants and young children. The incubation period is 1 to 3 days. A vaccine is now available. It is spread by the fecal–oral route. The peak incidence is in the fall and winter. *Salmonella* and *Shigella* would be less common in this age group. Adenovirus infection and Kawasaki disease do not present with diarrhea as the main symptom.

Atypical mycobacteria contrasts with tuberculosis infections by involving the cervical nodes; it has a PPD test that measures 0 to 15 mm and a normal chest x-ray. The therapy is the same as for TB, but the mainstay of treatment is excision.

20. **(B)** The pain pattern described is most suggestive of passing a ureteral stone. Characteristics are abrupt onset, severe flank pain that may radiate to the groin, and lack of increase in pain with palpation early in the course of illness. Patients do not seem to be able to remain still due to waves of ureteral colic.

21. **(C)** This scenario is most suggestive of ruptured diverticulitis, although a ruptured ectopic pregnancy may present similarly with accompanying hypotension in a woman of childbearing age. The acute onset of pain and subsequent peritonitis are characteristic of a ruptured viscus.

22. **(A)** The classic presentation of appendicitis is initial pain or obstruction of the appendiceal lumen, mediated by way of the foregut nerves, giving rise to poor localization of pain. When inflammation of the appendiceal surface finally causes pain in the parietal peritoneum of the abdominal cavity, better somatic localization results.

23. **(E)** Pain resulting from early pancreatitis is described in this scenario. If the process becomes more severe, diffuse abdominal pain and tenderness occur, which may mimic a ruptured viscus or ruptured abdominal aortic aneurysm (AAA).

24. **(D)** Pain associated with cholecystitis frequently awakens patients at night and radiates as described. The pain also characteristically lasts for hours and may be relieved by vomiting.

25–27. **(25-F, 26-E, 27-C)** ADHD involves a series of behaviors including restlessness, distractibility, impulsive behavior, excessive talking, interruptions, and engaging in dangerous activities. Children with ADHD present problems in school when they are expected to follow classroom routine. Ideally, these children need a team evaluation to rule out other medical problems and develop a treatment plan. There are no major neurological problems, although minor and soft signs may be present but have no significance. Routine CT or electroencephalogram (EEG) is not necessary for diagnosis. Treatment includes educational programs, family counseling, and, in many cases, medications such as methylphenidate (Ritalin). Intelligence may be normal, and that helps to rule out many of the other incorrect choices.

Autism consists of three primary characteristics: social indifference or failure to develop normal social responses; absent or abnormal speech and language development; and restricted, stereotyped responses to ob-

jects. Most autistic children have IQs of less than 70. The cause is unknown.

Lesch–Nyhan syndrome, a disorder of purine metabolism, is characterized by mental retardation, cerebral palsy, choreoathetosis, and self-destructive behavior. Children with this disorder classically bite themselves and can destroy lips or amputate fingers. The X-linked disease is produced by abnormal activity of the hypoxanthine guanine phosphoribosyl transferase (HGPRT) enzyme, which results in high levels of uric acid in the blood and urine, gouty arthritis, hematuria, and renal calculi.

28. **(C)** Venous stasis ulcers are usually located over the medial or lateral malleolus and are associated with incompetent perforating veins, which connect the superficial and deep venous systems. Prior DVT can contribute to the development of venous hypertension and, ultimately, a leg ulcer of this type.

29. **(F)** None of the medical diagnoses listed are treated primarily by antibiotic therapy. It may be adjunctive with the other lesions noted when an infection is present, but when used alone will not be curative.

30. **(A)** This patient has limb-threatening ischemia, with ischemic pain at rest and gangrenous changes of the toes. The presence of tissue loss with dry gangrene results in major amputation if blood flow to the extremity is not improved through revascularization with a bypass.

31. **(B)** A heel decubitus ulcer is usually the result of pressure applied to an area of decreased sensation or in an immobilized patient who is severely ill without appropriate heel protection.

32. **(E)** Tetanus prophylaxis should always be checked for currency with puncture wounds. These wounds are so-called "tetanus-prone."

33. **(D)** Recurrent lymphangitis and cellulitis are associated with chronic lymphedema.

34. **(D)** For both venous stasis disease and lymphedema, compression is the mainstay of therapy. Compression is inappropriate in patients with significant arterial insufficiency. Compression thrapy is not used for the management of a heel decubitus ulcer or a puncture wound.

35. **(C)** Pontine hemorrhage is associated with impaired oculocephalic reflexes and small, reactive pupils. It generally evolves over a few minutes, usually with coma and quadriplegia. The prognosis is poor, and death often occurs within hours.

36. **(B)** Cerebellar hemorrhage, when mild, may present with only headaches, vomiting, and ataxia of gait. Patients may complain of dizziness or vertigo. The eyes may be deviated to the side opposite the hemorrhage. Nystagmus is not common, but an ipsilateral sixth nerve palsy can occur. This is the only type of intracerebral hemorrhage that commonly benefits from surgical intervention.

37. **(B)** Intracerebral hemorrhage into the cerebellum, pons, and thalamus are usually due to spontaneous rupture of small penetrating arteries and are usually associated with hypertension, although hemorrhagic disorders and neoplasms are possible causes. Hypertensive encephalopathy is an unusual complication of chronic hypertension and nowadays is almost never the initial presentation of hypertension. Cocaine-related hemorrhage is caused by acute hypertension. Subarachnoid hemorrhage is more likely caused by an aneurysm, and lobar intracerebral hemorrhage is frequently caused by nonhypertensive factors such as amyloid angiopathy, AVM, and aneurysms.

38. **(G)** AVMs are more frequently seen in men and, although present from birth, do not usually become symptomatic until later in life. The peak incidence of symptoms is between ages 10 and 30. The headache can be similar to migraine or more diffuse. Presentation can also be seizure or rupture. Hemorrhage can be massive or minimal when rupture does occur.

39. **(E)** Diagnosing an acute hemorrhage. The MRI is insensitive to acute hemorrhage, but more sensitive to other symptoms.

40. **(C)** The thinning of the hair after a severe stress is due to the effect on hair follicles in the growing phase that are shifted into the resting phase. Hairs are shed when the growing phase resumes 2 to 3 months after the stress. The hair will return to a normal pattern of growth. Traction alopecia is incorrect, as this condition results from tight braiding or pulling of hair and would be more localized. Examination did not disclose evidence of fungal infection (tinea capitis). Alopecia areata results in hair loss in round patches. Trichotillomania is compulsive hair pulling, usually associated with irregular hair loss patches and psychiatric illness.

41. **(A)** Cancers of the rectum, like cancers of the colon, are thought to be related to diets rich in animal fat and are linked to a "Western" type of lifestyle.

42. **(D)** Exercise amenorrhea is the result of two independent factors: body fat below 22% and stress and energy use. Body fat greater than 22% is necessary to sustain menstruation. The hypothalamic dysfunction is not as severe as that seen in anorexia nervosa. Exercise decreases gonadotropins and increases prolactin (PRL), growth hormone (GH), TSH, and adrenocorticotropic hormone (ACTH). The thyroid hormones, including T_3, are suppressed. Estrogens are inactivated. Endorphins appear to suppress the secretion of GnRH. The effect on GnRH precedes menstrual irregularity.

43. **(E)** Psoriatic plaques, the typical presentation, are either not affected or slightly improved by sun exposure. Psoriasis is very common. Although it is can be confused with an occupational disorder because some patients develop psoriatic lesions at sites of injury or irritation (called Koebner's phenomenon), it is not related to any known occupational exposure.

44. **(C)** Because the disease is currently limited in area, choosing a topical agent makes the best sense. Parenteral corticosteroids should not be used because they may induce pustular lesions. PUVA is the treatment of choice when psoriasis involves more than 30% of the body surface. Etretinate is useful for treating pustular psoriasis. Cyclosporine is used, but the responses are not maintained and long-term safety is still an issue.

45. **(D)** An incubation period this short (5 minutes to 2 hours) almost certainly represents chemical food poisoning, since even staphylococcal food intoxication (preformed toxin), with its abrupt and sometimes violent onset, ordinarily has an incubation period of 30 minutes to 7 hours, usually 2 to 4 hours. In this case, the incriminated chemical was zinc, which is a major constituent of galvanized metal. On contact with acidic foods and beverages, it is converted to zinc salts, which are readily absorbed by the body.

46. **(B)** Nickel allergy is the most frequent cause of contact allergy in women. The development of allergy is frequently provoked by earrings, but metal buttons, bracelets, and watches are also frequent causes. Some studies suggest that about 10 to 15% of women become allergic to nickel. This sensitization is most commonly induced when nickel-containing posts are inserted at the time of the initial ear piercing.

47. **(A)** A STAT glucose is likely to show hypoglycemia in this patient with IDDM. While hyperthyroidism can also cause a psychotic episode, hypoglycemia is more likely in a patient taking insulin. An EEG would be useful to detect seizure activity or to determine the extent of encephalopathy, neither of which is indicated in this case. There are few, if any, findings on a CT scan that would be suggestive of a cause of an episode of psychosis.

48. **(B)** Because a hypoglycemic cause for this patient's psychosis is suspected, glucose administration would be most appropriate. Haloperidol would likely reverse some of her

psychotic symptoms, but the goal of therapy should always be reversal of the most primary cause of her psychosis. Haloperidol would not reverse the physiologic signs of her hypoglycemia (eg, diaphoresis and tremulousness). Similarly, lorazepam would not reverse the most primary cause of her symptoms. The patient does not have symptoms of depression, so neither fluoxetine nor amoxapine is appropriate.

49. **(C)** Maternal exposure to alcohol during pregnancy results in fetal alcohol syndrome associated with mental retardation, low birth weight, narrow palpebral fissures, microcephaly, and flattened nasolabial facies.

50. **(E)** Secondary amenorrhea in a woman who has been menstruating is defined as the absence of menses for a length of time equivalent to a total of at least six of the previous cycle intervals or 6 months. The initial steps in the work-up of amenorrhea include human chorionic gonadotropin (hCG) to rule out pregnancy, TSH to rule out thyroid disease, PRL to rule out hyperprolactinemia, and then a progesterone challenge to assess the level of endogenous estrogen and the competence of the outflow tract. A pelvic sonogram may be performed. An endometrial biopsy is useful in women over 35 with irregular bleeding to rule out endometrial hyperplasia. If she also has galactorrhea, then a serum prolactin and possible radiologic studies of the pituitary are indicated to rule out a microadenoma.

51. **(E)** The most likely cause of the new onset of trouble abducting and adducting the fingers on one hand is damage to the ulnar nerve. Falling asleep drunk, he did not feel the pain, and having his arm over the back of the chair for the night could have put enough pressure on the nerve to result in permanent or temporary dysfunction. Thiamine deficiency and alcohol intoxication give more generalized dysfunction. Brachial plexus damage would affect the whole arm, not just the fingers. B_{12} deficiency does not give an acute presentation but is primarily paresthesias in a stock-

ing-glove distribution and loss of fine touch and vibratory sensation.

52. **(A)** The combination of recent memory loss, ataxia, and confabulation are classic for Wernicke–Korsakoff syndrome, caused by thiamine deficiency. Alcohol intoxication can certainly give memory loss and ataxia, but the patient's speech is usually so dysarthric that confabulation is not a possibility. B_{12} deficiency usually presents with peripheral sensory changes. Alcohol withdrawal most commonly is accompanied by hallucinations and tremors. Folate deficiency mimics B_{12} deficiency in many ways.

53. **(B)** Prophylactic administration of librium in a withdrawing alcoholic can prevent or reduce severe symptoms such as delirium tremens. Prophylactic phenytoin and carbamazepine, however, are not helpful. A calm, quiet environment with close observation and frequent reassurance is very important. Vitamin administration (especially thiamine) is important, and frequently severe magnesium depletion will require treatment as well.

54. **(A)** Symptoms are highly suggestive of a group A streptococcal infection with several of the minor Jones criteria for rheumatic fever, such as fever and arthralgia. A throat culture for group A strep is warranted.

55. **(D)** Treatment of choice for group A streptococcal infections causing rheumatic fever is penicillin.

56. **(C)** Acute glomerulonephritis may follow a group A streptococcal infection and is manifested by hematuria, proteinuria, and RBC casts. The other manifestations are not directly associated with group A streptococcal infection.

57. **(C)** Follicular cysts are the most common cystic tumors of the ovary, followed by corpus luteum cysts and theca lutein cysts. Benign cystic teratomas may have solid components in their histology. Dysgerminomas are malignant, solid tumors of the ovary. Luteo-mas of pregnancy are hyperplastic reactions of ovarian theca lutein cells and are not true malignancies. Although they resolve spontaneously after delivery, they are relatively uncommon. The nodules do not arise from the corpus luteum of pregnancy. Luteomas may result in masculinization of the mother in 30% of cases.

58. **(B)** Kaposi's lesions are violaceous and reddish-brown plaques that occur most commonly on the skin and mucosa of patients with HIV. Bacillary angiomatosis is also seen in HIV infection, but the lesion is a friable vascular papule or subcutaneous nodule. It is much less common. As in most immunocompromised patients, melanomas are seen more often, but these lesions do not show the pigment changes or irregular borders of a typical melanoma. Mycosis fungoides presents with scaly patches and plaques. An infected excoriation would have more significant surrounding erythema.

59. **(E)** Kaposi's is associated with the herpesvirus 8, not parvovirus or HTLV-I. The incidence has been decreasing since homosexual men began practicing safe sex. It is a chronic disease when seen in its original form in Mediterranean men. It can spread beyond the skin to involve other organs.

60. **(E)** Because of the progression of the lesions, you need to assess the stage of the disease. Progression to visceral disease requires more aggressive treatment and is associated with a poorer prognosis. In the meantime, instituting antiretrovirals may improve the lesions and is indicated by the rapidly falling CD4 count. You might also want to order polymerase chain reaction (PCR) testing for viral load. The use of chemotherapeutic agents is an option, but not before adequate staging. Surgical resection is not useful apart from biopsy. Radiation is another treatment tool, but again one would want adequate staging and to treat the HIV first.

61. **(D)** Proguanil by itself has too high a resistance to be considered a good treatment op-

tion in a patient with this history. Clinical malaria developing in the face of chemosuppresion suggests probable drug resistance, for which the cinchona alkaloids (quinine and quinidine) and pyrimethamine–sulfadoxine (Fansidar) are probably the best options. Chloroquine in sufficient doses may also be useful.

62. **(B)** Ultrasound is reliable, noninvasive, and the preferred initial test in cases of asymptomatic AAA. A CT scan is accurate, but more expensive. CT scanning is useful in cases in in which aneurysmal leakage is suspected. Arteriography is reserved for selected cases where operation is planned in the near future. Doppler pressure indices do not diagnose aneurysmal disease and are used for the diagnosis of occlusive disease. MRI is currently more costly and without distinct advantage over CT scanning.

63. **(E)** All are established complications of infrarenal AAA repair.

64. **(A)** The mortality rate for elective infrarenal AAA repair is < 5%.

65. **(A)** The normal menstrual length is 28 days ± 7 days. The normal duration of flow is 4 days ± 2 days. The normal blood loss is 40 mL. The girl's menstrual cycles were within the normal range until recently.

66. **(B)** Endometrial carcinoma in a 15-year-old girl is extremely rare. The denial of sexual activity by the mother should not be taken at face value. An anovulatory cycle commonly results is a delayed heavy menstrual flow with pain from passage of clots. This picture could represent onset of sexual activity accompanied by chlamydial infection, accounting for the longer menses and then subsequent pregnancy. The diagnosis of PCO should be more strongly considered if there are other stigmata such as excess acne and hirsutism. A persistent functional cyst could also explain the recent event.

67. **(D)** A type and screen is repeated about every 48 hours to detect the development of alloantibodies before dispensing additional units. Many hospitals require, and most states mandate, a special consent for the transfusion of blood products, but it is not yet universal. Directed-donor blood is perceived as safer but may not be. Most blood donors are regulars whose blood has been screened multiple times, whereas a family member pressured to give may be a first-time donor or may not feel free to reveal any high-risk behaviors. Whole blood is the product of choice for replacing blood loss; however, whole blood is rarely stocked by most blood banks. As it is usually the oxygen-carrying capacity that is needed, packed RBCs are most often ordered. In large-volume loss, one must be careful to give platelets and plasma occasionally to prevent a washout phenomenon. Although a patient may need more than one unit, it is better to transfuse one unit and then reevaluate the situation. Especially in young patients, one unit may give good resolution of the symptoms. In older patients with compromised cardiac function, more than one unit at a time may be detrimental.

68. **(B)** The risk of contacting hepatitis C is approximately 1 in 5000 units transfused. The risk for hepatitis B is much lower, at about 1 in 200,000. The risk for other infections is:

HTLV	1/50,000
HIV-1	1/225,000
HIV-2	Very rare
Bacteremia	Rare
Cytomegalovirus (CMV)	Variable

69. **(A)** Febrile transfusion reactions are usually a reaction to WBCs contained in the RBC unit. Acetaminophen can minimize the reaction, and filtering can remove enough of the WBCs to eliminate the reaction. Irradiated blood decreases the incidence of graft-versus-host disease when administering blood products to immunocompromised patients but has no effect on febrile reactions. Bacterial contamination is very rare, whereas febrile

reactions are quite common. The use of directed-donor blood has no effect on the incidence of febrile reactions with the exception of children donating to their mothers when in fact the reaction rate may be higher.

70. **(B)** Regional suppurative lymphadenopathy is present in all of the diseases listed, and the lesions are almost indistinguishable from each other. However, given the travel history to an endemic area, *Yersinia* should be highly suspect.

71. **(E)** A patient with sickle cell disease commonly presents with symptoms of pain, fever, or a falling hemoglobin. A hemolytic or vaso-occlusive crisis may very well be the etiology; however, in this specific case, the probability of a crisis is decreased because of the given hematologic parameters. A patient who is carefully managed during her pregnancy must also have other potential etiologies for these symptoms aggressively ruled out. Pulmonary embolization of marrow is more common in sickle cell disease. Pneumonia and pyelonephritis are very common in patients with sickle cell disease. Sickle cell disease in pregnancy is increasingly managed by the use of prophylactic red cell transfusions, either by simple transfusion or by partial exchange transfusion. The goal of therapy is to keep the hemoglobin S level low enough to decrease the frequency or severity of sickle cell crises. The patient's morbidity is significantly decreased with these therapies. The fetal neonatal outcome may also be improved.

72. **(A)** Coccidioidomycosis, a mycotic infection, is extremely common in scattered, highly endemic arid and semiarid areas of the Western Hemisphere and is sometimes called valley fever after the Central Valley of California, an endemic area. Common symptoms are fever, chills, cough, and pleural pain.

73. **(C)** The disease is easily transmitted by dust fomites, and then spores are inhaled.

74. **(E)** *Trichomonas* vaginitis is a sexually transmitted vaginal infection that may cause vulvar itching, burning, and erythema. There is often copious discharge, which may be frothy and gray to yellow-green in color. There is no characteristic vulvar lesion. Condyloma lata are seen in 30% of patients with secondary syphilis, which occurs 4 to 8 weeks after the primary chancre appears. They appear as flat-topped, coalesced papules with a broad base and are highly infectious. The diagnosis is made with darkfield exam or serology. They will resolve spontaneously in 2 to 6 weeks. Hyperplastic dystrophy includes a variety of white lesions and is readily confused with atrophic lesions such as lichen sclerosis. Liberal use of vulvar biopsy is needed to distinguish among them and to rule out atypia and frank neoplasia. All may have pruritus as their chief symptom.

75. **(E)** *Trichomonas* can be treated with oral metronidazole, 2 g in one dose, 500 mg bid for 7 days, or 250 mg tid for 7 days. When one sexually transmitted disease is present, others should be screened for. The patient should return for follow-up, including vulvar biopsy in the event your initial suspicion about syphilis is incorrect and the white lesions remain present and undiagnosed.

76. **(B)** At autopsy, lung and pancreas are the most common primaries identified (about 40%). Generally, the prognosis is poor, but some subsets in which effective treatment is available can be identified by clinical criteria with only moderate investigations. These include peritoneal carcinomatosis in women (responds to treatment for ovarian cancer), predominant skeletal metastases in men (can reflect prostate cancer), and axillary lymphadenopathy in women (can reflect breast cancer). In the latter scenario, studies for estrogen and progesterone receptors are very useful in guiding therapy (ie, choosing tamoxifen as initial therapy versus cytotoxic agents).

77. **(D)** PSA is both sensitive and specific for abnormalities in the prostate. CA 125 is usually associated with ovarian cancer but can be elevated in any peritoneal or pleural process. Alpha-fetoprotein is useful in following germ cell tumors and hepatomas. CA 27.29 is a recognized marker for breast cancer but can be elevated in a number of other malignancies. CA 19-9 is most commonly elevated in malignancies of the biliary ducts, including the pancreas.

78. **(E)** Stage IB Hodgkin's disease is effectively treated with radiation alone. Some reports suggest that stage IIB can be similarly treated. Although physical examination and chest x-ray will initially suggest that 90% of patients with Hodgkin's have localized disease, by the end of staging, 60% will be stage III or IV. The purpose of staging laparotomy is to determine whether radiation alone will be used for treatment. As chemotherapy usage increases, the necessity for staging laparotomy decreases. Pruritus alone does not result in a B stage. B symptoms are drenching night sweats, fever greater than 38°C, or unexplained loss of greater than 10% of body weight within the preceding 6 months.

79. **(C)** The spleen is commonly involved in Hodgkin's but not in lymphocytic lymphoma. Hodgkin's is more likely to be localized and spreads via contiguous nodes, not by hematogenous or noncontiguous spread, which is characteristic of lymphocytic lymphoma. Marrow, central nervous system (CNS), and other non-nodal sites are commonly involved in lymphocytic lymphoma. Waldeyer's ring and epitrochlear nodes, occasionally involved in lymphocytic lymphoma, are almost never involved in Hodgkin's.

80. **(C)** Cyclophosphamide is associated with a hemorrhagic cystitis, not papillary necrosis, which is unusual in the moderate doses given in this regimen and can usually be prevented by adequate hydration during and shortly after administration. CHF begins to increase in incidence when doses of adriamycin rise over 400 mg/m². New agents are available which promise cardio-protection; their place in clinical practice is being defined. Vincristine is associated with peripheral neuropathy, which can manifest itself in decreased intestinal function—constipation, not diarrhea. Early intervention with diet, stool softeners, and laxatives can usually control this. Hypertension is not commonly seen with any of these agents.

81. **(D)** *Clostridium botulinum* will interfere with the cholinergic transmission of nerves by interfering with the release of acetylcholine in response to nerve stimulation. Epidemics have been associated with ingestion of honey and with breast feeding. Although polio may present with weakness and slow bowels, there will not be a dry mouth. Werdnig–Hoffman syndrome is a recessive anterior horn cell disease that presents with weakness and paradoxic breathing. Guillain–Barré syndrome presents with progressive muscle weakness, paresthesias in the legs, and diminished tendon reflexes. The usual incubation period for food-borne botulism is 12 to 36 hours (range 6 hours to 8 days). In infants, *C. botulinum* or toxin can be detected in stools. Toxin is found in only 10% of cases. Electromyography can also be used to demonstrate a characteristic pattern of brief, small, abundant motor action potentials.

82. **(B)** Treatment for this condition requires immediate admission to the ICU for observation and possible ventilatory support. Although botulinum antitoxin is available, it is not usually given to infants, because it might induce lifelong sensitivity to equine antigens and there is no evidence that it is effective in infants. Antibiotics do not improve the paralysis. Hyperbaric therapy and herbs will be of no help in treating botulism.

83. **(B)** Skin cancers are more common in patients living in southern latitudes of the northern hemisphere and in Australia, and in those with light complexions who burn easily. Although most people with blue or gray eyes have light complexions, it is not a one-

to-one correlation. These cancers are more common in sun-exposed areas of the body. They are more common in immunosuppressed patients, attesting to the importance of the immune surveillance system in the etiology of skin cancers. Living near power lines and having liver disease are not predisposing factors. The amount and intensity of exposure to ultraviolet light is a risk factor for developing skin cancers.

84. **(A)** Basal cell carcinomas have a substantial capacity for local destruction but rarely metastasize. They do not develop in long-standing scars or secondary to acid burns. They can be treated with radiation or surgery, depending on size and location.

85. **(B)** Squamous cell carcinomas differ from basal cells in a few ways. They do tend to metastasize and can develop in long-standing scars, hence the term "scar carcinomas." Like basal cells, both surgery and radiation are treatment options, but the margin of resection does not need to be 5 cm and the Mohs technique has quite good local control rates with very close margins. Basal cells can be part of the basal cell nevus syndrome, but squamous cell carcinomas are not associated with any particular syndrome.

86. **(C)** Patients with damage to part of the endopelvic fascia usually have multiple segments that are damaged. Prior to any repair, a careful inspection of the anterior vagina, uterine cervix, posterior cul-de-sac, posterior vagina, and the perineal body must be performed in order to determine all the damage. The patient's surgical options for correction of the cystocele may include all except the Burch procedure, which only repositions the urethrovesical angle.

87. **(E)** In genuine urinary stress incontinence, there is a hypermobility of the proximal urethra down into the pelvis so that it is no longer an intra-abdominal organ. This results in pressure being exerted onto the bladder but not the proximal urethra. The bladder

pressure then exceeds the urethra pressure, with loss of urine resulting.

88. **(A)** In the evaluation of urinary incontinence, the cystometrogram is used to detect the presence of uninhibited detrusor contractions, among other conditions not amenable to surgical therapy. It can be done simply and inexpensively by slowly filling the bladder with water through a catheter and syringe and closely watching the water level. The Q-tip test demonstrates a cystourethrocele.

89. **(E)** AIHA is the most likely diagnosis. Spherocytes are not typically seen in iron deficiency, liver failure, or splenomegaly, while congenital spherocytosis does not present in adulthood. Spherocytosis is seen as well in patients with extensive burns and in microangiopathic hemolytic anemia.

90. **(E)** Extravascular hemolysis usually occurs in the liver, spleen, or other reticuloendothelial sites and liberates unconjugated bilirubin. Causes of intravascular hemolysis are usually inherited and are a result of abnormalities of red cell membranes, enzymes, globins, or heme. Extravascular hemolysis is a result of mechanical forces, chemicals, microorganisms, antibodies, or sequestration in the monocyte–macrophage system.

91. **(C)** AIHA is a result of the development of autoantibodies and not a deficiency of iron or pyridoxine. Red cell survival is decreased as the antibodies expedite removal of the cells before they are senescent. The reticulocyte count is usually elevated as the bone marrow attempts to compensate for the destruction. RBC transfusion can be life saving, although cross-matching is often difficult because it is hard to distinguish an autoantibody effect from an incompatibility. "Least incompatible blood" is the best the blood bank can do.

92. **(E)** Unstable hemoglobins can precipitate and result in the formation of Heinz bodies. Hemoglobin E and beta-thalassemia classi-

cally give a microcytic anemia with normally shaped RBCs. ITP is not associated with RBC abnormalities, although thrombotic thrombocytopenic purpura is. Prosthetic valves, because of physical trauma to the RBC membranes, can cause an increased number of schistocytes to be present on the peripheral smear.

93. **(A)** The patient is in her second decade of IDDM, during which time renal disease becomes the major cause of death. During the first decade, the primary cause of death is ketoacidosis; after the second decade, it is renal and cardiovascular disease.

94. **(C)** Approximately 80 to 90% of patients with IDDM have some evidence of background retinopathy after having IDDM for at least 20 years.

95. **(B)** This generalized seizure disorder, also known as absence seizures, appears as momentary lapses in awareness, with amnesia. There is no warning or postictal state. The other answers are incorrect as they are not typical of absence seizures. (See Figure 2.12.)

96. **(D)** The definitive diagnosis must be made histologically. Although FNA can obtain cellular material for diagnosis, with a nonpalpable lesion this would be difficult without ra-

diologic guidance. An optimal course of therapy can be carried out when results of local tumor histology, size, degree of invasion, and receptor status has been obtained.

97. **(E)** The risk for breast cancer is increased by late menopause, nulliparity, late onset of first pregnancy, premenopausal breast cancer in a first-degree relative, alcohol consumption, and other factors. However, 50% of women with breast cancer have no obvious risk factors.

98. **(D)** A 1-mm tumor will have been present for approximately 6½ years, and a 1-cm tumor for approximately 10 years. Thus, this patient's use of hormone replacement therapy is unlikely to have caused her breast cancer.

99. **(B)** This red rash with satellite lesions in the intertriginous regions is most likely a *Candida albicans* infection, which favors warm, moist areas such as those between fingers, neck folds, corners of the mouth, and axilla. (See Figure 2.13.) Ringworm is incorrect, as this disorder usually has a circular appearance. Contact dermatitis may be red but does not have satellite lesions outside the contact area. Irritant diaper rash usually spares the intertriginous areas.

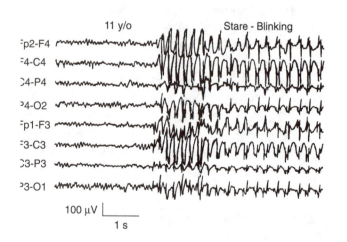

Figure 2.12

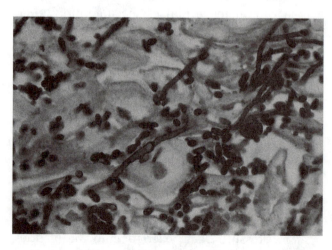

Figure 2.13

100. (B) The proper management for a cervical lesion is biopsy. The tissue necrosis may obscure the characteristics of malignancy of a Pap smear. A colposcopy-directed biopsy is may give a better yield. If microinvasion is diagnosed, a cold-knife biopsy is necessary to rule out coexisting invasive cancer. This distinction is important because management of these two entities differs from conservative to radical therapy. The other choices are inappropriate if invasion has not been reliably ruled out and would be open to criticism without having excluded or diagnosed invasion prior to surgery. Laser vaporization, as opposed to laser conization, does not provide a tissue sample for histologic interpretation. HIV disease is currently overrepresented in patients with carcinoma of the cervix.

101. (C) Cervical cancer staging is based on physical examination and selected endoscopic and radiologic imaging techniques. These include colposcopy, cystoscopy, proctoscopy, chest x-rays, IVP, and barium enema. Microinvasive cervical cancer (Stage IA-1) is the exception as only histology is used. Other diagnostic tests such as CT of the abdomen and pelvis, MRI, lymphangiography, or surgical staging may provide useful information for treatment individualization but not staging. The clinical stage may not change after treatment is started.

Stage I is confined to the cervix, stage II to the parametria, stage III to the pelvis, and stage IV to outside of the pelvis, including bladder or rectal mucosa or distant metastases. This patient has stage IIIB disease because of the hydronephrosis documented on IVP. The liver metastases seen on CT do change the staging.

102. (A) Mobitz type I, second-degree AV block (also called the Wenckebach phenomenon) is characterized by the progressive lengthening of the PR interval until there is a nonconducted P wave. The magnitude of the PR lengthening declines with each beat, so the RR intervals characteristically shorten prior to the dropped beat. The QRS complex is usually normal. Mobitz type II block occurs when there is a nonconducted P wave without previous lengthening of the PR interval. In complete heart block, there is no relationship between the P wave and the QRS complex. Parasystole is a second automatic rhythm existing simultaneously with normal sinus rhythm. The diagnosis of MAT can be made when there are at least three forms of P waves with varying PR and RR intervals.

103. (B) At the cellular level, exposure to excessive levels of cardiac glycosides, such as digoxin, causes increased automaticity and decreased conduction. These abnormalities are reflected in a broad array of rhythm disturbances (including the Wenckebach phenomenon) that are often difficult to distinguish from those caused by the underlying disease. First-degree and Mobitz type I blocks are seen as a side effect of digitalis, beta blockers, calcium channel blockers, and amiodarone. Because this phenomenon is relatively benign and often correctable, the placement of a pacemaker is not useful as the first intervention.

104. (B) Motor vehicle accidents are a leading cause of death for children aged 2 years and above. Most such fatalities are preventable by use of child restraints in automobiles. Counseling parents regarding use of a car seat, or safety belts for older children, is an important preventive measure. Lead toxicity, while a concern of this age, is rarely fatal. Tuberculosis, pneumonia, and influenza are not leading potential causes of death at this age.

105. (B) Treatment of disease that is already present to reduce the severity of its consequences is secondary prevention. Antiviral therapy for AIDS is direct treatment of the disease and thus is secondary prevention. Tertiary prevention would be limitation of disability through rehabilitation. Primary prevention could involve preventing exposure to the virus.

106. (B) The panic symptoms as described are limited to performance situations and do not generalize beyond them. The diagnostic use of a specific phobia is limited to nonsocial and performance stimuli, such as animals, environments, and situations. Patients with schizoid personality disorder would be noticeably asocial, a trait this patient does not have.

107. **(C)** The reported lifetime prevalence in the general population is 3 to 13%. Patients who present with anxiety complaints to outpatient clinics exhibit social phobia rates of 10 to 20%.

108. **(B)** The mechanism of tissue resistance to insulin appears to be primarily mediated through the increase of hPL. Estrogen and progesterone may have a role. The elevated level of hPL also increases lipolysis and circulating free fatty acid, which may further increase tissue resistance to insulin. These changes are consistent with the accelerated starvation state. The two primary effects of this are that the mother utilizes lipids for fuel, and therefore more glucose is available for the fetus. The pregnant woman is also prone to ketonemia. During a normal pregnancy, the postprandial response to glucose ingestion is prolonged hyperglycemia and hyperinsulinemia with greater suppression of glucagon. Facilitated diffusion of glucose by the placenta provides for a more rapid than expected transfer. Under this situation, the fetus has a steady postprandial supply of glucose, its principal caloric source.

109. **(B)** "Baby-bottle" tooth decay is most prevalent in the maxillary incisors. It is characterized by rapid development of caries in the primary teeth caused by prolonged tooth contact with cariogenic substances such as milk sweetened with sugar, sugared water, fruit juices, or carbonated beverages taken from a bottle or pacifier. Native Americans have an extremely high prevalence of "baby-bottle" caries.

110. **(B)** Although each of the questions listed is likely to be useful in the evaluation of this patient, who may suffer from borderline personality disorder, the urgency of the problem dictates that the degree of suicidality or homicidality of the patient be assessed imme-

diately. Such a question should be asked directly. It has been demonstrated that discussing suicide with patients does not increase their risk of suicide attempts.

111. **(D)** Patients with borderline personality disorder usually gain greater stability in relationships and vocational functioning during their 30s, 40s, and thereafter. There is not usually a progression to schizophrenia, but there is a higher-than-normal incidence of episodes of major depressive disorder and of self-harm in these patients.

112. **(D)** Calculations by the Centers for Disease Control and Prevention (CDC) focusing on years of potential life lost (YPLL) before age 65 goes beyond absolute causes of death to those that deprive people of the best years of their lives. "Unintentional injuries" include accidents and adverse effects.

113. **(C)** Lithium carbonate is prophylactic for episodes of mania and depression in bipolar illness. Carbamazepine is another prophylactic medication used in bipolar illness. Doses of lithium should be adjusted to reach serum levels between 0.8 to 1.2 mEq/L.

114. **(C)** This man is exhibiting psychotic symptoms; thus, an antipsychotic (neuroleptic) medication, such as haloperidol, is the treatment of choice. Clorazepate and lorazepam are anxiolytics (benzodiazepines). Amitriptyline and imipramine are antidepressants.

115. **(C)** Mercury poisoning can cause tremors and ataxia. It may also cause emotional lability, neurasthesias, and psychomotor disturbances. Organic mercury can cause visual field changes, while inorganic mercury can produce personality disturbances.

116. **(C)** This patient is likely experiencing a manic episode, symptoms of which include psychosis, a change in sexual desire, and decreased need for sleep. Unfortunately, the mood stabilizers (the traditional agent lithium, and antiepileptic agents such as valproic acid, carbamazepine) take several days

to have an effect. The antidepressant amitriptyline is contraindicated because it can induce rapid cycling in bipolar patients. Haloperidol is fairly rapid acting and can diminish psychotic symptoms while a mood stabilizer is taking effect.

117. **(C)** The typical recommended dose for maintenance treatment of patients with bipolar I disorder is 0.6 to 1.2 mEq/L. Lithium has a relatively low toxicity index, however, and can cause toxic effects at concentrations as low as 2.0 mEq/L.

118. **(C)** Pregnancy should be suspected. Other tests may be carried out to complete her evaluation.

119. **(D)** Failure rates are highest with Pomeroy-type tubal ligations done at cesarean and are estimated at 3/1000 (although preliminary findings from the CDC indicate a rate as high as 8/1000). However, this remains one of the most effective contraceptive methods. Failure rates are highest in the first year, when only 10% are ectopic. In later years, the ectopic rate remains constant, but the overall pregnancy rate decreases; thus, most pregnancies are ectopic. PID may be more difficult to diagnose, as there is less peritoneal spillage and infection remains confined to the endometrial cavity. The incidence of ovarian carcinoma appears to be decreased for at least 20 years after surgery.

120. **(A)** Bacterial vaginosis is currently thought to be a symbiotic anaerobic infection. For diagnosis, three of four signs should be present: clue cells, vaginal pH greater than 4.5, positive potassium hydroxide (KOH) whiff test, and thin homogeneous discharge adherent to the vaginal walls. Controversy continues about sexual transmission, and routine treatment of partners is not currently recommended. Treatment of asymptomatic women is not required except in pregnancy, where it has been associated with preterm labor and preterm rupture of membranes.

121. **(B)** Analgesic nephropathy (AN) mainly afflicts middle-aged women. Minimal cumulative ingestion of at least 3 to 5 kg of analgesic mixtures can cause AN. Caffeine intake, dehydration, and certain trace elements in water might facilitate renal injury. UTIs have dipstick findings of leukocytes, not protein. UTIs rarely lead to renal damage unless associated with diabetes, pregnancy, reflux, obstruction, or neurogenic bladder.

122. **(B)** For the diagnosis of major depression, either depressed mood or anhedonia must occur most of the day, nearly every day, for at least 2 weeks. In addition, at no time during the disturbance can there be delusions or hallucinations for as long as 2 weeks in the absence of prominent mood symptoms. Although not specified by the Diagnostic and Statistical Manual, 4th edition (DSM-IV), it would be highly unusual to have a major depression with psychotic features heralded by the psychotic components. Psychotic features may be mood congruent, but not necessarily so.

123. **(D)** The patient described experiencing auditory hallucinations, and they are a "symptom." Other choices are either not symptoms or are not present. Derailment consists of a pattern of incomprehensible speech. Loose associations are a hallmark of circumstantial, tangential, or illogical speech. Depersonalization is the sense that one's mind is being separated from one's body.

124. **(A)** Early in the course of viral meningitis, there may be equal numbers of polys and lymphocytes. In the first 6 hours, the lymphocytes increase, and eventually monocytes predominate. Glucose is normal, while protein may be slightly elevated.

125. **(D)** It is estimated that in approximately 20 to 40% of cases of maternal HIV infection, the virus is transmitted vertically to the infant. Administering AZT prenatally to the infected mother and postnatally to the infant has been reported to reduce HIV transmission substantially.

126. **(C)** In anorexia nervosa, the body is in a state of starvation. Signs of starvation include hypotension, bradycardia, dependent edema, and lanugo hair. T-cell lymphoma, a malignancy primarily of the skin, does not cause hypotension, bradycardia, dependent edema, or lanugo hair. CHF would be extremely rare in a 25-year-old person, and the symptoms in this young woman are not typical of CHF. An individual with untreated CHF will have hypertension and, rather than dependent edema, pitting edema that does not resolve with leg elevation. With an ovarian tumor, a woman may experience anorexia and loss of appetite, but would not have anorexia nervosa. Also, ovarian tumors may cause vague abdominal discomfort, and "clothes feeling tight around the abdomen." Classic signs of hyperthyroidism include tachycardia, brisk reflexes, fine tremor, and warm, smooth skin. Weight loss despite a good appetite and increased food intake is a classic symptom of hyperthyroidism.

127. **(D)** Obsessive–compulsive disorder is marked by the presence of obsessions or compulsions that cause distress, interfere with normal daily functioning, and are subjectively distressing to the individual experiencing them. Obsessions are recurrent or persistent thoughts, impulses, or images that cause marked anxiety or distress. Compulsions are repetitive behaviors, such as hand washing, or repetitive mental acts that an individual feels driven to perform in order to reduce anxiety or prevent something dreaded from happening. Unlike when an individual has obsessive–compulsive personality disorder, when an individual has obsessive–compulsive disorder, the individual is aware that he or she has a problem and is distressed by the symptoms. Tourette's disorder is characterized by multiple motor tics and at least one vocal tic. Asberger's disorder is a pervasive developmental disorder. "Anal-retentive personality disorder" is not a DSM-IV disorder.

128. **(E)** Once the patient is immunized with tetanus toxoid, the booster should occur every 10 years. With clean minor wounds, the 10-year schedule is satisfactory. If the wound is dirty, neglected, or had poor circulation in the area, tetanus toxoid should be given if the last toxoid was given 5 years ago.

129. **(B)** Important signs of bulimia nervosa include erosion of tooth enamel caused by acidic vomitus and abrasions on the dorsum of the hand due to scraping by the upper teeth as the individual pushes the hand to the back of the throat to induce vomiting. Coffee or tea consumption may cause brownish discoloration of teeth but does not cause erosion of tooth enamel. Caffeine dependence, like other drug dependence, is characterized by tolerance and withdrawal symptoms upon discontinuation of the drug. Pica is the eating of non-nutritive substances, such as soil or paper. Scratches on the back of the hand are not likely to be a sports injury of concern. Symptoms of multiple sclerosis include vision disturbance, fatigue, muscle weakness, and tingling or numbness in part of the body.

130. **(E)** Amiodarone is an antiarrhythmic agent used in the treatment of atrial firillation. A significant side effect of amiodarone that occurs in some individuals is hypothyroidism or hyperthyroidism. The most common psychiatric presentation for hypothyroidism is a retarded depression. Hyperthyroidism most commonly presents with anxiety, panic attacks, or agitated depression. Fosinopril and lisinopril are beta blockers. Hydrochlorothiazide and furosemide are diuretics. These medications do not cause hypothyroidism.

131. **(D)** Dermoid cysts or cystic teratomas in adolescent girls are the most common ovarian tumor in children or adolescents. These tumors contain tissue from all three germ layers, including skin, hair, and sebaceous glands. They may enlarge and produce symptoms of torsion or peritonitis.

132. **(D)** There is no specific test for ADHD. The diagnosis is a clinical one and can be made based only on a carefully taken history. A differential diagnosis includes temperamental characteristics, anxiety disorder, depressive disorder, conduct disorders, and learning disorders. Conduct or learning disorders are frequently comorbid with ADHD. Cognitive tests, such as the Continuous Performance Test, can help to confirm a diagnosis of ADHD.

133. **(C)** At this point, you have data to suggest impairment in social interactions with peers and a failure to seek out parents, as well as restricted and stereotyped behaviors. This suggests a pervasive developmental disorder, and questioning about language development will help to differentiate between a diagnosis of autistic disorder and Asperger's disorder, which is characterized by a lack of significant language and cognitive delays associated with autism.

134. **(D)** Ovarian cancers are divided into three major categories based on cell type. Epithelial tumors, the most common (85%), are derived from the mesothelial cells of the ovarian surface. Papillary serous adenocarcinoma is the most common malignant ovarian tumor. Other epithelial tumors are mucinous, endometrioid, clear cell, Brenner, mixed type, and undifferentiated. Germ cell tumors are the second most frequent class (10% of ovarian malignancies). These include dysgerminoma, endodermal sinus tumor, embryonal carcinoma, polyembryoma, choriocarcinoma, teratoma, mixed, and gonadoblastoma. Stromal tumors are the least common group (4% of ovarian malignancies). These include granulosa cell tumor, androblastoma (Sertoli–Leydig cell tumor), lipid cell tumor, gynandroblastoma, and unclassified. This latter group may or may not produce hormonal effects. CA 125 is associated with certain epithelial malignancies as well as benign conditions. It is frequently elevated in papillary serous carcinoma. It is not significantly elevated in mucinous tumors. Germ cell tumors such as dysgerminoma, choriocarcinoma, and embryonal cell carcinoma may have elevated beta-hCG. Alpha-fetoprotein may be associated with an endodermal sinus tumor.

135. **(C)** With nontender nodes and no symptoms of fever, plus the duration of the problem, it is unlikely that this represents an infection; therefore, antibiotics will not help. The chest will need to be evaluated, but a CT will provide more information. This is most likely a low-grade lymphoma, and therefore CT scan and referral to a surgeon for biopsy should be your next step. Thyroid cancer does not usually present with diffuse nodal involvement. A referral to radiation is premature; what is needed is tissue.

136. **(D)** Follicle center lymphomas are indolent lymphomas which, left untreated, still result in a survival of many years. Treatment is available and usually reserved for symptomatic disease. Bulky nodes would be an indication for treatment. Initial treatment is usually with relatively nontoxic oral agents, saving more aggressive treatments for later on, if ever, in the course. Aggressive treatment has not been shown to impact survival in older patients.

137. **(C)** Richter syndrome is a well-described entity wherein patients with indolent lymphomas develop a transformation in one area into a more aggressive process. Recurrence of the indolent lymphoma would be generalized and slower, as at the initial presentation. There is no evidence of infection, although all patients with lymphoma are to some degree immunocompromised, and this should be remembered. Although breast cancer is a common disease, the patient is at higher risk to have complications related to her lymphoma than a new disease process. Chlorambucil's main toxicity is to the bone marrow.

138. **(D)** From the information provided, this patient is normal. He is within the range of normal size, even though he is the shortest in his class. However, many parents want documentation of the diagnosis. This is done with a bone age radiograph, which demonstrates the sequential appearance of ossification of bones in the hand and knee area as the patient ages. This patient will have either a normal or slightly delayed bone age. If it is

slightly delayed, it shows that there is potential for growth. The major task is to observe him for determining further growth velocity and the growth achieved in a year. Giving growth hormone would not be the next most appropriate step. A complete blood count will not provide any information with respect to growth. Options A and C are incorrect because the child technically falls within normal growth charting.

139. (E) A barky cough in a 6-week-old infant is concerning for the diagnosis of a congenital disorder, such as a vascular ring. Vascular rings around the trachea and esophagus occur and produce varying degrees of compression. Other associated symptoms include wheezing and vomiting. Viral croup is usually seen in infants and children aged 3 months to 5 years. Classically, the patient presents with a barky cough and stridor. The diagnosis of tracheoesophageal fistula is typically made in the newborn period when the infant has choking, cyanosis, or coughing with an attempted feed. Of the five major forms, esophageal atresia with distal tracheoesophageal fistula occurs most often (seen in 87% of patients with tracheoesophageal fistula). Pulmonary sequestration refers to a nonfunctioning embryonic and cystic pulmonary tissue that receives its entire blood supply from the systemic circulation. On physical exam, patients with this lesion may have dullness to percussion and decreased breath sounds in the area of the sequestration. Bronchiolitis occurs during the first 2 years of life and is characterized by paroxysmal, wheezy cough; dyspnea; and irritability.

140. (A) Dermoid or mature (benign) teratoma is the most common ovarian neoplasm in the 0 to 19 age group, followed by serous cystadenoma, assuming follicle and corpus luteum cysts are not considered neoplasms.

141. (E) Serous cystadenocarcinoma of the ovary is the most common malignant neoplasm in all age groups; 33 to 66% are bilateral. It is rare in women under age 20.

142. (C) Mature cystic teratomas represent 20 to 25% of all ovarian neoplasms and occur in all age groups. They are bilateral 10 to 15% of the time, have a 46,XX karyotype, and contain elements of all three germ cell layers. Torsion is the most common complication, followed by rupture, infection, hemorrhage, and malignant degeneration.

143. (A) Most patients with endometriomas are asymptomatic. Endometriomas are not considered neoplasms by most investigators. There is no correlation between day of cycle and rupture. Endometriosis is classified as moderate when endometriomas are 2 cm or less; severe when endometriomas are 2 cm or greater.

144. (E) These symptoms reflect the immunodeficiency problems of children with HIV infection: abnormal B-cell function, relative hypogammaglobulinemia, decrease in CD4 cell count, and an abnormality in antibody-mediated immunity. Histiocytosis X is represented by three disorders, each of which involves an infiltrating histiocytosis. These disorders are eosinophilic granuloma of bone, Hand–Schuller–Christian syndrome (also bony lesions), and Letterer–Siwe syndrome (involving soft tissue, skin, liver, and lungs). Gaucher's disease is a disorder of glucosylceramide storage, with splenomegaly as the initial presenting symptom most often, along with pathologic fractures. Patients with IgG deficiency present with frequent infections. The disorder is very uncommon.

145. (A) The cause of trigeminal neuralgia (tic douloureux) is unknown, although some cases may be caused by compression of the trigeminal nerve by arteries or veins of the posterior fossa. The pain occurs in paroxysms and is strictly limited to one or more branches of the fith cranial nerve. Paroxysms may be brief or last up to 15 minutes. There is no objective sensory loss, but the patient may complain of hyperesthesia of the face. Watering of the eye on the involved side may occur during an attack.

146. **(D)** This anticonvulsant drug is given in doses varying from 400 to 800 mg/day. Phenytoin has also been used. The two drugs can also be used in combination. Operative procedures include alcohol injection of the nerve or ganglion, partial section of the nerve in the middle or posterior fossa, decompression of the root, and medullary tractotomy. Radiofrequency surgery can destroy pain fibers but spare motor fibers.

147. **(D)** Fetishism is a type of paraphilia in which intensely sexually arousing fantasies, urges, or behaviors involve nonliving objects. Dyspareunia is recurrent or persistent genital pain associated with intercourse. Pedophilia is a paraphilia involving sexual attraction to children; frotteurism is a paraphilia involving rubbing against others for sexual gratification; and exhibitionism is displaying oneself in a sexual manner for sexual gratification.

148. **(D)** This patient is exhibiting many of the signs of major depressive disorder: subjective depressed mood, inability to sleep, loss of appetite, diminished concentration, feelings of self-worthlessness, and guilt. However, because there is an identifiable life just before the onset of symptoms, DSM-IV suggests a diagnosis of adjustment disorder. For such a diagnosis, symptoms must appear within 3 months of the stressor and subside within 6 months of the event. However, this patient is only 4 months from the event, so the most appropriate diagnosis is adjustment disorder, depressive type.

149. **(B)** Weakness in the extremities, unilateral vision loss, uncoordination, and paresthesias are common presenting signs of multiple sclerosis (MS). Urinary frequency, retention, hesitance, or incontinence; hearing loss; vertigo; pain in the extremities, face, or trunk; and dysarthria, along with diminished intellectual function, are all less common initial features.

150. **(E)** MS is more common farther from the equator, where its incidence is less than 1 per 100,000, versus Northern Europe, where it is 30 to 80 per 100,000. Clusters of patients with MS have been seen, and it is more common in first-degree relatives, suggesting both an infectious etiology and a genetic predisposition, but the cause remains unknown. The average age of onset is in the mid-30s. Myelin dissolution is seen, but the axon remains intact.

Practice Test 3
Questions

DIRECTIONS (Questions 1 through 123): Each of the numbered items or incomplete statements in this section is followed by answers or by completions of the statement. Select the ONE lettered answer or completion that is BEST in each case.

Questions 1 Through 3

A 3-year-old girl is evaluated in the office. Her mother reports that the girl has had 2 weeks of continued fever, often spiking at night. On physical examination, she is noted to have dry, erythematous lips; strawberry tongue; bilateral conjunctivitis; erythema multiforme; cervical adenopathy; and splenomegaly. Laboratory studies demonstrate anemia and leukocytosis. Rapid strep screen is negative in the office. Tests for rheumatoid factor are negative, as is a heterophile, Lyme titer, antistreptolysin-O (ASO) titer, and an antinuclear antibody (ANA). Chest x-ray is normal. (See Figure 3.1.)

1. The MOST likely diagnosis is
   (A) mononucleosis
   (B) untreated Lyme disease
   (C) measles
   (D) Kawasaki disease
   (E) scarlet fever

2. The cardiovascular lesion MOST typically associated with this condition is
   (A) coronary artery aneurysms
   (B) myocardiopathy
   (C) second-degree heart block
   (D) aortitis
   (E) pulmonary hypertension

3. Once diagnosed, the next best treatment step (that also helps prevent cardiac sequela) is
   (A) radiation therapy
   (B) high-dose intravenous gamma globulin and aspirin
   (C) penicillin G
   (D) acetaminophen
   (E) doxycycline bolus

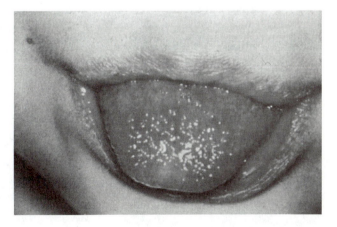

Figure 3.1

Questions 4 Through 6

A 27-year-old woman (P1000) presents for a prepregnancy counseling visit. She and her husband are of British Isle ancestry. Her son had a large meningomyelocele and died from postoperative meningitis. The baby had no other anomalies. She has several concerns relating to neural tube defects.

4. The usual karyotype of a baby boy with an open neural tube defect (NTD) is

    (A) 47,XY +13
    (B) 47,XX +13
    (C) 47,XX +18
    (D) 46,XY
    (E) 45,XO

5. NTDs result from the failure of the neural tube to close by

    (A) menstrual days 26 to 28
    (B) menstrual days 32 to 44
    (C) embryonic days 20 to 24
    (D) menstrual days 35 to 42
    (E) embryonic days 13 to 22

6. Prenatal screening for NTDs is available by using which of the following tests?

    (A) maternal serun acetyleholinesterase
    (B) maternal serum alpha-fetoprotein
    (C) basic sonography
    (D) directed magnetic resonance imaging (MRI)
    (E) amniocentesis

7. A patient is admitted to the emergency department in Cincinnati with suspected botulism. You would be particularly interested in a history of ingestion of

    (A) fish
    (B) pork
    (C) rice
    (D) home-canned vegetables and fruit
    (E) seafood

8. A 44-year-old man has been working as a boilermaker without adequate hearing protection. If an audiogram is performed, at which frequency will you expect to detect early hearing loss impairment?

    (A) 20 Hz
    (B) 16,000 Hz
    (C) 4000 Hz
    (D) 12,000 Hz
    (E) 8000- to 10,000-Hz range

9. A patient with cerebellar ataxia MOST likely will have had a recent infection with

    (A) chickenpox
    (B) strep
    (C) Lyme disease
    (D) rubella
    (E) parvovirus

Questions 10 Through 13

A 69-year-old man notices blood at the start of urination that clears as he continues to pass urine. Laboratory evaluation reveals a hemoglobin of 14.7 g/dL, with a mean corpuscular volume (MCV) of 90. The remainder of the blood studies are normal, including a prostate-specific antigen (PSA) of 1.2.

10. The bleeding is MOST likely due to

    (A) renal cell carcinoma
    (B) ureteral stone
    (C) severe bladder hemorrhage
    (D) urethral lesion
    (E) prostatic hypertrophy

11. The initial evaluation of his hematuria should include

    (A) acid phosphatase
    (B) transrectal biopsy of the prostate
    (C) intravenous pyelogram (IVP)
    (D) computed tomography (CT) of the pelvis
    (E) MRI of the pelvis

12. Because he is working and spending time with his grandchildren, he has trouble finding the time to complete his evaluation until about 2 months later. He returns to the office with more persistent hematuria and some new left flank pain. Physical examination reveals a fullness in the left flank. Laboratory investigation might now demonstrate

    (A) thrombocytopenia
    (B) hypocalcemia
    (C) polycythemia
    (D) leukocytosis
    (E) high renin hypertension

13. A renal arteriogram is done (see Figure 3.2). What is your diagnosis?

    (A) kidney contusion and laceration
    (B) transitional cell carcinoma
    (C) renal hematoma
    (D) renal cell carcinoma
    (E) renal hemangioma

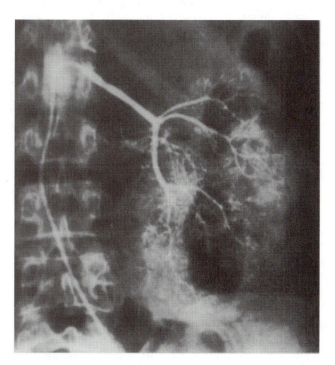

Figure 3.2

14. You have seen an employee from the laundry of another hospital because of low-back pain. He has responded well to anti-inflammatory therapy and after 3 days is ready to return to work. His supervisor asks you whether the patient has a past history of mental illness. You should

    (A) provide the information because it may expedite handling of insurance claims
    (B) provide the information because the supervisor has a need to know
    (C) decline to answer because you are employed by another hospital
    (D) decline to answer because the information is confidential
    (E) provide the negative information to protect the reputation of the patient from malicious gossip

Questions 15 Through 17

A 50-year-old divorced woman presents for psychiatric evaluation in January. She complains of depressed mood since the previous October, becoming progressively worse. In addition, she complains of tearfulness, impaired sleep, impaired concentration, anxiety, overeating with weight gain, anhedonia, and loss of libido. She adds that she has experienced similar symptoms each year from October through May since moving to the Midwestern United States five years ago. Prior to 5 years ago, she lived in the Southwestern United States and was asymptomatic.

15. Which of the following is the MOST appropriate diagnosis?

    (A) major depressive disorder, single episode
    (B) chronic adjustment disorder with depressed mood
    (C) major depressive disorder, recurrent, with seasonal pattern
    (D) bipolar II disorder, depressed, with seasonal pattern
    (E) posttraumatic stress disorder (PTSD), chronic

16. Which of the following medications would be MOST appropriate as pharmacotherapy for this patient?

    (A) alprazolam
    (B) sertraline
    (C) lithium
    (D) benztropine
    (E) haloperidol

17. After 6 weeks of treatment with the above medication, the patient experiences some improvement, but severe depressive symptoms persist. Which of the following treatment modalities would be the FIRST choice as an adjunct to her pharmacotherapy?

    (A) electroconvulsive therapy (ECT)
    (B) psychoanalysis
    (C) psychostimulant therapy
    (D) psychosurgery
    (E) phototherapy

Questions 18 and 19

A 23-year-old woman has had several episodes of severe wheezing over several years. She is a non-smoker and feels well between episodes. The wheezing usually occurs in the spring.

18. The major underlying factor in this woman is

    (A) elevated immunoglobulin E (IgE) levels
    (B) mast cell instability
    (C) nonspecific hyperirritability of the tracheobronchial tree
    (D) disordered immediate hypersensitivity
    (E) disordered delayed hypersensitivity

19. The MOST likely food to precipitate an asthmatic reaction in this woman is

    (A) red meat
    (B) egg whites
    (C) green salad
    (D) gluten
    (E) mayonnaise

Questions 20 Through 23

A 40-year-old woman presents with upper abdominal pain and hyperamylasemia.

20. All of the following disorders are associated with hyperamylasemia EXCEPT

    (A) acute pancreatitis
    (B) pernicious anemia
    (C) perforated peptic ulcer
    (D) ruptured aortic aneurysm
    (E) parotiditis

21. All of the following criteria are predictive for the severity of an episode of pancreatitis EXCEPT

    (A) age
    (B) serum low-density lipoprotein (LDH)
    (C) white blood cell (WBC) count
    (D) amylase level
    (E) Pa_{O_2}

22. All of the following are indications for surgery EXCEPT

    (A) unresolving mature pancreatic pseudocyst (> 12 weeks)
    (B) pancreatic sepsis
    (C) an amylase greater than 1000 units
    (D) to correct associated biliary tract disease
    (E) progressive clinical deterioration

23. The patient is initially treated without surgery but 10 days later develops leukocytosis, fever, and increasing abdominal pain. A CT scan is obtained and indicates the presence of a 5-cm pancreatic abscess. Treatment may include all of the following EXCEPT

    (A) antibiotic therapy
    (B) external drainage
    (C) debridement of necrotic pancreatic material
    (D) near total pancreatectomy
    (E) open packing

24. Which of the following coagulation factors undergoes the greatest change in pregnancy?

    (A) factor I (fibrinogen)
    (B) factor VII
    (C) factor VIII
    (D) factor XI
    (E) factor XIII

Questions 25 and 26

An obese 19-year-old woman with nephrotic syndrome is pictured in Figure 3.3. She recently noted increasing abdominal girth. A fluid wave and shifting dullness were noted upon physical examination of her abdomen.

25. Which of the following would be expected if laboratory analysis of the patient's ascitic fluid were performed?

    (A) protein content of 5 g/dL
    (B) 1500 WBC/mm^3
    (C) thick, cloudy ascitic fluid
    (D) bloody fluid
    (E) none of the above

26. Which of the following would MOST likely be found in this patient?

    (A) elevated total serum protein
    (B) marked proteinuria

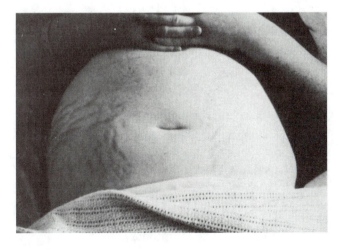

Figure 3.3

(C) decreased serum cholesterol
(D) decreased serum triglycerides
(E) decreased aldosterone production

Question 27 Through 29

A 65-year-old man was admitted to the hospital with congestive heart failure (CHF). He responded with a rapid diuresis after receiving digoxin and furosemide with potassium supplementation. His breathing improved markedly, but he complained of a pain in his left great toe. On examination, his toe was slightly swollen, markedly erythematous, and exquisitely tender to touch.

27. Which of the following MOST likely describes his condition?

    (A) septic joint
    (B) gout
    (C) Janeway lesion
    (D) osteomyelitis
    (E) arterial embolism

28. On examination under a polarizing microscope, joint fluid from the same patient would reveal

    (A) weakly positive birefringence
    (B) strongly positive birefringence
    (C) weakly negative birefringence
    (D) strongly negative birefringence
    (E) no birefringence under polarized light but gram-positive bacteria under light microscopy

29. Initial treatment of this patient might include

    (A) colchicine, PO
    (B) methotrexate, IV
    (C) methotrexate, PO
    (D) allopurinol
    (E) gold

30. A 26-year-old nulliparous woman with a history of irregular menses, obesity, and acne has an increased possibility over the normal population of

    (A) normal fertility
    (B) polycystic ovarian disease
    (C) alopecia
    (D) twin pregnancy
    (E) ovarian tumor

Questions 31 and 32

A 56-year-old man presents to his internist with complaints of difficulty in beginning urination, dribbling after micturition, and nocturia. He denies pain or obvious blood in his urine. The symptoms have gradually worsened over the past 6 months, but he does not feel ill. He states he would not have sought medical attention, but his wife is irritated at being awakened several times each night when he gets out of bed. There is no family history of prostate cancer. He assures you that he is monogamous.

31. Which of the following should be part of the initial evaluation?

    (A) sigmoidoscopy
    (B) urinalysis and culture
    (C) ultrasound of the prostate
    (D) carcinoembryonic antigen (CEA)
    (E) serum VDRL (Venereal Disease Research Laboratory)

32. The patient's PSA level is 11 ng/mL (normal is < 4 ng/mL). Which of the following statements is correct?

    (A) This patient has a 95% likelihood of having prostate cancer.
    (B) This patient's symptoms are not consistent with benign prostatic hypertrophy (BPH).
    (C) This patient's symptoms are not consistent with prostate cancer.

    (D) Having BPH does not appear to be causally related to the development of prostate cancer.
    (E) Prostate cancer is the most common cause of cancer-related death in men in the United States.

33. A patient is in active labor. She is 9 cm dilated and the vertex is at +1 station. Repetitive late decelerations are present. The fetal heart rate is 155 bpm with decreased variability. She is in a left lateral position, with oxygen administered by mask. Her blood pressure is normal. Her labor is spontaneous. The fetal scalp pH just reported to you is 7.21. Your plan is

    (A) to perform a forceps delivery
    (B) immediate cesarean section
    (C) to continue in utero resuscitative measures and repeat scalp pH in 1 hour
    (D) to continue in utero resuscitative measures and repeat scalp pH in 30 minutes
    (E) to obtain a second opinion

Questions 34 Through 36

A 22-year-old mentally retarded woman with a history of a seizure disorder is evaluated by a dermatologist because of the presence of wartlike lesions on her cheeks and forehead. The individual lesions are about 0.1 to 1 cm in size; they are elevated and pink-yellow. Several other family members have similar disorders.

34. This patient MOST likely has

    (A) Down syndrome
    (B) tuberous sclerosis
    (C) secondary syphilis
    (D) congenital rubella
    (E) congenital toxoplasmosis

35. This patient's skin lesions are referred to as

    (A) adenoma sebaceum
    (B) neurofibromatosis
    (C) condyloma acuminata
    (D) condyloma lata
    (E) basal cell carcinoma

36. Which of the following statements is true of this condition?

    (A) This disease is inherited as an autosomal dominant trait.
    (B) Few patients suffer from seizures.
    (C) Cystic lung disease is common.
    (D) Mental retardation occurs in over 90%.
    (E) No specific genetic mutation has been identified.

Questions 37 and 38

Your patient is a 25-year-old woman at term in active labor. The internal monitoring of the fetal heart rate shows a normal baseline of 130 bpm and normal variability. The last two contractions are associated with a sharp drop to 90 bpm lasting less than 30 seconds. The heart rate recovers promptly at the end of the contraction.

37. The MOST likely physiologic event associated with this pattern is

    (A) fetal acidemia causing cardiac depression
    (B) fetal hypoxia due to umbilical vein occlusion
    (C) fetal hypertension from umbilical artery occlusion
    (D) compression of the fetal head
    (E) maternal hypotension resulting from supine positioning

38. The patient is progressing normally in labor and has reached 7 cm cervical dilatation. The baseline heart rate is 165 bpm, and the variability is decreased. Moderate to severe variable decelerations have been present for the last 20 minutes. The BEST response to this situation is to

    (A) get the ultrasound machine for a biophysical profile
    (B) perform an amnioinfusion
    (C) perform a scalp pH
    (D) proceed to cesarean section
    (E) continue to watch the fetal heart rate without intervening

39. Which of the following patterns is considered to be reassuring?

    (A) baseline heart rate, 158 bpm; variability, normal; decelerations, moderate variable
    (B) baseline heart rate, 116 bpm; variability, decreased; decelerations, none
    (C) baseline heart rate, 128 bpm; variability, normal; decelerations, none
    (D) baseline heart rate, 174 bpm; variability, absent; decelerations, late
    (E) baseline heart rate, 144 bpm; variability, normal; decelerations, mild variable

Questions 40 Through 42

A 47-year-old woman with cancer phobia comes to your office for counseling. She wants to spend time reviewing her risks and what screening tests are appropriate for her.

40. Which statement is true?

    (A) Cancer is the most common cause of death in the United States.
    (B) Cancer is the most common cause of death in middle-aged women.
    (C) Incidence rates for cancer are generally higher in women than men.
    (D) Colon and rectum cancers have the highest mortality rate when considering both women and men.
    (E) About 25% of all cancers in the United States are due to environmental factors.

41. Recommended screening tests include

    (A) Papanicolaou (Pap) smear for standard risk patients every year
    (B) colonoscopy for people over age 50
    (C) mammogram every year for women over the age of 50
    (D) PSA blood test yearly for men over 50
    (E) yearly serum cholesterol levels for men over 35 and women over 45

42. Which of the following statements is true about specific environmental factors associated with cancer?

    (A) Alcoholic beverages are associated with cancer of the mouth and liver only in the presence of concomitant tobacco use.

    (B) Asbestos increases risk of lung cancer twofold, and cancer of the peritoneum 100-fold, but only in association with tobacco use.

    (C) Human papillomavirus (HPV) is linked to cancer of the cervix, vulva, and penis.

    (D) Tobacco smoke has not been conclusively linked to the development of cancer.

    (E) The highest rates for breast, uterus, and ovarian cancer are seen in African Americans.

Questions 43 and 44

43. An 18-year-old primigravid woman at 36 weeks' gestation develops intrapartum vaginal bleeding and abdominal pain, accompanied by late decelerations of the fetal heart rate. Her admission blood pressure was 180/107 mm Hg. It is now 127/100 mm Hg. The uterus is contracting every 2 minutes. The bleeding is assessed to be 200 mL every 10 minutes. The MOST likely diagnosis is

    (A) vasa previa
    (B) uterine rupture
    (C) placenta accreta
    (D) placenta previa
    (E) abruptio placenta

44. A 36-year-old woman (P5005) at 34 weeks' gestation presents with painless vaginal bleeding starting at 1:00 A.M. She has a history of two prior cesarean sections and two vaginal births after cesarean section. Her pulse is 115 beats per minute. Her blood pressure is 90/60 mm Hg. The MOST likely diagnosis is

    (A) vasa previa
    (B) uterine rupture
    (C) placenta accreta

    (D) placenta previa
    (E) abruptio placenta

45. A 33-year-old woman requests elective surgery for tubal ligation. She gives a history that 8 weeks previously she suffered a severe urticarial reaction to a condom and collapsed shortly afterwards. To proceed to definitively diagnose her condition, you should next obtain

    (A) skin patch testing with appropriate allergens

    (B) radioallergosorbent testing (RAST) for appropriate antibodies

    (C) skin prick testing with appropriate antigens

    (D) a complete blood count (CBC)

    (E) an eosinophil count

46. A 28-year-old man has had repeated conflicts with the law and frequently gets into arguments. He has a poor employment history. Which of the following might BEST describe this man?

    (A) autistic
    (B) antisocial personality
    (C) obsessive–compulsive personality
    (D) histrionic personality
    (E) none of the above

47. A 49-year-old man presents with detailed complaints of difficulty thinking, which have been of short duration. He reports memory gaps, but his attention and concentration are well preserved. He makes little effort to perform simple tasks in the mental status examination. The MOST likely diagnosis is

    (A) delirium
    (B) dementia
    (C) pseudodementia
    (D) schizophrenia
    (E) mental retardation

48. A 9-year-old girl is evaluated in the emergency department. She is known to have a history of asthma. The parents report that the child had a "cold" several days earlier, after which her asthma worsened. Her medications include theophylline and a albuterol inhaler via home nebulizer along with cromolyn sodium (Intal). A CBC is performed and is noted to be fairly unremarkable. Chest x-ray is negative for pneumonia. You make a tentative diagnosis of status asthmaticus. Which blood gas results are MOST typical of status asthmaticus?

   (A) $pO_2 = 80$, $pCO_2 = 40$, pH = 7.47
   (B) $pO_2 = 100$, $pCO_2 = 42$, pH = 7.45
   (C) $pO_2 = 70$, $pCO_2 = 58$, pH = 7.32
   (D) $pO_2 = 80$, $pCO_2 = 38$, pH = 7.33
   (E) $pO_2 = 60$, $pCO_2 = 42$, pH = 7.47

Questions 49 Through 51

You see an 18-year-old college student for the first time in the emergency department at 1:00 A.M. complaining of abdominal pain. Her boyfriend is in the exam room waiting with her. On reviewing her record, you observe that she has had repeated similar visits. You suspect abuse and are even more concerned when you notice bruises on her upper arms and back; however, she does not say anything about it.

49. A woman's lifetime risk of being battered is

   (A) 5%
   (B) 10%
   (C) 15%
   (D) 20%
   (E) 25%

50. Girls are MOST likely to be sexually abused by

   (A) date rape
   (B) a stalker
   (C) a family member
   (D) a stranger
   (E) a teacher

51. Victims of abuse

   (A) avoid medical care
   (B) almost always remember that they have been abused
   (C) usually volunteer this information in the course of giving a medical history
   (D) have more frequent premenstrual syndrome, headaches, asthma, and gastrointestinal problems
   (E) have more frequent endometriosis

Questions 52 and 53

A 72-year-old man complains of increasing abdominal pain and an inability to void for 48 hours. He has a history of BPH, for which he takes terazosin at bedtime. On physical examination, the suprapubic region is very tender to palpation. An ultrasound of the abdomen reveals a hugely expanded bladder with significant bilateral hydronephrosis.

52. Placement of a catheter into the bladder results in the rapid drainage of 3200 cc of clear yellow urine. Cultures are sent. Over the next few days, he continues to put out large quantities of urine. The urine is likely to be

   (A) low in sodium
   (B) dilute and alkaline
   (C) concentrated
   (D) acidic
   (E) none of the above

53. In a normal kidney, the largest volume of water is reabsorbed at the

   (A) collecting ducts
   (B) proximal tubules
   (C) distal tubule
   (D) ascending loop of Henle
   (E) descending loop of Henle

54. A mother has been found to have 20 parts per billion (ppb) polychlorinated biphenyls (PCBs) in her breast milk, and she comes to you for advice as to whether she should continue breast feeding. You decide

    (A) no, because 20 ppb is an insignificant trace amount of a chemical
    (B) no, because PCBs are potentially toxic to infants and young children
    (C) no, because there is no breast cancer hazard from PCBs
    (D) further information is required on the safe level in milk
    (E) yes, because the psychologic benefits of breast feeding are more important than potential adverse effects

55. A 25-year-old worker has developed contact dermatitis from working with glue. He has been diagnosed as having an allergy to acrylates. Which of the following is true of his condition?

    (A) Cross-sensation will not occur.
    (B) A clinical reaction will usually occur 48 to 72 hours after he contacts the causal substance.
    (C) This condition will be provoked only by considerable amounts of the allergen.
    (D) The allergen is likely to be a high-molecular-weight molecule.
    (E) Gloves will never prevent this condition.

56. A 52-year-old woman developed fever and a dry cough after traveling to a convention. On examination, there are some signs of consolidating pneumonia. Sputum culture grows *Legionella pneumophila*. This condition

    (A) has a fatality rate of almost 90% if untreated
    (B) is virtually never fatal
    (C) is best treated with erythromycin
    (D) occurs as a result of hotel food
    (E) almost always occurs in epidemics associated with specific buildings

57. A 30-year-old medical resident is noted to be especially frugal, rigid, and punctual. In most areas of his life, he is meticulous, but his desk and bedroom are very messy. He tends to be obsequious with superiors and rather sadistic with the medical students in his control. Occasionally, he has temper tantrums. From a psychoanalytic point of view, these characteristics are derivatives of which stage of development?

    (A) oral
    (B) anal
    (C) phallic
    (D) oedipal
    (E) latency

58. A 24-year-old woman is reported to the police as a missing person by her parents. Her fiance had recently broken their engagement, and she had been extremely despondent. When found by the police in another state, she was noted to be suffering from amnesia. Which of the following BEST characterizes her situation?

    (A) extinction
    (B) fugue
    (C) autosuggestion
    (D) schizoid personality
    (E) introversion

Questions 59 and 60

A 10-year-old boy is evaluated in the office. He is complaining of diarrhea and abdominal pain along with flatus and nausea. He denies blood in his stool and is found to be afebrile. Examination discloses diffuse lower abdominal tenderness without guarding or rigidity. His bowel sounds are somewhat hyperactive. No peritoneal signs are present. On reviewing the patient's history, you are made aware of the fact that he lives in a rural area where there are animals, and well water and insecticides are used.

59. The MOST likely cause of his problem is

    (A) *Shigella*
    (B) insecticide poisoning

(C) *Salmonella*

(D) enterocytopathogenic human orphan (ECHO) virus

(E) *Giardia*

60. The next appropriate treatment step in this case would be the administration of

(A) an enema

(B) tetracycline

(C) amoxicillin

(D) an anticholinergic

(E) quinacrine hydrochloride (Atabrine) or metronidazole (Flagyl)

Questions 61 Through 63

A 20-year-old man falls, striking his head. He is briefly unconscious and then awakens. His pupils are equal. He is taken to the emergency department. While there, he complains of a headache and becomes lethargic, then comatose. He vomits and is noted to have unequal pupils (left pupil dilated and nonreactive to light). His CT scan is shown in Figure 3.4.

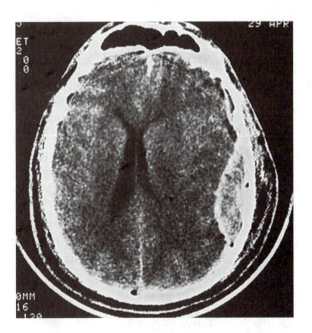

Figure 3.4

61. The dilation of the pupil is caused by

(A) injury to the eye

(B) elevated intracranial pressure effect on a cranial nerve

(C) direct nerve injury in the accident

(D) hyperventilation treatment

(E) a congenital lesion

62. The MOST important intervention for the treatment of this patient is

(A) observation

(B) intubation and hyperventilation

(C) mannitol

(D) surgical decompression

(E) elevation of the head of the bed

63. All of the following measures decrease intracranial pressure EXCEPT

(A) increasing Pa_{CO_2}

(B) removing brain tissue

(C) removing cerebrospinal fluid (CSF)

(D) decreasing cerebral blood flow

(E) decreasing Pa_{CO_2}

Questions 64 Through 66

64. A patient presents for her second prenatal visit at 12 weeks. Her history is significant for the presence of "anemia," which was treated by her family physician with iron and B_{12} shots. She was last treated approximately 1 year ago. Her hemoglobin is 8.5 g/dL. The indices show a hypochromic microcytic anemia. The MCV is 68. Her sickle prep is negative. A ferritin level is very low. Prior to this pregnancy, she had a hemoglobin electrophoretic pattern of hemoglobin A, 97%; hemoglobin A_2 2%; and hemoglobin F, < 1%. The MOST likely diagnosis is

(A) normal hemoglobin and hematocrit

(B) polycythemia

(C) megaloblastic B_{12} deficiency anemia

(D) anemia with beta-thalassemia trait

(E) iron-deficiency anemia

65. Assuming the patient now has a normal hemoglobin, which of the following is the MOST correct statement about iron metabolism during pregnancy?

    (A) Approximately 3000 mg are transferred to the fetus and placenta.
    (B) Approximately 500 mg are required for the expanding maternal hemoglobin mass.
    (C) Iron utilization occurs evenly over the entire pregnancy.
    (D) Ascorbic acid may facilitate iron absorption.
    (E) At least 300 mg of elemental iron per day should be added to the diet in the latter half of pregnancy.

66. The pregnant patient's need for folic acid is

    (A) decreased from 1000 µg to 400 µg
    (B) decreased from 1 mg to 0.4 mg
    (C) unchanged
    (D) increased from 180 µg to 400 µg
    (E) increased from 400 µg to 1000 µg

67. Temporary threshold shift

    (A) is age dependent
    (B) never becomes permanent hearing loss
    (C) usually lasts a few days
    (D) occurs after a loud noise
    (E) is usually one-sided

68. Which of the following was in the top five causes of death in both 1900 and 1985?

    (A) heart disease
    (B) tuberculosis
    (C) accidents
    (D) cancer
    (E) diabetes

69. A 35-year-old man being treated for a psychiatric disorder by his primary care practitioner is referred to you for a "pharmacologic tune-up." The patient reports that he has suffered from a dry mouth, constipation, light-

headness, and fatigue since starting on his medication 6 weeks ago. The patient was MOST likely prescribed

    (A) fluoxetine
    (B) amitriptyline
    (C) valproic acid
    (D) lorazepam
    (E) phenelzine

70. A 12-year-old boy whom you have been seeing for 6 months reports to your office one day wearing sunglasses. Because this is strange behavior for the boy, who has always been cooperative, open, and truthful in your sessions, you are surprised when he refuses to remove the sunglasses. Instead, he says he has a headache and that the light bothers him. He reports no other symptoms, but appears more anxious as the session comes closer to an end. Finally, with 5 minutes left in the session, he begins crying. After you gently ask him to remove the sunglasses, he does so, revealing a black eye. "My father did this to me," he sobs, "but don't tell anyone 'cause he says he'll do it to my other eye." Your obligation at this point is to

    (A) respect the patient's wishes and tell no one of the incident
    (B) recommend that the patient go to the emergency department and have a spinal tap to rule out meningitis
    (C) demand that the boy's father speak with you
    (D) notify a child services agency in your state
    (E) wait a month, and if there is no further evidence of abuse, tell no one of the incident

71. A 42-year-old woman is diagnosed with stage IB-1 squamous cell carcinoma of the cervix. Which of the following is the BEST management option?

    (A) cold-knife cone biopsy
    (B) vaginal hysterectomy

(C) total abdominal hysterectomy, bilateral salpingo-oophorectomy, and bilateral pelvic lymph node dissection

(D) radical hysterectomy and bilateral pelvic lymph node dissection

(E) total abdominal hysterectomy and bilateral salpingo-oophorectomy

72. The treatment recommended for stage IIB cervical cancer diagnosed during the first trimester of pregnancy should be

(A) immediate radical hysterectomy and bilateral pelvic lymph node dissection

(B) radiation

(C) termination of pregnancy followed by radical hysterectomy and bilateral pelvic lymph node dissection

(D) await spontaneous delivery and begin radiation therapy 10 days postpartum to allow for uterine involution

(E) total abdominal hysterectomy followed by radiation therapy

Questions 73 and 74

A 45-year-old man who has been a coal worker for 20 years presents with dyspnea that started 6 months ago and has grown progressively worse. He is a nonsmoker. He has had a chronic cough for nearly 12 months. He is a poor historian and unaware of what previous examinations have shown. He states that he had always felt fine up until about 1 year ago. Examination of the lungs shows mild wheezing on forced expiration, with a slightly increased expiratory phase.

73. A chest x-ray is performed. What findings are likely, on the basis of the history and examination?

(A) lobar infiltrates in the lower lung fields

(B) pleural thickening laterally

(C) hilar and mediastinal adenopathy

(D) multiple small, rounded opacities

(E) granulomatous disease

74. For what additional pulmonary pathology is this man at increased risk?

(A) pleural effusion

(B) mesothelioma

(C) adenocarcinoma of the lung

(D) *Mycobacterium tuberculosis* infection

(E) pneumonia

Questions 75 and 76

A 45-year-old man is admitted with his third episode of upper gastrointestinal hemorrhage. He has had two prior ulcer operations.

75. You suspect Zollinger–Ellison syndrome. All of the following would support your suspicions EXCEPT

(A) a fasting gastrin level of 450 pg/mL

(B) suppression of hypergastrinemia by secretion given intravenously

(C) past operative notes detailing ulcers in the duodenum and jejunum

(D) liver metastases on CT scan

(E) a history of diarrhea

76. On further probing of the family history, you learn that his mother had a parathyroidectomy at age 52. You now are concerned that the patient has multiple endocrine neoplasia type I (MEN I). All of the following are consistent with MEN I EXCEPT

(A) it is inherited as an autosomal dominant gene

(B) it is asociated with pituitary tumors

(C) it is associated with parathyroid tumors

(D) it is associated with hyperparathyroidism

(E) it is associated with the presence of a pheochromocytoma

Questions 77 Through 79

A 57-year-old man presents with fatigue and back pain. Evaluation reveals a normochromic, normocytic anemia.

77. An IVP must be performed with caution in this patient if he has

(A) hyperparathyroidism
(B) pyelonephritis
(C) nephrolithiasis
(D) hypernephroma
(E) multiple myeloma

78. Further evaluation reveals an immunoglobulin G (IgG) paraprotein. He is likely to develop renal involvement resulting in

(A) nitrogen retention
(B) hypertension
(C) retinitis
(D) edema
(E) hematuria

79. Amyloid is detected on rectal biopsy. Which statement concerning his renal evaluation is correct?

(A) It is caused by primary amyloidosis.
(B) Hypertension is present.
(C) Nephrotic syndrome is likely.
(D) There is impaired tubular function.
(E) Hematuria is present.

80. All of the following are associated with congenital lung cysts EXCEPT

(A) they become infected
(B) they resemble a pneumothorax or emphysema on chest x-ray
(C) they compress normal lung tissue
(D) they undergo malignant change
(E) they fill with fluid

81. For siblings of a child with insulin-dependent diabetes mellitus (IDDM), the probability of developing the disease is

(A) 0%
(B) 5 to 10%
(C) 25%
(D) 40 to 50%
(E) 100%

82. An investment banker whose avocation is cooking has developed hand dermatitis from frequent immersion in liquids and exposure to detergents and strong cleaning agents. She has been advised to use powdered rubber gloves to help limit her exposure. Which condition will NOT occur as a complication from using rubber gloves?

(A) anaphylaxis
(B) pneumoconiosis
(C) rhinitis
(D) allergic contact dermatitis
(E) urticaria

83. A young woman who is being treated with medication for an atypical depression goes to a party, where she eats chicken liver paté and cheese. She develops a severe headache. Her physical examination is normal except for a blood pressure of 200/130 mm Hg. The woman probably has been taking

(A) a butyrophenone
(B) a phenothiazine
(C) a monoamine oxidase inhibitor (MAOI)
(D) a tricyclic antidepressant
(E) lithium carbonate

84. A 58-year-old man has just had a lung biopsy, which shows carcinoma of the bronchus. He has smoked one pack of cigarettes a day for 30 years. Twelve months ago, he took a job as an asbestos removalist, in which he was lax in taking the required precautions. Two months ago, he took a job as a chemical technician, where he uses

chromium compounds under a properly functioning fume hood. The MOST likely cause of his lung cancer is

(A) chromium

(B) chromium interacting with tobacco smoke

(C) tobacco smoke

(D) asbestos

(E) asbestos interacting with tobacco smoke

85. All of the following are associated with hemoptysis EXCEPT

(A) mitral stenosis

(B) bronchiectasis

(C) pneumonia

(D) empyema

(E) bronchogenic carcinoma

86. A 15-year-old overweight girl is evaluated in the emergency department. She reports that she felt fine until sustaining a fall while playing tennis the previous afternoon. The patient reports that she cannot walk. She has pain in the left hip and knee. On examination, you find the patient's hip to be held in external rotation. (See Figure 3.5.) The MOST likely diagnosis is

(A) fracture of the head of the femur

(B) intracapsular hip fracture

(C) contusion of the hip capsule

(D) slipped femoral epiphysis

(E) patellar fracture

87. On the first day following a cesarean section, the patient complains of acute shortness of breath and anxiety. Her respiratory rate is 26 breaths per minute. Her pulse is 112 beats per minute. Her oxygen saturation is 85% on room air. Her lungs are clear. Homan's sign is negative. What is the MOST likely diagnosis?

(A) atelectasis

(B) popliteal thrombosis with pulmonary embolization

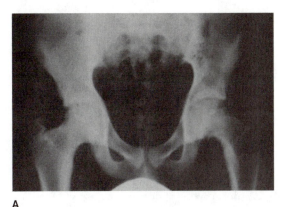

A

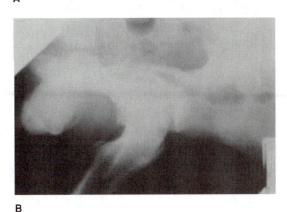

B

Figure 3.5

(C) iliofemoral thrombosis with pulmonary embolization

(D) pulmonary edema

(E) pulmonary infarction

Questions 88 and 89

88. A 34-year-old woman complains of recent numbness in the fingers. On examination, tapping over the dorsum of the wrist produces paresthesias in the distribution of the median nerve. A clinical feature you would NOT expect her to exhibit is

(A) clumsiness and dropping some objects

(B) awakening at night with numbness and tingling in the hand

(C) pain over the lateral epicondyle

(D) sensory loss in the hand

(E) positive Tinel's sign

89. Which of the following would NOT be likely to contribute to causing this condition?

    (A) diabetes
    (B) pregnancy
    (C) working with small parts in automobile assembly
    (D) working as a receptionist
    (E) rheumatoid arthritis

90. Which of the following does NOT characterize hyperacute organ rejection following transplantation?

    (A) presence of preformed antibodies to donor cells
    (B) graft destruction by 24 to 48 hours
    (C) tolerance to a second transplant from the same donor
    (D) no effective method for treatment
    (E) may be eliminated by pretransplant crossmatch testing

Questions 91 Through 95

A 70-year-old man comes to the office with a generalized scaling eruption of the skin. The itching is severe. He denies exposure to any new medications.

91. This disorder usually

    (A) is secondary to a systemic disorder
    (B) is benign and self-limited
    (C) requires systemic therapy
    (D) has a malignant etiology
    (E) worsens with oral corticosteroids

92. Physical examination reveals diffuse lymphadenopathy. This finding points to

    (A) viral infection
    (B) pyoderma
    (C) lymphoma
    (D) leukemia
    (E) nothing specific

93. Once hospitalized, a CBC is performed. The hematology technician calls you to report unusually large monocytoid cells. You review the smear with the pathologist and find large mononuclear cells with cerebriform, clefted nuclei. The MOST likely diagnosis is

    (A) leukemia
    (B) visceral B-cell lymphoma
    (C) primary cutaneous T-cell lymphoma
    (D) viral infection (usually Epstein–Barr)
    (E) paraneoplastic syndrome secondary to lung cancer

94. Prognosis for this syndrome is

    (A) rapidly downhill
    (B) determined by the type of medical care
    (C) rarely fatal
    (D) remissions and exacerbations, but with eventual progression to a fatal outcome
    (E) eventual complete recovery, regardless of the treatment

95. The treatment of this syndrome requires

    (A) antibiotics
    (B) antiviral medication
    (C) aggressive systemic chemotherapy
    (D) symptomatic treatment
    (E) early use of high-dose systemic steroids

96. A 4-year-old girl is evaluated because of a skin lesion. You feel that the lesion represents a form of hemangioma. The lesion is noted to be well demarcated. It is an elevated, bright red mass composed of numerous coalescing papules or nodules, which blanch incompletely upon pressure. This type of lesion's deep segment often presents as an ill-defined subcutaneous mass with a bluish hue. What type of hemangioma is this?

    (A) nevus flammeus
    (B) port-wine stain
    (C) strawberry hemangioma
    (D) hemangiosarcoma
    (E) cavernous hemangioma

Questions 97 Through 99

A 65-year-old morbidly obese woman is postoperative day 4 from a left hemicolectomy for colon cancer. You are called to evaluate her for sudden shortness of breath and pain when trying to take a deep breath, which occurred suddenly after getting her out of bed. On initial examination, she is tachypneic (respiratory rate, 40/min) and her lips are cyanotic. Her lungs are clear to auscultation, with diminished breath sounds at the bases bilaterally. Her chest x-ray is clear. Her arterial blood gas demonstrated a PO_2 of 50.

97. The MOST likely diagnosis is

   (A) pneumonia
   (B) pulmonary embolus (PE)
   (C) atelectasis
   (D) bronchiectasis
   (E) pneumothorax

98. Given your diagnosis, an appropriate diagnostic test would be

   (A) lower-extremity venous duplex ultrasound examination
   (B) lower-extremity arteriogram
   (C) CT scan of the chest without contrast
   (D) bronchoscopy
   (E) none of the above

99. All of the following statements regarding prophylaxis against DVT in postoperative patients are true EXCEPT

   (A) pneumatic compression stockings are an effective mode of DVT prophylaxis
   (B) unfractionated heparin is an effective mode of DVT prophylaxis
   (C) aspirin is the superior agent for DVT prophylaxis
   (D) low-dose warfarin has been shown to be effective for DVT in hip fracture patients
   (E) low-molecular-weight heparin is an effective mode of DVT prophylaxis

100. A child is brought into your office for a routine examination. He is a new patient to you and has not had the benefit of medical care in the past because the family lacked health insurance. On examination, you make note of frontal and parietal bossing, enlarged maxilla, and protruding front teeth along with marked malocclusion. The child appears pale. The MOST likely diagnosis is

   (A) sickle cell trait
   (B) thalassemia
   (C) craniostenosis
   (D) cleidocranial dysostosis
   (E) Pierre Robin syndrome

101. A primigravida at 20 weeks is concerned about harming her unborn baby by caring for her sister's infant after vaccination. Which of the following vaccinations is contraindicated for the child of a pregnant woman?

   (A) diphtheria–pertussis–tetanus (DPT)
   (B) measles–mumps–rubella (MMR)
   (C) hepatitis B
   (D) all of the above
   (E) none of the above

Questions 102 Through 105

An 18-year-old man of Italian heritage is found to have a hypochromic microcytic anemia of 10 g/dL. In addition, there is a fair degree of anisocytosis, poikilocytosis, and targeting on the peripheral smear. The white count is 9500, the platelet count is 240,000, and the reticulocyte count is 7%. The spleen is palpated 5 cm below the left costal margin.

102. The MOST likely diagnosis is

   (A) sickle cell trait
   (B) thalassemia minor
   (C) hemoglobin sickle cell disease
   (D) iron-deficiency anemia
   (E) hereditary spherocytosis

103. Which of the following would be most helpful in distinguishing this case from one of pure iron-deficiency anemia?

    (A) peripheral blood smear
    (B) osmotic fragility test
    (C) Ham's test
    (D) hemoglobin electrophoresis
    (E) serum ferritin determination

104. One would expect to find which of the following in this man?

    (A) an increased amount of fetal or A2 hemoglobin
    (B) increased osmotic fragility of the red cells
    (C) absent bone marrow iron
    (D) increased macroglobulins in the serum
    (E) small amounts of hemoglobin S

105. The present treatment of choice for this man is

    (A) splenectomy
    (B) removal of the abnormal hemoglobin pigment
    (C) supportive
    (D) plasmapheresis
    (E) intramuscular iron

106. A 15-month-old child is evaluated in your office for rectal bleeding. The MOST common cause of rectal bleeding at this age is

    (A) rectal fissure
    (B) intestinal polyp
    (C) inflammatory bowel disease
    (D) arteriovenous malformation
    (E) intussusception

107. When preparing a trial that will evaluate two surgical techniques (eg, inguinal hernia repair, technique A, the standard technique; and inguinal hernia repair, technique B), which of the following statements would be appropriate to state the nondirectional alternative hypothesis?

    (A) Surgical technique A is better than surgical technique B.
    (B) Surgical technique B is not better than surgical technique A.
    (C) Surgical technique A is different than surgical technique B.
    (D) Surgical technique B is not different than surgical technique A.
    (E) Surgical technique A is not different than surgical technique B.

108. You are called to evaluate a 4-month-old infant with constipation. On examination, you find the child to be alert and fussy. His abdomen is distended. No stool is noted in the rectum upon rectal examination. There is no blood noted. The child has had a poor weight gain. Which of the following diagnoses is MOST consistent with your findings?

    (A) botulism
    (B) functional megacolon
    (C) rectal fistula
    (D) aganglionic megacolon
    (E) tethered cord

109. If an oral thermometer were to break in the mouth, swallowing the inorganic mercury would cause

    (A) hypochromic microcytic anemia
    (B) no health effects
    (C) central and peripheral neuropathy
    (D) deafness and vision problems
    (E) acute renal failure

110. A blood type O-negative patient received a 300-µg intramuscular dose of anti-D immunoglobulin (Rh immunoglobulin) on the second day following the delivery of an anemic and hypovolemic type O-positive baby. Four years later, Rh sensitization was diagnosed and the baby required an exchange transfusion. A 300-µg dose of anti-D immunoglobulin will neutralize approximately

how many milliliters of Rh-positive red blood cells in the maternal circulation?

(A) 5

(B) 10

(C) 15

(D) 20

(E) 25

Questions 111 and 112

A 63-year-old woman with diabetes develops a sudden deterioration in renal function. An IVP reveals papillary necrosis.

111. This is likely due to

(A) diabetes mellitus

(B) glomerulonephritis

(C) pyelonephritis

(D) hypertension

(E) cortical necrosis

112. Papillary necrosis is associated with

(A) morphine use

(B) pregnancy

(C) obesity

(D) peripheral vascular disease

(E) alpha-thalassemia

113. The three major foci for Health People 2000, a set of national priorities for public health, are

(A) access, equity, and comparison

(B) access, protection, and prevention

(C) protection, prevention, and promotion

(D) education, primary care, and rehabilitation

(E) managed care, cost effectiveness, and equal access

114. A psychiatric consult is requested for a 63-year-old woman to determine the etiology of her dementia. She had been admitted to the hospital appearing extremely malnourished and emaciated. She had already been evaluated by a dermatologist and a gastroenterologist for some of her medical problems. Which of the following vitamin deficiencies did the psychiatrist suspect?

(A) vitamin A deficiency

(B) vitamin B_1 (thiamine) deficiency

(C) vitamin B_2 (riboflavin) deficiency

(D) vitamin B_3 (niacin) deficiency

(E) vitamin C deficiency

115. A 54-year-old Vietnam veteran with considerable combat experience, on questioning by a psychiatrist, appeared to have forgotten and was reluctant to discuss certain events. With the help of a psychiatrist, he was able to recall these experiences. He felt relieved after some previously repressed incidents were recalled. The emotional release the patient underwent is called

(A) abreaction

(B) acting out

(C) adaptation

(D) compensation

(E) parapraxis

116. A 78-year-old woman is brought to the emergency department because the family felt "she was going crazy." On examination, she has a deep voice, her face is somewhat puffy, her skin is dry, her hair is thin, and she is hard of hearing. Which of the following is the MOST likely diagnosis?

(A) hyperthyroidism

(B) hypothyroidism

(C) hyperparathyroidism

(D) hypoparathyroidism

(E) Addison's disease

117. A 19-year-old primigravid woman had an uncomplicated vaginal delivery 3 weeks ago. She is breast feeding. She has a 2-day history of fever, chills, myalgia, and breast pain. On examination, the right breast is erythematous, with a 3-cm localized area of tenderness and edema in the right upper outer quadrant. There are no palpable nodules or masses in either breast. The MOST appropriate next step is to

(A) instruct the patient to discontinue breast feeding

(B) obtain a mammogram

(C) prescribe a 7-day course of dicloxacillin, 500 mg PO qid

(D) observe and follow up in a week

(E) schedule immediate incision and drainage

118. A 3-year-old child is referred to you because he has been observed to eat paint and is living in a house where another child has been diagnosed with lead poisoning. Laboratory results show his blood lead is 12 μg/dL (reference < 10 μg/dL), hematocrit 44%, and free erythrocyte protoporphyrin (FEP/RBC) is 412 μg/dL (reference 25 to 75 μg/dL). You interpret from these results that

(A) his current lead absorption is higher than his absorption in the past several months

(B) the lead and FEP results may be influenced by anemia

(C) his current lead absorption is lower than his lead absorption in the past several months

(D) his lead absorption has been static for a number of months

(E) his lead level is normal

119. A 39-year-old woman has recently started dating again after divorcing her husband of 14 years. She reports that she becomes sexually excited by her new partner but that when they try to have intercourse it is very painful for her and they are not able to. She had never experienced this with her ex-husband. You suspect that she has involuntary muscle contraction of the outer third of the

vagina sufficient to prevent penile insertion, a condition known as

(A) vaginismus

(B) dyspareunia

(C) anhedonia

(D) frigidity

(E) anorgasmia

120. A 34-year-old Malaysian man suddenly bursts into a wild rage and kills an innocent bystander. Which of the following conditions would BEST describe the episode?

(A) susto

(B) acute paranoia

(C) amok

(D) amentia

(E) none of the above

121. You admit to the hospital a patient with a 6-month history of marked thought disorder, inappropriate affect, and auditory hallucinations. His level of consciousness is clear, and his orientation and memory good. Making a diagnosis of schizophrenic disorder, you prescribe trifluoperazine, 5 mg qid. The next day, he develops a painful spasm of the sternocleidomastoid muscle, which twists his head to the right. He has developed

(A) acute dystonia

(B) tardive dyskinesia

(C) akathisia

(D) akinesia

(E) parkinsonism

Questions 122 and 123

A patient presents to the emergency department with a 6-week history of amenorrhea, 1 week of irregular vaginal bleeding, a 1-day history of abdominal and pelvic pain, and 3 hours of lightheadedness while sitting and shoulder pain when lying flat. The beta-subunit was 9324 mIU/mL. A transabdominal ultrasound did not show any evidence of an intrauterine pregnancy. The right adnexa was noted to be approximately 5 cm in its greatest dimension.

122. The MOST likely diagnosis is

(A) acute pelvic inflammatory disease
(B) ruptured corpus luteum
(C) tubal ectopic pregnancy
(D) cervical ectopic pregnancy
(E) abdominal pregnancy

123. The MOST common etiology for ectopic pregnancy is

(A) menstrual reflux
(B) prior operation on the tube
(C) prior ectopic pregnancy
(D) salpingitis with peritubal adhesions
(E) developmental abnormalities

DIRECTIONS (Questions 124 through 150): Each group of items in this section consists of lettered headings followed by a set of numbered words or phrases. For each numbered word or phrase, select the ONE lettered heading that is most closely associated with it. Each lettered heading may be selected once, more than once, or not at all.

Questions 124 Through 126

Match the following oncologic diseases with the associated laboratory finding.

(A) chromosomal anomalies
(B) destruction of bone in pelvis
(C) low T-cell count
(D) elevated acid phosphatase
(E) ecchymosis of eyelid
(F) hyperglycemia
(G) elevated amylase

124. Acute myelogenous leukemia (AML)

125. Neuroblastoma

126. Ewing sarcoma

Questions 127 Through 130

Match the following choices with the numbered cases.

(A) right colon cancer
(B) left colon cancer
(C) rectal cancer
(D) epidermoid anal cancer
(E) cancer of the appendix

127. Treated primarily by radiation and chemotherapy

128. Often found incidentally during another procedure

129. May grow to large size and not obstruct bowel lumen

130. May cause colonic perforation remote from the site of tumor

Questions 131 Through 135

(A) polyarteritis nodosa (PAN)
(B) Churg–Strauss disease
(C) Henoch–Schönlein purpura
(D) Wegener's granulomatosis
(E) giant cell arteritis
(F) Kawasaki disease
(G) Behçet syndrome

131. A 38-year-old man has pulmonary involvement and peripheral eosinophilia.

132. A 58-year-old woman has aneurysms and renal involvement.

133. A specific serum test is positive when the disease is active.

134. A 10-year-old girl has several episodes and then a spontaneous remission.

135. A 30-year-old man has oral and genital ulcerations.

Questions 136 and 137

Match each one of the following household settings with the most common mental health problem associated with it.

    (A) dormitory suburbs

    (B) slums

    (C) single-room rented apartments

136. Schizophrenia

137. Depression

Questions 138 Through 141

Match the compound with the clinical symptoms.

    (A) iron

    (B) carbon monoxide

    (C) lead

    (D) insecticide (parathione)

    (E) lidocaine

    (F) vitamin C

    (G) acetaminophen

138. Headache, nausea, confusion, and syncope

139. Nausea and vomiting of blood, followed by an asymptomatic period; later, abdominal pain, severe bleeding, metabolic acidosis, and shock

140. Cyanotic patient with headache, dizziness, nausea, and dyspnea

141. A patient with "congestive heart failure" with a decreased sensorium

Questions 142 Through 145

    (A) Draw-a-Person Test

    (B) Stanford–Binet IQ Test

    (C) Minnesota Multiphasic Personality Inventory

    (D) Sentence Completion Test

    (E) Wechsler Scale of Intelligence

    (F) Rorschach Test

    (G) Test of Early Written Language

    (H) Thematic Appreception Test (TAT)

142. Most useful for judging motivational aspects of behavior

143. May be used to tap specific conflict areas; generally, reveals more conscious, overt attitudes and feelings

144. Useful for detecting psychomotor difficulties correlated with brain damage

145. Especially revealing of personality structure; most widely used projective technique

Questions 146 Through 150

Match the developmental milestones with the given ages.

    (A) walks alone

    (B) stands holding on

    (C) waves bye-bye, plays patty cake

    (D) says two- to three-word phrases

    (E) sits without support, transfers objects

146. 8 months

147. 10 months

148. 12 months

149. 15 months

150. 2 years

Answers and Explanations

1. **(D)** Kawasaki disease is a disorder of unknown etiology, most often affecting children under the age of 5. Presenting symptoms and findings include prolonged high (and often spiking) fevers for 1 to 3 weeks along with injected oropharyngeal mucosa, cervical lymphadenopathy, and skin lesions. The skin lesions may take the form of polymorphous, macular, erythematous rashes. Poststreptococcal disease is part of the differential diagnosis, but the negative ASO titer and rapid strep test make this choice less likely in this particular scenario. With a negative Lyme test and heterophile, Lyme disease and mononucleosis are obviously incorrect.

2. **(A)** Some patients with Kawasaki disease experience serious cardiac disease, including coronary arteritis, myocarditis, and arrhythmias. Within the first 2 weeks of the illness, 10 to 40% of affected children will have evidence of coronary vasculitis. The cardiovascular lesions most typically associated with this disorder are coronary artery aneurysms. Second-degree heart block is very uncommon in children.

3. **(B)** Treatment protocols have included high-dose intravenous gamma globulin along with aspirin. Antibiotics have not been shown to be of benefit, nor have radiation or acetaminophen.

4. **(D)** The majority of neural tube defects are the result of multifactorial or polygenic inheritance. Remember, only 15% have a prior history of NTDs. Trisomy 21 (Down syndrome) is not associated with an open NTD. Trisomy 13 and trisomy 18 occasionally will have associated open NTDs. The recurrence risk for most multifactorial disorders is 2 to 5%. The unknown/polygenic/multifactorial disorders are responsible for approximately 65 to 70% of all recognized developmental defects in humans. Most NTDs and congenital heart defects are mulitfactorial. Mendelian disorders are responsible for 20%. These include enzyme deficiencies. Chromosomal abnormalities are recognized in 5%. Drugs, medications, and environmental chemicals are responsible for approximately 5%.

5. **(D)** The neural tube forms a midline thickening of embryonic ectoderm. The fusion starts in the midportion and proceeds rostrally and caudally at about 22 embryonic days (36 menstrual days) and is completed by 28 embryonic days (42 menstrual days). Most patients have not yet had their pregnancy diagnosed by this point. NTDs result from the failure of the neural tube to close. Anencephaly results from failed anterior closure, and lumbosacral NTDs result from failed rostral closure.

6. **(B)** Prenatal screening is performed by assessing the mother for an elevated level of alpha-fetoprotein in her serum or by utilizing directed sonography in the at-risk patient. The NTD allows excessive quantities of AFP to enter the amniotic fluid and the maternal serum. The presence of amniotic fluid acetylcholinesterase is a diagnostic test. Some centers utilize directed sonography as either a screening or a diagnostic test. MRI does not play a role in the prenatal diagnosis of NTDs. Amniocentesis is used as a diagnostic test.

Folic acid supplementation (1 to 4 mg/day) has been shown to significantly decrease the incidence of babies with NTDs in women who have previously delivered a baby with a neural tube defect. Neural tube defects are examples of multifactorial inheritance; therefore, more than one factor is necessary to allow expression of the problem.

7. **(D)** The great majority of incidents of botulism have been associated with home-canned vegetables in the United States. In the former Soviet Union, Canada, and Japan, most outbreaks are associated with fish or fish products. Pork is the most common vehicle for *Staphylococcus* infection. Rice has been associated with *Bacillus cereus* intoxication.

8. **(C)** Noise-induced hearing loss first becomes apparent in audiometric examinations in the 4000-Hz range.

9. **(A)** Acute cerebellar ataxia and acute cerebritis often follow varicella, mycoplasma, and other viral infections such as enterovirus, influenza virus, and myxovirus. It may also be secondary to acute labyrinthitis and drug intoxication. Brain tumors and hydrocephalus are rare causes; however, they must be considered in the differential diagnosis. Patients with these later conditions will have papilledema and headaches. In those problems associated with varicella and other viruses, the duration of ataxia is limited in time. There is no evidence of papilledema and no characteristic laboratory abnormalities. The other options are incorrect as they would not result in cerebellar ataxia.

10. **(D)** Urethral lesions may cause hematuria that presents as initial bleeding only. Renal cell carcinoma, ureteral stone, and bladder hemorrhage should present blood throughout micturition. Prostatic hypertrophy alone is not associated with hematuria.

11. **(C)** Routine evaluation of hematuria includes urinalysis, complete blood count (CBC), IVP, and cystoscopy. Acid phosphatase is not useful in evaluating this process. MRI or CT of the pelvis and transrectal prostate biopsy are not routinely done unless something in the initial work-up is suggestive.

12. **(C)** This patient is likely to have a renal cell carcinoma (hypernephroma). Polycythemia is caused by the production of erythropoietin-like factors. There is no relationship to hypertension.

13. **(D)** This is a renal cell carcinoma. There is marked hypervascularity of the left kidney. The arteries are irregular and tortuous, following a random distribution. There are small vessels within the renal vein that indicate the blood supply of the neoplastic thrombosis involving the renal vein. The kidney is enlarged and abnormally bulbous in the lower pole.

14. **(E)** This information is not related to the back injury and is confidential. No need to know has been established. Your employment is not relevant to this issue.

15. **(C)** By fulfilling the criteria for major depressive disorder, with a regular temporal relationship between the onset of the episode and a particular time of year for more than 2 years, this patient best meets criteria for a major depressive disorder, with a seasonal pattern. Chronic adjustment disorder does not exist; any persistence of symptoms over 6 months is no longer adjustment disorder. The patient has no evidence of manic episodes, nor does she have any of the classic symptoms of PTSD, including an identifiable stressor event.

16. **(B)** Sertraline, a member of the selective serotonin reuptake inhibitor (SSRI) family of antidepressants, is the best choice of those listed. Alprazolam, a benzodiazepine, is contraindicated, because it would most likely cause further depression and this patient does not exhibit symptoms of anxiety. The patient is neither psychotic nor manic, so neither haloperidol nor lithium is indicated, respectively. Benztropine is given prophylactically

with high-potency antipsychotics such as haloperidol to minimize the risk of dystonias and tardive dyskinesia.

17. **(E)** Phototherapy has been shown to be effective in treating symptoms of seasonally mediated major depressive disorder. ECT, while useful in patients who have failed trials of multiple medications and psychotherapy, is not indicated in this patient at present. Psychoanalysis is geared more toward examining conflicts, and may or may not be useful in the presence of an obvious environmental stressor known to the patient. Psychostimulant therapy is usually reserved for those patients who cannot tolerate antidepressants' side effects. Finally, psychosurgery has been shown to be effective only in intractable obsessive–compulsive disorder and in certain types of intractable epilepsy.

18. **(C)** There is a constant state of hyperreactivity of the bronchi, during which exposure to an irritant precipitates an asthmatic attack. A following subacute phase has been described that can lead to late complications. The presence of inflammation in the airways has resulted in increased usage of inhaled corticosteroids for maintenance therapy. Many cases of asthma have no discernible allergic component.

19. **(C)** Sulfites, used to keep salad greens fresh, can cause severe asthmatic reactions. Other sulfite-containing foods include fresh fruits, potatoes, shellfish, and wine. Aspirin, tartrazine (a coloring agent), and beta-adrenergic agonists also commonly provoke asthmatic attacks.

20. **(B)** Hyperamylasemia is most commonly seen with pancreatic disorders; however, high false-positive and false-negative rates are present. In an acute hospital setting, nearly one third of elevations in amylase are unrelated to the pancreas. A multitude of disorders cause hyperamylasemia; some common disorders include perforated peptic ulcer, ruptured abdominal aortic aneurysm (AAA), intestinal obstruction, and parotiditis.

21. **(D)** Although serum amylase is useful in the diagnosis of acute pancreatitis, the actual level does not correlate with the severity of the disease. Eleven criteria (Ranson's criteria) that predict the severity of the episode are obtained within 48 hours of admission.

22. **(C)** The degree of amylasemia is not a reliable predictor of the severity of the pancreatitis or whether surgery should be done. A mature, nonresolving pseudocyst (6 to 12 weeks) should undergo a drainage procedure. Pancreatic abscess formation can develop in necrotic pancreatic tissue, requiring drainage and often debridement. Biliary pancreatitis usually resolves quickly, and cholecystectomy can be performed within 5 to 7 days. If clinical deterioration persists despite optimum support, exploratory laparotomy may be indicated to exclude the presence of a surgically correctable cause.

23. **(D)** The treatment includes antibiotic therapy and drainage. Infected necrotic pancreatic material often requires operative debridement. In severe cases, open packing of the abscess allows multiple packing changes until the necrotic material is cleared and the infection controlled. Anatomic pancreatectomy should not be performed in patients with pancreatic abscess.

24. **(A)** The coagulation factors in pregnancy undergo significant change. The greatest change is in the fibrinogen, which increases by approximately 50%. Factors VII, VIII, and X increase significantly. The increase in factor VIII is responsible for the decreased severity of von Willebrand's disease during pregnancy. The activities of factors XI and XIII are mildly decreased.

25. **(E)** Patients with nephrotic syndrome may develop a transudate-type ascites. Ascites occurs only when the serum albumin is very low, usually less than 2 mg/dL. The fluid is clear and straw-colored and usually contains less than 100 WBC/mm^3. The protein content is usually less than 3 g/dL. Bloody ascitic

fluid may be found in patients with tumors or tuberculosis.

26. **(B)** Most patients with nephrotic syndrome develop heavy proteinuria (over 3 g/day protein loss). Hypoalbuminemia and thus a decreased total protein level results in decreased plasma oncotic pressure and fluid transudation into the interstitial spaces. A decrease in plasma volume results in elevated production of aldosterone. Hyperlipidemia and hypercholesterolemia are common in the nephrotic syndrome and are inversely proportional to the serum albumin concentration.

27. **(B)** Uricosuric agents may induce gouty attacks by lowering synovial fluid urate levels and favoring shedding of synovial crystals during dissolution. An acute attack can be incapacitating, with at least half of them involving the metatarsophalangeal joint of the great toe (podagra). Within minutes to hours, the affected joint becomes hot, dusky red, and exquisitely painful. A septic joint or arterial embolism could have a similar physical examination but the clinical setting is more consistent with gout. Janeway lesions occur in endocarditis and are found on the palms and soles of the feet. Osteomyelitis generally occurs at spots of trauma, which can be external or at sites of infarction in patients with systemic sclerosis disease. Again, this is not the right clinical setting.

28. **(D)** Urate crystals are water soluble, but when tissues are treated with nonaqueous fixatives (ie, absolute alcohol), the crystals are preserved and are strongly negatively birefringent in compensated light.

29. **(A)** The affected joint should be rested and an anti-inflammatory administered promptly. Three options are colchicine, nonsteroidal anti-inflammatory drugs (NSAIDs), and glucocorticoids. Allopurinol, which is of no value in the treatment of the acute attack, is used in the management of chronic gout. Methotrexate (in either form) and gold are used in the treatment of rheumatoid arthritis.

30. **(B)** Polycystic ovarian disease (hyperandrogenic chronic anovulation) presents as amenorrhea secondary to abnormal ovarian function. It is the most common cause of hirsutism. Luteinizing hormone (LH) : follicle-stimulating hormone (FSH) is elevated. Estrone level is greater than estradiol. Testosterone and androstenedione are borderline elevated. The patient may have elevated local and systemic levels of androgens, which leads to follicular atresia and amenorrhea. This leads to infertility, abnormal bleeding patterns, hirsutism, and acne. Elevated androgen levels increase the risk of cardiovascular disease. Without ovulation, progesterone levels are low and the endometrium is exposed to prolonged unopposed estrogen stimulation, which increases the risk of endometrial carcinoma. In addition, if the patient desires children, fertility is impaired due to anovulation.

31. **(B)** The differential for this presentation includes infection (bladder and prostate), for which a urinalysis is useful. A digital rectal exam and PSA would also be helpful in evaluating the prostate. An ultrasound is unnecessary at this point but could be a useful second-line evaluation. Sigmoidoscopy and CEA are not indicated for these symptoms. The serum VDRL will tell you only if the patient has been exposed to the agent of syphilis (*Treponema pallidum*) in the past, since it is an antibody test. It cannot tell you if the current symptoms are caused by untreated syphilis.

32. **(D)** Measurements of serum PSA are not sufficiently accurate to diagnose men with early prostate cancer. Approximately 15 to 20% of men with BPH have PSA values greater than 10 ng/mL. Symptoms due to BPH can be obstructive (hesitancy, straining, dribbling, and retention) or irritative (frequency, nocturia, dysuria, urgency, and incontinence). Early carcinoma of the prostate is asymptomatic. As the disease spreads into the urethra, it may cause symptoms of obstruction indistinguishable from those of BPH. The etiology of prostate cancer is un-

known, though the disease does not occur in men castrated before puberty. Multiple factors, including viral and environmental, have been postulated, but BPH alone does not appear to be a specific risk factor. Although prostate cancer is only the fourth most common cancer in the world (and as a cause of malignancy-related death, only second behind lung cancer), it is the most common cancer diagnosed in men in the United States and Northern Europe.

33. (D) The fetal heart rate assessment is concerning; late decelerations are always ominous, but the presence of variability and a normal baseline heart rate provide partial reassurance. The fetal scalp pH is in an indeterminant range. Under these circumstances, a reassessment to determine the progression of the fetal acidosis is most appropriate. The intrauterine resuscitation is already in progress and should be continued. If the continuous monitoring showed significant deterioration, the plan should be modified.

34. (B) The earliest skin lesions in patients with tuberous sclerosis are whitish spots, which develop over the extremities and trunk and can be visualized using a Wood's lamp as a source of ultraviolet light. A shagreen patch (leathery plaque of subepidermal fibrosis) of rough, thickened, yellow skin may develop over the lower back. This disorder is inherited as an autosomal dominant trait, but about 80% of cases occur spontaneously.

35. (A) Rather than being true adenomas, the skin lesions in patients with tuberous sclerosis are actually angiofibromas. They may, on occasion, be vascular, with a telangiectasia-like appearance.

36. (A) The disease is inherited as an autosomal dominant trait, but about 80% of cases are sporadic, secondary to new mutations. Recently, the gene has been mapped to the long arm of chromosome 11. Mental deficiency may be mild or severe, but one third of affected individuals have normal or even superior intelligence. Seizures occur in 80% of cases, usually starting before age 5. Cystic lung disease is uncommon.

37. (C) The fetal heart rate changes described are variable decelerations. Compression of the umbilical cord produces an abrupt deceleration of the fetal heart rate. The decrease in fetal heart rate is mediated by baroreceptors responding to the increase in peripheral resistance rsulting from occlusion of the umbilical arteries. Chemoreceptors respond next to the increase in carbon dioxide and decrease in oxygen.

38. (B) Variable decelerations are often caused by umbilical cord compression, which may be corrected by amnioinfusion of sterile saline to "float" the cord. BPP and acoustic stimulation are not helpful in managing most labors. A scalp pH may be performed when the fetus does not respond to in utero resuscitative measures. Scalp sampling may be repeated as indicated by fetal heart rate. Fetal acidosis occurs in only 50% or less of fetuses with variable decelerations; therefore, emergency delivery of a patient progressing normally in labor is not generally warranted.

39. (C) A reassuring fetal heart rate has a baseline rate between 120 and 160 beats per minute, the presence of normal variability, and the absence of decelerations. The presence of a normal reassuring fetal heart rate pattern almost always ensures a normal oxygen and acid–base status of the fetus. The normal pattern can be affected by benign as well as adverse factors. Prolonged periods of hypoxia resulting in tachycardia, loss of variability, and late decelerations may result in acidemia sufficient to cause permanent damage.

40. (B) When men and women of all ages are considered, cardiovascular diseases are the most common cause of death. However, among women aged 35 to 74, cancer is the leading cause of death. Lung cancer is the number one cause of death from cancer when both men and women are considered. Men

generally have higher rates for cancer: breast, gallbladder, and thyroid cancer are the exceptions. It is felt that 75 to 80% of all cancers in the United States are due to environmental factors. This does not mean just pesticides and fertilizers, but also tobacco and alcohol. The environmental contribution is estimated by comparing age-adjusted U.S. rates of specific cancers to the rates for the country with the lowest risk.

41. **(E)** Controversy surrounds many screening recommendations. Pap smears continue to be performed yearly in high-risk women (sexually active with multiple partners), but a minimum of every 3 years is recommended for all women. Occult blood testing and sigmoidoscopy continue to be the norm and have been shown to decrease the mortality from colon and rectal cancer. Some studies suggest the benefits of performing a colonoscopy instead, but it has not become standard. The mammogram topic has been very controversial, with many physicians still claiming that the benefits of mammograms are most dramatic in women over 50 and therefore efforts should be placed there. Data does support a decreased mortality rate for women in the 40- to 50-year-old age group but at the cost of 25% false positives and a significantly higher cost per life saved. Current recommendations from the National Cancer Advisory Board in March 1997 are for mammogram every 1 to 2 years in women over the age of 40. No universally agreed-upon guidelines have been established for PSA levels.

42. **(C)** Alcoholic beverages by themselves are associated with an incrased risk of cancer, but tobacco use increases the risk. Asbestos exposure by itself increases the risk of lung and peritoneal cancer. The use of tobacco increases the risk of lung cancer beyond that induced by asbestos alone. HPV has been conclusively linked to the development of all three cancers listed. Tobacco use has without doubt been linked to the development of a multitude of cancers. The highest rates for the development of breast, uterine, and ovarian cancers are seen in Caucasian women.

43–44. **(43-E, 44-D)** All of the choices may cause third-trimester bleeding. Third-trimester bleeding and uterine tenderness are hallmarks of placental abruption. Risk factors include smoking, cocaine, chronic hypertension, and severe preeclampsia. Decreased uterine perfusion and placental surface area coupled with vasospasm may lead to profound hypoxia and acidemia relatively quickly, depending on the size of the abruption. Prompt and aggressive neonatal resuscitation is necessary in these cases for optimal outcome. Nonetheless, placental abruption is an independent risk factor for late neurologic sequelae. Uterine rupture is unlikely in the first pregnancy. Placenta previa is seen more often in multiple gestation, prior cesarean section, multiparity, and prior placenta previa. Vasa previa is associated with the rupture of a fetal (umbilical) blood vessel, resulting in the loss of fetal blood. Frequently, there is a velamentous insertion of the umbilical cord. The risk of placenta accreta is increased in the presence of placenta previa, especially if the patient also had a prior cesarean section.

45. **(B)** The patient has a history strongly suggestive of an immediate hypersensitivity reaction to latex. If she has latex allergy, she will be at serious risk of an anaphylactic reaction if she comes into contact with latex rubber during her surgery. The first step is to obtain a RAST, which will be positive in about 90% of cases. Skin prick testing will be positive in slightly more cases but carries a risk of anaphylaxis, so RAST should be performed first. Patch testing is appropriate for delayed hypersensitivity reactions rather than immediate hypersensitivity.

46. **(B)** Individuals with antisocial personality disorders have difficulty getting along with others and often have problems such as those experienced by this man. Antisocial personality disorder is characterized by a pervasive pattern of disregard for and violation of the rights of others, beginning by age 15. Autistic disorder is a pervasive developmental disorder characterized by impairment in social in-

teraction and communication and restricted, repetitive patterns of behavior. The individual with autistic disorder is generally not functional enough to engage in arguments or obtain work. Obsessive–compulsive personality disorder is characterized by a pervasive pattern of preoccupation with orderliness, perfectionism, and control. Typically, the individual with obsessive–compulsive personality disorder would not break laws or perform poorly at work. Histrionic personality disorder is characterized by a pervasive pattern of excessive emotionality and attention-seeking behavior. The histrionic person is dramatic but easily influenced by others and not likely to get into arguments or into trouble with the law.

47. **(C)** Pseudodementia is a presentation of depressive illness in which the patient complains of difficulty thinking but makes little effort to perform well on the mental status examination. It is important to recognize pseudodementia because depression is treatable. Delirium is characterized by fluctuating clouding of consciousness, including reduced ability to concentrate or sustain attention. Dementia is characterized by difficulty remembering or thinking despite great effort. Individuals with schizophrenia often have poor insight, not recognizing the extent of their thought disorder. Mental retardation is a developmental disorder; thus, an adult would not complain of new-onset difficulty in thinking.

48. **(E)** Status asthmaticus indicates that a person with asthma is unresponsive to initial therapy or is at risk for respiratory failure. There is airway narrowing and varying degrees of airway obstruction, resulting in ventilation–perfusion mismatch and subsequent hypoxemia. In moderate cases, hyperventilation leads to respiratory alkalosis and hypocapnia.

The blood gas in option B is a normal blood gas. Option C represents combined respiratory and metabolic acidosis as well as hypoxemia. This is a blood gas one might see in a burn victim who suffers from volume

loss and smoke inhalation. In option D, there is evidence of hypoxemia and a metabolic acidosis, as may be seen in a patient with sepsis.

49. **(E)** Twenty-five to fifty percent of women will be battered at some time. Too often in our society, the victim is blamed for causing the abuse. Ten percent of adolescents were victims of severe parental abuse. Forty-seven percent of women who experienced severe violence had three or more episodes that year. One in five women seeking emergency department care have been abused by their partners.

50. **(C)** A male relative is the most frequent perpetrator, although all of the above groups have members who have committed sexual abuse. Socioeconomic class does not limit it. The severity and duration of the abuse correlate with long-lasting sequelae.

51. **(D)** Abuse victims have 3 to 5 times as many visits for medical care. Thirty-eight percent in one study did not recall abuse verified by old hospital records. Five percent tell their physicians, but, when they are asked directly, the rate increases considerably. The perpetrator frequently accompanies the patient on the visit, and insists on being present in the exam room.

52. **(B)** The diuresis that ensues after relief of obstruction results in urine that is typically dilute, alkaline, and high in sodium. Careful attention must be paid to electrolytes in the postobstruction period to prevent hyponatremia as well as hypokalemia, hypomagnesemia, and volume depletion.

53. **(B)** The largest volume of water is reabsorbed in the nephron at the proximal convolution. Maximally concentrated urine depends on antidiuretic hormone (ADH), which allows distal convoluted tubules and collecting ducts to become permeable to water.

54. **(D)** Without more information on safe levels, the significance of this level cannot be determined. We would be concerned in this decision with toxic effects on the infant, rather than whether PCBs caused breast cancer (which in any case is not a known hazardous effect).

55. **(B)** The reaction of allergic contact dermatitis characteristically occurs 48 to 72 hours after contact. Cross-sensitization to related molecules is possible. Small amounts of allergen may provoke a reaction. The allergen is usually a relatively low-molecular-weight compound. Suitable gloves will help prevent the condition, provided they are impermeable to the particular allergen involved.

56. **(C)** Legionellosis is best treated with erythromycin. Untreated, it has a fatality rate of 3 to 30%. Most cases are nonepidemic in nature, although it can occur in epidemics originating in buildings, such as among hotel guests, hospital inpatients, office building workers, and factory workers. Legionnaires' disease is acquired by inhaling aerosolized water containing *Legionella* organisms or possibly by pulmonary aspiration of contaminated water.

57. **(B)** Frugality, punctuality, meticulousness, sadistic rage, problems with control, submission, and defiance are common with people fixated at the anal stage. In psychoanalytic theory, fixation at any stage of early development is believed to lead to particular personality characteristics. The fixation may occur either because of excessive gratification or because of deprivation, as experienced by the child in terms of individual needs. Characteristics derived from the oral stage of development include excessive optimism, narcissism, pessimism in depressive states, and demandingness. Characteristics derived from the phallic and oedipal stages of development include focus on castration in men and on penis envy in women. Characteristics derived from the latency stage of development include lack of interest in learning or in developing skills.

58. **(B)** A fugue is defined as a state of dissociation or a personality separation, during which normal life patterns are totally repressed. The state may last for days or months, even years, during which the individual may initially have total amnesia, leaving home and wandering about for days. The subject may appear quite normal, or may be confused and disoriented. Extinction is the weakening of a conditioned response that occurs if the response is not maintained by reinforcement. Autosuggestion is self-conditioning that involves repeating ideas to oneself in order to change a habit or psychological state, such as anxiety. Schizoid personality disorder is characterized by emotional coldness to others, lack of close friends, lack of response to praise or criticism, and inability to enjoy activities or relationships. Introversion is a personality trait characterized by interest in oneself with lack of interest in the outside world.

59. **(E)** The hint about the well water and lack of significant findings on abdominal examination, along with the lack of blood in the stool, should make you investigate the stools for *Giardia*. *Giardia* is the most frequent identifiable agent of water-borne diarrhea. Cysts may be seen in the stool, although it may take three stool examinations to find the cysts.

60. **(E)** The most effective treatment is Atabrine or Flagyl. Antibiotics are not indicated for mild cases of *Salmonella*. *Shigella* may be better treated with trimethoprim–sulfamethoxazole.

61. **(B)** A unilateral dilated pupil and a decreasing level of consciousness are suggestive of elevated intracranial pressure. In this scenario, intracranial hemorrhage is high on the list of differential diagnoses. Either epidural or subdural hemorrhage may produce this problem. However, his history describes the classic "lucid interval" seen with an epidural hematoma, occurring after the brief loss of consciousness directly after injury and before the clinical deterioration. The CT scan in Figure 3.4 demonstrates an epidural hematoma.

Direct eye injury and congenital eye lesion are unlikely due to his history. Most epidural hematomas are arterial in origin, but they can also arise from torn meningeal veins or venous sinuses.

62. **(D)** Early surgical decompression is the most important intervention in the management of an epidural hematoma. Observation is not appropriate. The other interventions are directed at decreasing intracranial pressure and are useful in limiting secondary brain injury due to edema.

63. **(A)** Increasing $Paco_2$ acutely increases cerebral blood flow and, thereby, elevates intracerebral pressure (ICP). All other noted maneuvers lead to a decrease in ICP.

64. **(E)** Although this patient has a history of being treated with iron and B_{12}, the current indices are most consistent with an iron deficiency. Thalassemia minor has been ruled out by the prior hemoglobin electrophoresis. Women of African-American, Mediterranean, and Italian descent are at risk for beta-thalassemia. Management of this patient is to continue prenatal vitamins with folic acid and administer adequate amounts of iron (200 mg elemental), and then reassess the hemoglobin and hematocrit in approximately 2 to 4 weeks. A significant rise in her hemoglobin will be present if she is taking the iron and your diagnosis is correct.

65. **(B)** Iron stores and dietary iron are inadequate to meet the demands of a normal pregnancy for the average patient. Approximately 300 mg of elemental iron is transferred from the maternal compartment to the fetus and placenta. An additional 500 mg are utilized to expand the maternal red cell mass. A patient's need for iron is predominantly in the second half of pregnancy. Ascorbic acid does not facilitate iron absorption. During pregnancy, it is recommended that the average woman consume an additional 30 mg of elemental iron per day. Iron is actively transported in the placenta.

66. **(D)** The normal nonpregnant requirement of folic acid is 180 µg per day. During pregnancy, this is increased to 400 µg. Most prenatal vitamins, however, contain 800 to 1000 µg. Folic acid supplementation prior to pregnancy reduces the risk of neural tube defects. During pregnancy, it facilitates hematopoieses.

67. **(D)** Temporary threshold shift is a partial hearing loss that occurs after sudden exposure to a loud noise. It usually lasts a few hours, but hearing loss can be permanent.

68. **(A)** Disease of the heart was among the top five leading causes of death identified in both 1900 and 1985. In the early 1900s, the leading cause of death was infectious diseases. In 1985, the major cause of death was the chronic diseases of an aging population.

69. **(B)** Differentiating the side effect profiles of psychoactive medications can be difficult, as many profiles overlap. The anticholinergic effects of fluoxetine (an SSRI), amitriptyline (a tricyclic antidepressant), and phenelzine (a traditional antipsychotic) all include dry mouth. Fatigue is a fairly nonspecific symptom, although SSRIs are more likely to cause anxiety and restlessness than fatigue. The symptom of constipation, however, in the setting of dry mouth, lightheadedness, and fatigue points to amitriptyline, because the other medications listed are more likely to cause diarrhea than constipation.

70. **(D)** Psychiatrists are required by law to report any situation in which they suspect child abuse. This obligation supersedes any obligation to the patient's confidentiality. In addition, the physician herself must report the abuse.

71. **(D)** Radical hysterectomy with bilateral pelvic lymph node dissection is the standard surgical therapy for stages IB-1 and IIA cervical cancer. A radical hysterectomy attacks the pattern of local spread in cervical cancer. The en bloc dissection of the upper vagina, cervix, uterus, and parametrial tissue removes the

tissue site of local disease. The pelvic lymph nodes are removed because 15% of patients with stage IB-1 disease will have lymphatic disease. The cure rate for stage IB-1 cervical cancer is approximately 85% when treated by either radition therapy or appropriate surgery. Surgery has the advantage of preserving ovarian and vaginal function.

72. **(B)** The therapy of cervical cancer during pregnancy balances the maternal needs, the fetal needs, the stage of the disease, size of the lesion, number of weeks to fetal viability, and the mother's desire for the pregnancy. In the first half of pregnancy, immediate treatment should be offered. The treatment is dependent on the stage of the disease. Radiation therapy will result in fetal death. Stage IIB is treated with radiation therapy. Radical hysterectomy has the same indications in the nonpregnant patient. There is no evidence that pregnancy has a negative effect on the 5-year survival rates of women treated appropriately for their stage of disease. Summary of various series in the literature shows similar survival rates for pregnant and nonpregnant patients. The stage of the disease at the time of diagnosis is the only determining prognostic factor. Therapy may be delayed awaiting viability if the diagnosis is made after the late second trimester. Most patients are delivered by cesarean section even though the mode of delivery does not affect survival.

73. **(D)** Coal worker's pneumoconiosis has two forms: simple and complicated (which is also called progressive massive fibrosis [PMF]). Symptoms do not usually occur in nonsmokers until PMF develops. In this case, there will be a background of small, rounded opacities (which are seen early), generally with at least one shadow over 1 cm in diameter. Subsequently, as the disease progresses, large conglomerate shadows may be seen.

74. **(D)** Coal worker's pneumoconiosis puts one at increased risk of developing *Mycobacterium tuberculosis* infection. It does not increase the risk of the other diseases mentioned.

75. **(B)** Zollinger–Ellison syndrome is manifested by gastric acid hypersecretion secondary to a gastrinoma. Secretin causes a marked increase in the serum gastrin. This is a diagnostic test for Zollinger–Ellison syndrome. All other findings suggest this diagnosis.

76. **(E)** The positive family history for parathyroid disease in a patient with a gastrinoma should alert the physician to the presence of a MEN I. The three tumor types associated with MEN I are: parathyroid gland, pancreatic islet, and pituitary gland. Statements A through D are consistent with MEN I. Pheochromocytoma is consistent with MEN II.

77. **(E)** The danger of acute renal failure after IVP has led to caution, especially in patients with multiple myeloma. The patient should be well hydrated if the IVP is necessary.

78. **(A)** Nitrogen retention is characteristic of renal involvement in multiple myeloma. Hypercalcemia may produce transient or irreversible renal damage, as do amyloid and myeloma cell infiltrates.

79. **(C)** Renal amyloidosis can occur in primary and secondary amyloidosis. The hallmark finding, nephrotic syndrome, is present in 25% of patients at presentation, and probably develops in over 50%.

80. **(D)** The cysts do not undergo malignant change. All the other options are usually associated with these cysts.

81. **(B)** Siblings of a child with IDDM have a 5 to 10% risk of developing diabetes.

82. **(B)** Use of rubber gloves is associated with latex allergy, which causes anaphylaxis, rhinitis, and urticaria. Allergic contact dermatitis can also occur from additives to rubber used in making rubber gloves. Pneumoconiosis is not a potential complication.

83. **(C)** When a person who is taking an MAOI eats food containing the amino acid tyramine, he or she may have a hypertensive crisis. Foods to be avoided include red wine, beer, fava beans, aged cheeses, smoked meats, liver, and yeast. In addition, over-the-counter medicines containing pseudoephedrine or similar sympathomimetics can also cause problems. Butyrophenones, phenothiazines, tricyclic antidepressants, and lithium carbonate do not cause hypertensive crises as MAOIs can.

84. **(C)** Tobacco smoke is the likely cause, although asbestos and chromium are also known to cause lung cancer. The latent period has not been sufficient to see a development cancer from his asbestos exposure or from a synergistic effect between smoking and asbestos. The same is true for chromium, and his actual exposure to chromium has been small.

85. **(D)** Empyema, purulent material in the pleural space, does not usually cause hemoptysis. Pneumonias, bronchiectasis, and cancer may lead to empyema.

86. **(D)** This condition of teenagers is bilateral in 30% of cases. The epiphysis falls posteriorly and medially, and there is proximal and anterior migration of the femoral metaphysis. The cause is unknown. This may represent a local manifestation of a more general disorder of endochondral ossification. Radiographs of anterior posterior and lateral views confirm the diagnosis with the characteristic "ice cream falling off the cone" appearance. In Figure 3.5, there is subtle medial displacement, best appreciated by drawing a line up the lateral side of the normal and abnormal femoral neck. The frog-leg view clearly demonstrates posterior displacement. Treatment is with spica cast and careful rehabilitation. Some cases may require surgery. Fracture of the head of the femur and intracapsular hip fracture would be uncommon in a young individual with simply a fall while playing tennis. Patellar fracture would

have presented with knee pain and swelling. Contusion of the hip capsule would more likely result in a limp rather than an inability to walk.

87. **(C)** Pregnancy is a hypercoagulable state. After a cesarean section, a patient may also have endothelial injury and stasis, thus predisposing her to deep venous thrombosis and possible pulmonary embolization. Approximately 50% of pulmonary emboli originate in the iliofemoral system. A high index of suspicion, arterial blood gas, and a ventilation–perfusion scan are typically used in making the diagnosis. The radiation exposure of a ventilation–perfusion scan is low. Venography and pulmonary arteriography via the brachial route are associated with less than 50 millirads of exposure each. A pulmonary arteriogram via the femoral route has the highest exposure of 200 to 300 millirads.

88. **(C)** The numbness together with the positive Tinel's sign are characteristic of carpal tunnel syndrome. Clumsiness and dropping objects and awakening at night with numbness and tingling in the hand are common in this condition. Sensory loss in the median nerve distribution is common. Pain in the lateral epicondyle is not caused by median nerve compression in the wrist and is not a feature of carpal tunnel syndrome.

89. **(D)** Regular work as a receptionist should not contribute to this condition. Soft-tissue swelling from diabetes or pregnancy can cause compression of the contents of the carpal canal and contribute to carpal tunnel syndrome. Repetitive trauma associated with fine motor work in automobile assembly and inflammation of the wrist in rheumatoid arthritis could also impair the median nerve.

90. **(C)** A second organ from the same donor (not usually possible) would also undergo hyperacute rejection. Pretransplant crossmatch testing between donor and recipient should identify patients with preformed antibodies.

91. (C) Exfoliative dermatitis is a rare skin condition, but because of its severity, patients with this syndrome are often admitted to the hospital. The syndrome can be primary, appearing in otherwise healthy individuals, or secondary to a malignancy, contact dermatitis, drugs, or other dermatologic diseases (eg, psoriasis). Even mild cases require systemic therapy for the severe itching. Antihistamines are usually the first choice.

92. (E) Most cases of exfoliative dermatitis will have widespread lymphadenopathy, whether they are primary or secondary forms. Biopsy will usually reveal lipomelanotic reticulosis (dermatopathic lymphadenopathy) and is not diagnostically specific.

93. (C) These cells are typical of Sézary syndrome. This is frequently an early presentation of mycosis fungoides or cutaneous T-cell lymphoma. There may be a relationship to Epstein–Barr virus (and human T-lymphotropic virus [HTLV] types I and II), but it is not universal.

94. (D) The typical course of mycosis fungoides is an initial erythematous stage (which might become diffuse and cause an exfoliative dermatitis, as in this case), a plaque stage, and a tumor stage. The course is usually progressive through these stages, but all stages can be bypassed. The early stages may progress slowly with remissions or exacerbations. The disease can be rapidly progressive, particularly when the tumor stage is reached. The disease is invariably fatal.

95. (D) There is no curative therapy, and most experts provide treatment only when symptoms occur. Therapy includes topical treatments such as tar cream plus ultraviolet light or local nitrogen mustard, and systemic treatment with steroids and radiation therapy. Chemotherapy regimens are used but not with great success.

96. (C) This hemangioma sits on the skin as if a lump of putty were put there. It typically be-

comes larger, gets a grayish-blue frosting, and then involutes. Size and location do not affect prognosis. Port-wine stains are lesions with dilated capillaries in the dermis. Cavernous hemangiomas are soft, subcutaneous, often bluish, ill-defined masses, often referred to as a "bag of worms."

97. (B) This patient is at high risk for the development of a PE secondary to deep venous thrombosis (DVT). The major risk factors for DVT that pertain to this patient are obesity, carcinoma, immobility, and major intra-abdominal surgery. The clinical history of sudden onset of tachypnea, hypoxia, and pleuritic chest pain are consistent with PE. The other diagnoses are less likely, given the sudden onset of symptoms and the relatively normal chest x-ray.

98. (A) Given the presumed diagnosis is a PE secondary to DVT, a lower-extremity venous duplex scan may demonstrate a DVT and, therefore, identify the likely cause. A ventilation–perfusion scan is an appropriate next step and is fairly reliable if there is a high- or low-probability scan. The definitive diagnostic test would be a pulmonary arteriogram. A lower-extremity arteriogram is irrelevant because it would not demonstrate information about the venous system. The chest CT scan and bronchoscopy would be noncontributory.

99. (C) While some studies show aspirin to be superior to no treatment in regard to DVT prophylaxis following hip replacement surgery, aspirin is not generally thought to be as good a venous prophylactic agent as the other modes available. Aspirin's antiplatelet actions appear to be much more effective in preventing arterial than venous thrombosis. Pneumatic compression hose, leg elevation, and ambulation are means of increasing venous flow and decreasing stasis. Heparin acts through amplification of the naturally occurring antithrombin III. The so-called "mini-dose" heparin regimen acts by inhibiting activated factor X, the common pathway for intrinsic and extrinsic coagulation systems. Low-dose warfarin and low-molecular-weight heparin are also effective modes for DVT prophylaxis.

100. **(B)** Thalassemia stems from the abnormal synthesis of one of the globulin polypeptide chains. Alpha-thalassemia is usually caused by deletion of one or more globulin genes, while beta-thalassemia may also be due to gene deletion. The chronic hemolysis causes the bone marrow to produce more red blood cells. This increase in production leads to hypertrophy of the bone marrow and cosmetic changes of prominent forehead and maxillary bones as well as malocclusion problems. As the hemolysis progresses, the spleen enlarges, causing abdominal pain, lumbar lordosis, and anorexia. The chronic anemia will strain the heart, producing cardia dilation. Pierre Robin syndrome consists of micrognathia and a high arched or cleft palate. Cleidocranial dysostosis or dysplasia includes bony hypoplasia (clavicles, sacral rami) along with delayed anterior fontanelle closure, frontal bossing, and dental abnormalities (delay in dentition).

101. **(E)** MMR, DPT, or hepatitis B vaccination is not contraindicated for a pregnant woman's baby or children. Most vaccinations are acceptable in pregnancy. Inactivated virus vaccines (eg, influenza, rabies, and hepatitis B) should be given whenever indicated. Live virus vaccines are contraindicated in most situations. Selected use of inactivated bacterial vaccines, toxoids, hyperimmunoglobulins, and pooled immune serum globulins may also be administered to selected pregnant women.

102. **(B)** Thalassemia minor (also called beta-thalassemia) usually represents a heterozygous state and is often asymptomatic. Symptoms may develop during periods of stress such as pregnancy or severe infection. Hemoglobin values are usually in the 9 to 11 g/dL range. The red cells are small and poorly hemoglobinized.

103. **(E)** A serum ferritin determination would be most helpful. Iron stores in thalassemia are normal or increased. Some of the increase may be secondary to injudicious iron therapy or secondary to frequent blood transfusions. In the past, one of the complications of beta-thalassemia was iron overload. This is now aggressively handled with chelation therapy from the start. A hemoglobin electrophoresis can be helpful by demonstrating an elevated hemoglobin A2, but its presence does not rule out the additional complication of iron deficiency as a cause of a microcytic anemia.

104. **(A)** An increased amount of fetal or A2 hemoglobin would be expected. As beta chains are decreased, the alpha chains combine with gamma and delta chains to produce hemoglobin F and hemoglobin A2. There is no effect on the red cell membrane to give increased fragility. Iron stores are most commonly normal or increased. Macroglobulinemia is associated with myeloma. Hemoglobin S is seen only in patients carrying the abnormal gene and not in otherwise normal individuals.

105. **(C)** The present treatment of choice for thalassemia minor is supportive. Care is taken to watch for anemia during intercurrent illness, to avoid iron overload, and to provide counseling concerning reproductive risks.

106. **(B)** In children, juvenile intestinal polyps are the most frequent cause of intestinal bleeding in the 2- to 5-year-old age group. In the first year of life, the leading cause of rectal bleeding is anal fissures, usually associated with passage of large stools. Gastrointestinal infections at any age may cause bleeding.

107. **(C)** Generally, one of two conclusions can be drawn after comparing two (or more) different techniques (or therapies, etc.) in a study. The researcher may or may not find a difference between the techniques (or therapies). The researcher should state the study question in the form of statistical hypotheses. These hypotheses should specifically reflect the two potential conclusions: the null hy-

pothesis and the alternative hypothesis. The null hypothesis states that no difference exists between the items being compared; the alternative hypothesis states that a difference does exist between the items being compared. The alternative hypothesis can be directional or nondirectional. A directional alternative hypothesis not only states that a difference exists, but also states the expected direction of the difference (ie, repair technique A is better than repair technique B). More frequently, however, no specific direction of the difference will be noted (ie, a difference exists between surgical technique A and surgical technique B). In this case, the alternative hypothesis is nondirectional.

108. **(D)** Congenital aganglionic megacolon (Hirschsprung disease) may present in the newborn period with bowel obstruction but is usually diagnosed in childhood because of failure to thrive, irritability, poor feeding, and constipation. The rectal examination will show an empty rectum. Barium enema will show a narrowed area where there are no ganglion cells. Biopsy of the involved area will help establish the diagnosis.

109. **(B)** Contrary to common fears, swallowing inorganic mercury, such as would occur if an oral thermometer were to break while in the mouth, poses virtually no health threat. Such mercury simply passes through the gastrointestinal tract and is excreted through the kidneys in a few days.

110. **(C)** A single dose of Rh immunoglobulin will neutralize approximately 15 mL of Rh (D) positive red blood cells or 30 mL of fetal blood. The principal reason for the significant fall in D isoimmunization is the aggressive use of anti-D immunoglobulin. The 2% failure rate for postpartum administration is accounted for by a fetal–maternal bleed of greater than 15 mL of red blood cells (RBCs) at delivery or silent antepartum fetal–maternal transfusion. An excessive fetomaternal transfusion is suspected because of the neonatal anemia and hypovolemia and the immunoglobulin failure. The administration

of Rh immunoglobulin at 28 weeks reduces the sensitization risk from 2% to 0.07%.

111. **(A)** Papillary necrosis is prone to occur in diabetes mellitus. Infection of the renal pyramids in association with vascular disease or obstruction leads to papillary necrosis. Radiologic findings include calyceal clubbing, papillary cavities, and calyceal filling defects (secondary to a sloughed papilla, the ring sign).

112. **(D)** Analgesic abuse (eg, phenacetin), chronic alcohol use, peripheral vascular disease, and sickle cell anemia all have effects on the vasculature or are directly toxic to the renal papillae and predispose to papillary necrosis. Morphine use, pregnancy, obesity, and alpha-thalassemia have no such effects.

113. **(C)** The 1990 goals, the National Health Objectives, defined a set of national priorities for public health. The goals are grouped into three major foci: prevention, protection, and promotion.

114. **(D)** Frequent manifestations of niacin deficiency (pellagra) are dementia, diarrhea, and dermatitis. Pellagra psychosis formerly resulted in a relatively high incidence of admissions to mental hospitals but, due to the addition of niacin to most breads, its occurrence is uncommon at present. Patients with niacin deficiency invariably are deficient in other vitamins as well. Both delirium and seizures may occur early, with motor abnormalities developing later. Vitamin A, riboflavin, and vitamin C deficiencies do not cause dementia. Vitamin A deficiency causes stunted growth and night blindness. Vitamin C deficiency causes scurvy. Thiamine deficiency can cause nerve damage but is not associated with skin and gastrointestinal manifestations.

115. **(A)** Becoming aware of previous unpleasant incidents, which the patient has repressed, can result in an emotional release or abreaction. This discharge of unpleasant emotion can assist patients and allow them to gain in-

sight into the problem areas, with some resultant desensitization. Acting out is direct expression of an unconscious wish, often manifest as impulsive behavior. Adaptation is the phenomenon of a gradually diminishing response to a continuous or repetitive stimulus. Compensation is the act of making up for a deficiency. Parapraxis is an unconsciously motivated lapse from logical thought, known as a freudian slip. Parapraxis is part of normal thinking.

116. **(B)** Many endocrinopathies, including hypothyroidism, can result in mental changes. The presence of such disorders should be considered in patients presenting with psychiatric manifestations. Severe cases of hypothyroidism may result in what has been referred to as "myxedema madness." Slow, hoarse speech; periorbital and peripheral edema; pale, dry skin; coarse, thin hair; and deafness are clinical features of hypothyroidism. This constellation of signs is not seen in hyperthyroidism, hyperparathyroidism, hypoparathyroidism, or Addison's disease.

117. **(C)** The patient presents with clinical signs and symptoms of puerperal mastitis. In the absence of an abscess, it is reasonable to initiate a 7-day course of antibiotic therapy. An oral agent effective against *Staphylococcus aureus* is the most appropriate choice. Breast feeding may be continued. If an abscess is present, drainage and appropriate antibiotics are usually effective.

118. **(C)** The child has a slightly elevated blood level. He is not anemic (hematocrit is 44%). The fact that his FEP is elevated much more than his lead reflects that his lead level was higher in the past than it is currently.

119. **(A)** Vaginismus is the involuntary contraction of the outer vagina, preventing intercourse. Dyspareunia is pain on intercourse. Anhedonia is lack of pleasure in activities that were once enjoyable, a symptom common in individuals with depression. Frigidity is lack of sexual desire. Anorgasmia is the inability to reach orgasm.

120. **(C)** The phrase "to run amok" is derived from the culturally specific disorder known as amok, which is seen primarily in Malaysian men. Amok is characterized by sudden rampage, usually including homicide or suicide. Physicians should be aware of practices and beliefs found in cultures different from their own that may impact upon a patient's health. Susto is a syndrome characterized by severe anxiety, restlessness, and fear of black magic, seen in Latin American individuals. In a state of acute paranoia, an individual is suspicious or believes he or she is being persecuted or controlled, but generally that person does not exhibit impulsive homicidal behavior motivated by the paranoia. Amentia is another term for mental retardation or mental deficiency, a state characterized by intellectual deficit, not sudden homicidal rage.

121. **(A)** An acute dystonic reaction, such as painful spasm of the sternocleidomastoid muscle, is an involuntary sustained contraction of a skeletal muscle that develops suddenly within the first few days of initiating treatment with an antipsychotic medication. Tardive dyskinesia, akathisia, akinesia, and parkinsonism are other side effects of antipsychotic medication use. Tardive dyskinesia is characterized by slow choreiform or tic-like movements, usually of the mouth and facial muscles, and develops over months to years of antipsychotic medication use. Akathisia is a subjective feeling of muscular tension, causing one to be fidgety and restless, which develops within 1 month of initiating or increasing antipsychotic medication. Akinesia is lack or slowing of physical movement, also seen in catatonic schizophrenia. Parkinsonism, manifest by tremor, rigidity, or akinesia, develops within a few weeks of initiating or increasing medication.

122. **(C)** Patients with ectopic pregnancy most frequently present complaining of abdominal and pelvic pain (95%). Amenorrhea or abnor-

mal vaginal bleeding is seen in approximately 60 to 80%. The absence of an intrauterine gestation in a patient with a beta-subunit above the discriminatory zone places ectopic pregnancy at the top of the differential. Acute pelvic inflammatory disease (PID) is a common cause of pelvic pain. A ruptured corpus luteum may have a similar presentation except for the ultrasound findings. The presence of the signs and symptoms associated with hypovolemia add urgency to the need for prompt definitive therapy. Ninety-five percent of ectopic pregnancies are tubal in location. The other 5% are interstitial (involving the interstitial portion of the uterus), cervix, ovary, and the abdomen. Cervical, ovarian, and abdominal pregnancies are rare and are associated with diagnostic and therapeutic challenges.

123. **(D)** The incidence of tubal ectopic pregnancy has progressively risen in the United States. The risk of death has decreased significantly. Between 1970 and 1987, ectopic pregnancies increased by a factor of 4.9. Although the mortality has diminished, ectopic pregnancy represents the second leading cause of maternal mortality in the United States. All of the factors mentioned are risk factors. The most significant factor appears to be salpingitis with peritubal adhesions. The salpingitis results in tubal narrowing and blind pocket formation. The peritubal adhesions kink and narrow the tube. Prior ectopic pregnancy is associated with approximately a 7 to 15% chance of recurrence.

124–126. **(124-A, 125-E, 126-B)** Chromosome abnormalities are found in almost 100% of AML cases. In the adult form of chronic myelogenous leukemia, the Philadelphia chromosome is present in 90% of the cases. These genetic characteristics correlate with the treatment success of some subtypes of these forms of leukemia. Most of the cases of leukemia in children are acute lymphoblastic leukemia. When periorbital metastasis occurs, proptosis and periorbital ecchymosis ("black eyes") occurs.

Neuroblastoma, arising from the neural crest tissue, is the most common extracranial solid tumor in childhood. It commonly arises in either the adrenal gland or in the paraspinal area. The other common abdominal tumor, Wilms' tumor, arises in the kidney. Neuroblastoma metastasizes to lymph nodes, bone marrow, liver, skin, the orbits, and bone. It produces catecholamines such as vanillylmandelic acid (VMA) and homovanillic acid (HVA).

Ewing sarcoma, the second most common bone tumor in children, accounts for about 30% of primary bone tumors. Osteogenic sarcoma, or osteosarcoma, is the most common bone tumor. The most common sites of involvement in Ewing sarcoma are the pelvis, proximal extremities, upper tibia, and rib. The patients present with pain and soft-tissue mass. If the lesions are in the vertebrae, there may be neurologic defects. The classic radiologic finding is a lytic, destructive bone lesion with laminar periosteal reaction, which results in the classic onionskin appearance.

127. **(D)** A combination of radiation and chemotherapy with fluorouracil and either mitomycin or cisplatin is the preferred treatment. Abdominoperineal resection is reserved for unresponsive tumors.

128. **(E)** These tumors are rare, with carcinoid being the most common type. About half of adenocarcinomas of the appendix appear as appendicitis. Tumors less than 2 cm are generally cured by appendectomy alone.

129. **(A)** The cecum is the largest part of the colon. Tumors may grow to a fairly large size before producing obstructive symptoms.

130. **(C)** An obstructive left-sided colon cancer may cause perforation at the cecum because the wall tension is greatest there (LaPlace's law).

131. **(B)** Churg–Strauss can be very similar to PAN, except renal involvement is less common and less severe. Pulmonary involvement often dominates the clinical presentation, and peripheral eosinophilia is common.

132. **(A)** PAN is a multisystem, necrotizing vasculitis of small and medium-sized muscular arteries. Aneurysmal dilations of the arteries are characteristic. Nonspecific signs and symptoms are the usual method of presentation. Renal involvement is clinically present in 60% of cases, and is the most common cause of death.

133. **(D)** A high percentage of patients with Wegener's develop antineutrophil cytoplasmic antibodies (ANCAs). In particular, cytoplasmic or c-ANCAs are both sensitive and specific of Wegener's.

134. **(C)** Henoch–Schönlein purpura, characterized by palpable purpura, arthralgias, gastrointestinal symptoms, and glomerulonephritis can be seen in any age group but is most common in children. It can resolve and recur several times over a period of weeks or months, and can resolve spontaneously.

135. **(G)** Behçet syndrome is a leukocytoclastic venulitis characterized by episodes of oral ulcers, genital ulcers, iritis, and cutaneous lesions.

136–137. **(136-B, 137-C)** Studies have shown the association between mental health disorders and urban living conditions. Schizophrenia and alcoholism have maximum prevalence in slums and skid-row districts. Depression is clustered in neighborhoods where a high proportion of the people live in single-room rented apartments. Adolescent delinquency, vandalism, and underachievement at school have a high prevalence in dormitory suburbs occupied by low-paid workers.

138. **(B)** Carbon monoxide exposure (in cars, poorly ventilated homes with house heaters, or house fires) may produce symptoms ranging from mild headache to coma. There may be hypotension, encephalitis, and cardiac arrhythmias. Cherry red lips are uncommonly seen.

139. **(A)** Iron poisoning will cause early changes of hemorrhagic gastroenteritis followed by a quiet period of up to 12 hours. Then, in ingestions of large amounts, the third phase will develop, with circulatory collapse, hepatic and renal failure, bleeding, and coma. The iron pills can be seen on radiographs as radiodense particles in the gastrointestinal tract. Serum iron levels will confirm the diagnosis. Treatment with desferoxamine, if used early, will help reverse the poisoning.

140. **(E)** Methemoglobinemia, the oxidized form of hemoglobin that is incapable of carrying oxygen, may result from local anesthetics, sulfa drugs, nitrites, and aniline dyes. The cyanotic appearance stems from the dark brown color of the blood containing methemoglobin. A drop of blood from the patient placed on filter paper next to a normal patient's blood will demonstrate the brown color. Treatment is with methylene blue.

141. **(D)** Insecticides containing organophosphates (anticholinesterases) will cause excessive salivation and sweating, mimicking some symptoms of heart failure. They also produce diarrhea, urination, and muscle fasciculation. The problems may be reversed with atropine, 2-PAM, or protopam.

142. **(H)** The TAT contains a series of 30 pictures and one blank card that the subject uses to create a story. TAT card have different stimulus values and can be assumed to elicit data pertaining to different areas of functioning. The TAT is most useful as a tool for judging motivational aspects of behavior.

143. **(D)** The Sentence Completion Test responses have been shown to be useful in creating a level of confidence with regard to predictions of overt behavior and may be used to tap specific conflict areas of interest to the psychologist.

144. **(A)** The Draw-A-Person Test, initially used to measure intelligence in children, is now also used in adults. The test assumes that the person drawn represents the expression of the body of the person in the environment. Many clinicians use the drawings as a screen-

ing technique for the detection of brain damage.

145. **(F)** The Rorschach Test is a standard set of 10 inkblots that serve as the stimuli for associations. It is especially helpful as a diagnostic tool and is one of the most commonly used individual tests in clinical settings throughout the country.

146–150. **(146-E, 147-C, 148-B, 149-A, 150-D)** These answers reflect the upper limits of the normal range by which the milestones should be reached. Most children will achieve these milestones earlier. These answers reflect the time after which the child may be demonstrating a developmental delay.

Practice Test 4
Questions

DIRECTIONS (Questions 1 through 131): Each of the numbered items or incomplete statements in this section is followed by answers or by completions of the statement. Select the ONE lettered answer or completion that is BEST in each case.

Questions 1 Through 3

A 48-year-old man with a history of exploratory laparotomy with a bowel resection 3 years prior presents with a 12-hour history of nausea and vomiting. His last bowel movement was 48 hours prior and he has not passed any flatus for the past 24 hours. On physical examination, his abdomen is distended, with high-pitched bowel sounds, and his rectal vault is empty. His abdominal series is shown in Figures 4.1 and 4.2.

1. All of the following are true regarding the findings on his x-ray series EXCEPT

   (A) dilated loops of small bowel with air fluid levels on the upright x-rays
   (B) if these findings do not resolve, the patient will require an exploratory laparotomy
   (C) findings consistent with a colonic obstruction
   (D) no evidence exists of a pneumoperitoneum
   (E) findings consistent with a small bowel obstruction

2. All of the following statements regarding bowel obstruction are true EXCEPT

   (A) abdominal distention usually noted on physical examination and dilated loops of bowel usually present on abdominal x-ray
   (B) likely to require operation if not resolved promptly
   (C) treated by bowel stimulants (eg, neostigmine)
   (D) characterized by high-pitched, tinkling bowel sounds
   (E) characterized by intermittent spasms of pain interspersed with relatively pain-free periods

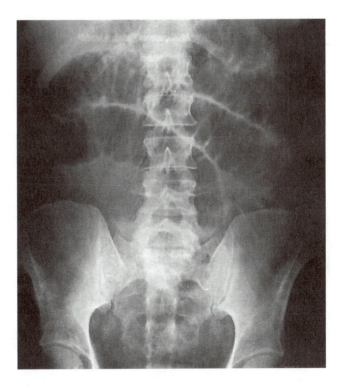

Figure 4.1

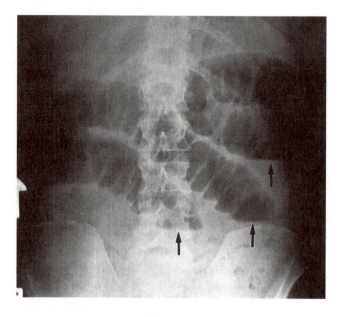

Figure 4.2

3. The MOST common cause of a small bowel obstruction is

    (A) incarcerated hernia
    (B) intussusception
    (C) neoplasm
    (D) volvulus
    (E) adhesions

Questions 4 and 5

4. A woman (P2002) at 30 weeks presents to labor and delivery complaining of not feeling fetal movements for 4 days. Fetal heart tones are not auscultated. An ultrasound is ordered. Which of the following is most likely present if the presumptive diagnosis of intrauterine fetal demise (IUFD) is confirmed?

    (A) fetal spine overlapping maternal spine
    (B) Spalding sign
    (C) positive fetal limb and body movement
    (D) gas in fetal vessels
    (E) reduced fetal heart movement

5. What is the risk that this patient will develop disseminated intravascular coagulopathy (DIC) secondary to the intrauterine fetal demise?

    (A) 0%
    (B) < 5%
    (C) 5 to 6%
    (D) 15%
    (E) 30%

Questions 6 Through 9

A 37-year-old newspaper editor comes to the office with a rash that she noticed after spending the weekend at her family's home in Connecticut. She feels well, although she has a few muscles aches because she spent most of the weekend clearing brush. (See Figure 4.3.)

6. The rash pictured is classic for the illness it represents. This disease is caused by

    (A) a fungus that lives on the keratin of the stratum corneum, nails, and hair
    (B) dry skin or underlying infections
    (C) an adverse reaction to a medication
    (D) a spirochetal infection passed through a tick bite
    (E) a fungus transmitted through puncture wounds from rose thorns

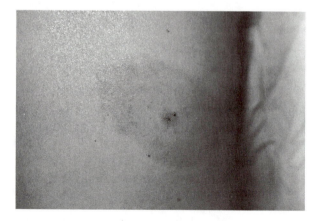

Figure 4.3

7. Which of the following is a louse-borne illness?

    (A) Lyme disease
    (B) ehrlichiosis
    (C) tularemia
    (D) epidemic typhus
    (E) babesiosis

8. Which of the following is a possible manifestation of the early form of this disease?

    (A) diffuse, maculopapular rash
    (B) acrodermatitis chronica atrophicans
    (C) vasculitis
    (D) cranial neuropathy
    (E) hematuria

9. Which of the following is an effective treatment for this disease?

    (A) trimethoprim–sulfamethoxazole
    (B) amoxicillin
    (C) metronidazole
    (D) ibuprofen
    (E) prednisone

Questions 10 Through 12

An 18-month-old infant is referred to you for failure to thrive and chronic diarrhea. There is a family history of celiac disease. You consult the texts to familiarize yourself with this disease and plan a work-up. (See Figure 4.4.)

10. Which of the following is the LEAST likely cause for this presentation?

    (A) secondary disaccharidase deficiency
    (B) cystic fibrosis
    (C) cow's milk protein sensitivity
    (D) celiac sprue
    (E) chronic nonspecific diarrhea of infancy

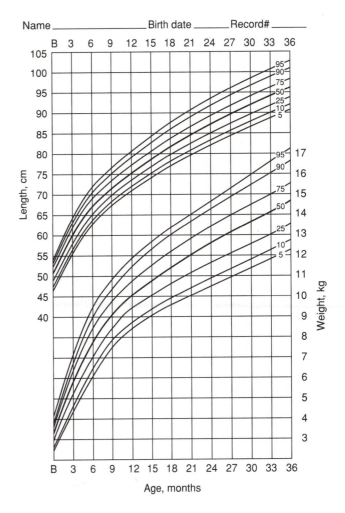

Name _____ Birth date _____ Record# _____

Figure 4.4

11. Clinical manifestations of celiac disease include

    (A) unresponsive iron deficiency
    (B) normal stools
    (C) normal abdominal examination
    (D) weight gain
    (E) increased appetite

12. Which of the following is a true statement about the treatment of this condition?

    (A) Oral iron may be indicated.
    (B) Fat-soluble vitamins K and D should not be supplemented.
    (C) Steroids frequently aid in more rapid resolution of the disease.
    (D) Resolution of symptoms may take several years.
    (E) The normal range for weight is usually not reached.

13. A patient at 34 weeks' gestation presents, complaining of weakness and burning numbness in the left hand greater than right hand, and decreased sensation in the thumb and first two fingers. Your recommendation is

    (A) neurologic evaluation
    (B) neurosurgical evaluation
    (C) orthopedic consultation
    (D) release of the flexor retinaculum
    (E) wrist splints

14. There are a variety of drugs available for inhibiting uterine activity and treating preterm labor. Ritodrine and terbutaline are considered effective because they

    (A) inhibit the development of oxytocin receptors in the myometrium
    (B) decrease concentraion of prostaglandin synthetase
    (C) are beta-1-adrenergic receptor agonists
    (D) are beta-2-adrenergic receptor agonists
    (E) are beta-2-adrenergic receptor antagonists

Questions 15 Through 17

A 22-year-old woman is 6 days status post appendectomy for appendicitis with perforation and peritonitis.

15. All of the following factors may predispose this patient to having a prolonged postoperative ileus EXCEPT

    (A) hypokalemia
    (B) opioid medications

    (C) intraperitoneal inflammation
    (D) hunger
    (E) hypomagnesemia

16. All of the following statements regarding ileus are true EXCEPT

    (A) abdominal distention usually noted on physical examination and loops of bowel with gas throughout the gastrointestinal tract present on abdominal x-ray
    (B) usually responds to supportive measures and correction of underlying disorders
    (C) treated by bowel stimulants (eg, neostigmine)
    (D) characterized by hypoactive bowel sounds
    (E) not characterized by intermittent spasms of pain interspersed with relatively pain-free periods

17. The standard treatment of paralytic ileus includes all of the following EXCEPT

    (A) intravenous fluids
    (B) nasogastric suction
    (C) correction of electrolyte imbalance
    (D) cessation of oral intake
    (E) early operation

Questions 18 and 19

A 2-year-old boy is brought into your office with a 12-hour history of pruritus over his extremities. On physical examination, he is found to have linear streaks of vesicles surrounded by erythema over his arms and lower legs. Further history reveals that he was playing in the local forest 36 hours earlier. (See Figure 4.5.)

18. The MOST likely cause for this rash is

    (A) poison ivy
    (B) Lyme disease
    (C) abrasions by thorn bushes
    (D) varicella
    (E) pemphigus

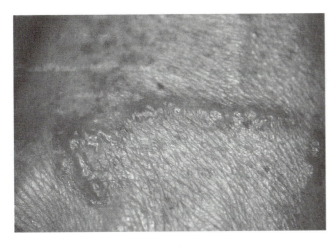

Figure 4.5

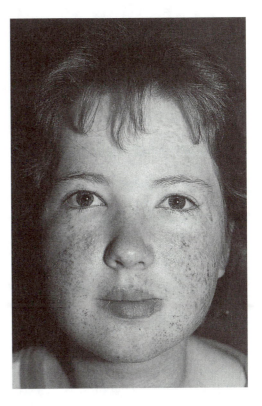

Figure 4.6

19. This is an example of

(A) type I hypersensitivity reaction, immunoglobulin E (IgE)-mediated
(B) type II hypersensitivity cytotoxic reaction
(C) type III immunopathic reaction
(D) type IV cell-mediated hypersensitivity reaction

Questions 20 Through 24

A 22-year-old woman develops a rash over her cheeks (see Figure 4.6). She also has pain and swelling in both knees as well as several small joints in her hands. Laboratory evaluation initially reveals thrombocytopenia and neutropenia as well as 3+ proteinuria.

20. The MOST specific test for diagnosis is

(A) lupus erythematosus (LE) cells
(B) antinuclear antibodies (ANA)
(C) anti-Sm antibodies
(D) anti-Ro antibodies
(E) antiphospholipids

21. In the course of this disease, the MOST common symptoms are related to

(A) renal pathology
(B) cardiopulmonary pathology
(C) musculoskeletal pathology
(D) thrombotic events
(E) gastrointestinal pathology

22. The MOST likely cardiac manifestation is

(A) pericarditis
(B) myocarditis
(C) aortic regurgitation
(D) nonbacterial endocarditis
(E) myocardial vasculitis with infarction

23. The MOST diagnostically helpful eye finding would be

(A) microaneurysm
(B) cytoid bodies
(C) Argyll–Robertson pupil
(D) macular degeneration
(E) nystagmus

24. Which of the following statements concerning renal disease in this patient is correct?

(A) Evidence of any pathologic change on renal biopsy indicates a poor prognosis.
(B) Rapidly deteriorating renal function and an active urine sediment require prompt renal biopsy.
(C) About 50% of patients with this disease have immunoglobulins in glomeruli.
(D) The presence of anti-DNA antibodies is associated with active nephritis.
(E) Mesangial involvement suggests a poor prognosis.

25. If a statistically significant difference is found between two therapies, what else is known?

(A) The type II error was probably low.
(B) Alpha was set at 0.05 or 0.01.
(C) The null hypothesis was accepted.
(D) The alternative hypothesis was accepted.
(E) The null hypothesis was rejected.

26. A patient develops dyspnea and shortness of breath during labor. Her labor is complicated by severe preeclampsia, treated with magnesium sulfate, and chorioamnionitis, treated with ampicillin and gentamicin. Her temperature is 102.4°F. Her intake is greater than her output during her course of labor. An arterial blood gas shows a PO_2 of 45 mm Hg, while breathing 100% oxygen. She has diffuse rales and rhonchi in both lung fields. A chest x-ray shows a pattern of bilateral diffuse infiltrates. Her MOST likely diagnosis is

(A) asthma with respiratory failure
(B) community-acquired pneumonia
(C) aspiration pneumonia
(D) adult respiratory distress syndrome (ARDS)
(E) pneumocystis carinii (PCP) pneumonia

Questions 27 Through 29

A 30-year-old African-American woman had the x-ray seen in Figure 4.7 done during a hospitalization for a routine cholecystectomy. She has no pulmonary symptoms. A later x-ray was found to be normal.

27. The MOST likely diagnosis is

(A) pulmonary embolism
(B) pneumonitis
(C) tuberculosis
(D) sarcoidosis
(E) primary pulmonary hypertension

28. Of the following skin lesions, which would have been more likely to have been present in this patient?

(A) erythema marginatum
(B) erythema multiforme
(C) erythema nodosum
(D) erythema bullosum
(E) erythema annulare centrifugum

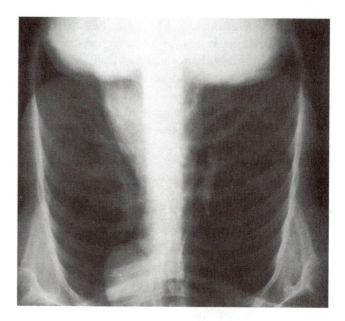

Figure 4.7

29. Which of the following is true of this process?

    (A) It is treated with corticosteroids.
    (B) Chloroquine is used in treating mildly symptomatic patients.
    (C) Spontaneous remissions of this sort are unusual.
    (D) Hemoptysis rarely occurs and is easily controlled.
    (E) Surgery can be helpful in the early stage.

30. Caput succedaneum is characterized by which of the following?

    (A) A diffuse, edematous swelling of the soft tissues of the scalp, involving the portion presenting during vertex delivery
    (B) never extends across the midline
    (C) does not extend across suture lines
    (D) edema that usually disappears within 2 to 3 days
    (E) the scalp overlying the area should not show mild bruising

Questions 31 Through 33

A 19-year-old college student presents to his family physician during the Thanksgiving break with complaints of malaise, fever, sore throat, and diminished appetite of about 2 weeks' duration. He thought he had "the flu that is going around" because his girlfriend was similarly ill several weeks ago. He tried taking some extra ampicillin that he had lying around from a previous ear infection. He has a mild cough but denies shortness of breath, genitourinary symptoms, or changes in bowel habits. He does complain of a vague "fullness" in his abdomen but denies constipation. On examination, he is febrile to 102.2°F orally; other vital signs are normal. His exam is significant for tender cervical lymphadenopathy bilaterally, enlarged tonsils without exudate, mild tender hepatomegaly, splenomegaly, and a scattered macular rash. His skin is not icteric. A rapid heterophile test done in your office is highly positive.

31. The MOST likely diagnosis, based on the history and physical examination, is

    (A) varicella viral infection
    (B) recurrent streptococcal infection of the throat

    (C) infectious mononucleosis
    (D) acute human immunodeficiency virus (HIV) infection
    (E) acute hepatitis B infection

32. The patient's girlfriend comes to visit him and requests that you test her for evidence of recent Epstein–Barr virus (EBV) infection. Which of the following tests would you MOST expect to be elevated?

    (A) immunoglobulin G (IgG) viral capsid antigen (VCA)
    (B) Epstein–Barr nuclear antigen (EBNA) titer
    (C) immunoglobulin M (IgM) VCA
    (D) early antigen (EA)
    (E) CMV titre

33. Despite advising him to avoid contact sports, the patient is cajoled into a game of touch football on the front lawn. The game becomes rowdy, and he is tackled hard, landing under a pile of people. He does not get up. You are called to see him in the emergency department of the local hospital. His blood pressure is low, his pulse is rapid, and his abdomen is rigid. What is the MOST likely explanation for his condition?

    (A) He is dehydrated from fever and exertion.
    (B) He has ruptured his liver.
    (C) He has ruptured his spleen.
    (D) He has had an allergic reaction to the ampicillin.
    (E) He has ruptured his appendix.

34. Which of the following is characteristic of a single umbilical artery?

    (A) It occurs in about 5 of 100 births.
    (B) About 80% of such infants have congenital abnormalities.
    (C) Trisomy 21 is frequently found.
    (D) Among twins, the rate of occurrence is 350 per 1000.
    (E) The associated congenital abnormalities may involve the respiratory tract.

35. A 29-year-old woman (P3013) at 20 weeks' gestation is in your office for a routine prenatal visit. She states that she noticed a lump in her breast approximately 1 month ago and it has not gone away. Your examination reveals a round, freely mobile mass, measuring approximately 2 cm, in the perangulum of the breast. Your recommendation is to

    (A) observe
    (B) observe for the duration of the pregnancy and reassess with mammography at 6 weeks postpartum
    (C) perform breast ultrasound
    (D) perform mammography and fine-needle aspiration or open biopsy
    (E) perform a partial mastectomy

Questions 36 Through 38

A 22-year-old man presents to the county sexually transmitted disease (STD) clinic complaining of an odorless discharge from his penis for the past week. He has had two sexual partners in the past month. He has been in touch with both, and neither has had any genitourinary symptoms.

36. Which of the following is a likely pathogen in this case and the most common sexually transmitted infection?

    (A) *Neisseria gonorrhoeae*
    (B) *Chlamydia trachomatis*
    (C) *Treponema pallidum*
    (D) herpes simplex, type 2
    (E) *Trichomonas vaginalis*

37. What is the treatment of choice for this condition?

    (A) penicillin
    (B) acyclovir
    (C) metronidazole
    (D) doxycycline
    (E) tinidazole

38. Which of the following is a serious long-term complication of this infection?

    (A) heart damage
    (B) degeneration of the anterior horn cells in the spinal column
    (C) blindness secondary to uveitis
    (D) chronic persistent hepatitis
    (E) infertility in sexual partners

39. A 25-year-old Chinese man, who has just arrived in the United States, complains that his penis is retracting into his abdomen and fears that this will kill him. He mentions that several young men in his Chinese village had the same complaint when he left China. The MOST likely diagnosis is

    (A) hysterical koro
    (B) antisocial personality disorder
    (C) alcohol intoxication
    (D) amphetamine intoxication
    (E) schizophrenia

40. A 20-year-old man who recently moved to the area came to a general medical clinic complaining of insomnia, lack of appetite, vague muscular aches, lack of zest, and feelings of sadness and loneliness. The examining student made the diagnosis of adjustment disorder with depressed mood and sympathized with the patient for his not yet having made new friends. Two weeks later, the young man returned, reporting, "I did like you said, and now do we have trouble!" He said that he had found a friend, a young girl who was a minor and the local sheriff's daughter. On their first date, they proceeded to have intercourse in the living room of the sheriff's home and made enough noise to get caught. The examining student would MOST appropriately respond at this time as follows:

    (A) "What do you mean we?"
    (B) "I didn't tell you to do anything."
    (C) "You sure goofed up."
    (D) "Tell me more about what happened."
    (E) "How are we going to get out of this mess?"

41. In a child with a year-round stuffy nose, which of the following is the BEST approach to diagnosing allergy?

    (A) Tell the child's mother to clean the room, cover the mattress, and get rid of the stuffed animals.
    (B) Take a good history and make a smear of nasal secretions.
    (C) Get a serum IgE level.
    (D) Order a radioallergosorbent test (RAST).
    (E) Use direct skin testing methods.

Questions 42 Through 44

A 39-year-old nulliparous woman presents for advice on contraception. She has been with her new sexual partner for 6 months and anticipates that they will marry and want a family. She has a maternal history of breast cancer with onset at age 65. She has a 15 pack-year smoking history but stopped 4 years ago.

42. The failure rates during the first year of attempted contraceptive use from lowest to highest are

    (A) injectable progestin, combination oral contraceptive, intrauterine device (IUD), condom, diaphragm
    (B) combination oral contraceptives, injectable progestin, progestin-only pill, IUD, diaphragm
    (C) combination oral contraceptives, IUD, withdrawal, diaphragm, condom
    (D) combination oral contraceptives, withdrawal, condom, periodic abstinence (rhythm), IUD
    (E) combination oral contraceptives, diaphragm, condom, IUD, douche

43. Advantages of injectable progestins include

    (A) regular menses
    (B) rapid return of ovulation after discontinuation
    (C) amenorrhea

    (D) effectiveness
    (E) decreased risk of thromboembolism compared to estrogen–progestin oral contraceptives

44. Absolute contraindications to the oral contraceptive include

    (A) migraine headaches
    (B) age > 35
    (C) diabetes
    (D) epilepsy
    (E) heavy smoking

Questions 45 Through 48

A 50-year-old woman comes to your office for a first visit. She was referred to you by her primary care physician, who said she was concerned about her patient's mood and self-reported performance at work. The patient appears well dressed but somewhat distracted at her appointment. Upon questioning, she says that she has felt somewhat depressed for about 4 months, since her youngest son was killed in an automobile accident, and she has not slept or eaten well for several weeks. She says that she feels unable to concentrate at work, although her coworkers have been sympathetic and cut her enough slack. "I don't deserve to be treated well," she says tearfully. "How could I let this happen?" The patient denies suicidal ideation.

45. The MOST appropriate diagnosis at this time is

    (A) major depression, single episode
    (B) major depression, chronic
    (C) benzodiazepine dependence
    (D) adjustment disorder, depressive type
    (E) bipolar disorder, depressive episode

46. The MOST appropriate intervention at this time is

    (A) lithium administration
    (B) electroconvulsive therapy (ECT)
    (C) fluoxetine administration
    (D) short-term supportive psychotherapy
    (E) hospitalization for benzodiazepine taper

The patient undergoes treatment, with some improvement. However, 6 months later, at a regularly scheduled appointment, she reveals that she has begun to think of ways to kill herself. "Nothing's going well," she reports, although she has just finished telling you that she was recently promoted at work and that she has regained her appetite.

47.   The MOST appropriate diagnosis at this time is

   (A) major depression, single episode
   (B) schizophrenia, paranoid type
   (C) benzodiazepine dependence
   (D) adjustment disorder, depressive type
   (E) bipolar disorder, depressive episode

48.   The MOST appropriate intervention at this time is

   (A) immediate hospitalization for suicidality
   (B) fluoxetine administration
   (C) electroconvulsive therapy
   (D) haloperidol administration
   (E) assessment of nature and magnitude of suicidal ideation

Questions 49 and 50

The following questions concern the epidemiology and prevention of HIV/acquired immune deficiency syndrome (AIDS).

49.   The HIV/AIDS epidemic has followed several distinct courses in its spread around the world. In which of the following cities is intravenous drug use the most important route for the spread of the infection?

   (A) New York
   (B) San Francisco
   (C) Kampala, Uganda
   (D) Manila, Philippines
   (E) Key West

50.   The use of zidovudine (AZT) monotherapy is a significant means of preventing HIV transmission in which of the following settings?

   (A) given prophylactically prior to transfusion with blood from unscreened donor

   (B) given during pregnancy and delivery to prevent vertical transmission
   (C) given to an HIV-positive mother to prevent breast milk transmission
   (D) given for 6 weeks following needle-stick injury to prevent infection in the occupational setting
   (E) given to a hemophiliac child during infusion of factor VIII concentrate

51.   A pregnant woman at 24 weeks' gestation presents with a history of Graves' disease. She is not on medication, her pulse is 76, sensitive thyroid-stimulating hormone (TSH) is 0.8, T_4 is 14.2, and T_3 resin uptake is decreased. Your diagnosis is

   (A) primary hypothyroidism, active
   (B) primary hypothyroidism, in remission
   (C) Graves' disease, active
   (D) Graves' disease, in remission
   (E) no thyroid disease

Questions 52 Through 54

One day after a ladies' charity brunch, 43 of the 78 guests developed symptoms of nausea, vomiting, abdominal cramps, diarrhea, fever, and headache. The menu included the following items: iced tea, made-to-order omelets, fresh fruit compote, raspberry sorbet, and coffee cake.

52.   Knowing nothing else, which food is the MOST likely source of the trouble?

   (A) iced tea
   (B) omelets
   (C) fruit compote
   (D) raspberry sorbet
   (E) coffee cake

53.   What is the MOST likely pathogen?

   (A) *Vibrio cholerae*
   (B) *Vibrio parahaemolyticus*
   (C) *Salmonella enteritidis*
   (D) *Shigella*
   (E) *Giardia lamblia*

54. If the illness had been due to staphylococcal food poisoning, in which of the following ways would the outbreak have presented differently?

(A) higher attack rate
(B) milder symptoms
(C) gradual onset
(D) less prominent nausea and vomiting
(E) shorter incubation period

Questions 55 and 56

As college health service director, you are notified that a 19-year-old sophomore has just been hospitalized with fever, headache, nuchal rigidity, prostration, and widespread purpuric rash. She felt mildly ill yesterday, but her condition rapidly deteriorated overnight. She has not been off campus for the past 3 weeks and has had no known contact with infected persons.

55. What is the likely cause of this illness?

(A) *Pneumococcus*
(B) *Neisseria meningitidis*
(C) coxsackievirus
(D) *Haemophilis influenzae*
(E) *Cryptococcus neoformans*

56. Which of the following should be part of the college's response to this case?

(A) cancel sports teams' travel to other campuses
(B) screening of students, faculty, and staff for carrier status
(C) immunization of all susceptible individuals
(D) chemoprophylaxis for close contacts
(E) increase chlorination in college pool

Questions 57 and 58

A 26-year-old primigravida presents to labor and delivery for evaluation. She has noted many hours of irregular contractions and increased vaginal secretions and bloody show. She first noted the show 2 days ago. She is assessed for fetal well-being, labor, and rupture of membranes. The fetal assessment is reassuring. The nitrazine test is positive, and ferning is negative. There is no pooling of fluid in the vagina.

57. What conclusion can be made from the positive nitrazine test?

(A) It is unequivocal evidence of rupture of the membranes.
(B) It is presumptive evidence of rupture of the membranes.
(C) It is unequivocal evidence of intact membranes.
(D) It is equivocal evidence of intact membranes.
(E) It is unrelated to the bloody show.

58. Uterine contractions that are irregular in frequency, brief in duration, more common in late pregnancy and multiparous women, and with pain located in the lower abdomen or groin are commonly called

(A) Braxton–Hicks contractions
(B) false labor
(C) protracted labor
(D) active-phase labor
(E) latent-phase labor

Questions 59 and 60

A 19-year-old African-American woman is referred for evaluation when she is found to have a significant anemia on her college physical. She gives a history of anemia treated unsuccessfully in the past with iron pills. She notes that most of the women in her family are on iron pills. Her complete blood count (CBC) shows a white blood cell (WBC) count of 3200, hemoglobin of 9 g/dL, mean corpuscular volume (MCV) of 68, red cell distribution width (RDW) of 13, and platelet count of 320,000. A hemoglobin electrophoresis is normal.

59. What is the MOST likely diagnosis?

(A) alpha-thalassemia trait
(B) inadequately treated iron deficiency
(C) beta-thalassemia minor
(D) lead toxicity
(E) hereditary spherocytosis

60. Counseling of this patient regarding her diagnosis should include which of the following?

(A) Single gene deletions are very common and asymptomatic.
(B) Double gene deletions are very rare and of two types.
(C) There is no in utero testing available.
(D) Hydrops fetalis is almost exclusively seen in Africans.
(E) She need not be evaluated for iron deficiency.

Questions 61 Through 65

An agitated, 24-year-old, unmarried white man is brought to the emergency department by the police. He has a 5-year history of multiple drug use. He does not work, and lives with people he meets on the streets. In the past, he has supported himself through dealing drugs and shoplifting. He reports having no friends. About 5 years ago, he began to develop feelings of vague suspicion. He recognized that this was just his way of perceiving the world, rather than reality. However, 3 days ago, his suspi-

ciousness increased, and he has become convinced that his neighbor is a member of the Mafia and is plotting to kill him. He is unable to sleep. This evening, the patient went to his neighbor's house in an attempt to eavesdrop. The neightbor, seeing him, came to the door, at which point the patient shot him.

61. The axis IV diagnosis is

(A) none
(B) threat of job loss
(C) partner relational problem
(D) unemployment and homelessness
(E) illiteracy

62. If this syndrome were alcoholic hallucinosis, the clinical history would include

(A) auditory hallucinations
(B) clouding of consciousness
(C) "rum fits"
(D) family history of alcoholism
(E) prominent paranoid delusions

63. If this syndrome were amphetamine-induced psychotic disorder with delusions, the clinical history would likely include

(A) aggressiveness and hostility
(B) visual hallucinations
(C) psychomotor retardation
(D) bulimia
(E) strephosymbolia

64. The immediate treatment of choice for this patient is

(A) insight-oriented psychotherapy
(B) antipsychotic and supportive therapy
(C) barbiturates
(D) ECT
(E) methadone

65. The patient's attorney could argue that his client is not legally responsible for shooting his neighbor because

    (A) he was suffering from a substance-induced psychotic disorder
    (B) the neighbor was, in fact, a member of the Mafia
    (C) he is incompentent to stand trial
    (D) he did not know the gun was loaded
    (E) none of the above

66. In autosomal dominant inheritance, the trait will be found in one parent and

    (A) 25% of daughters and 75% of sons
    (B) 25% of sons and 75% of daughters
    (C) 50% of daughters and 50% of sons
    (D) only in daughters
    (E) only in sons

67. A "controlled" trial is so named because

    (A) the experimenter is overseeing the assignment of subjects
    (B) the experimenter has included a therapy or procedure with a known or expected outcome to compare to the experimental therapy or procedure
    (C) the study is designed in a prospective fashion to permit full oversight over the collection of data
    (D) the experimenter is minimizing bias by including a randomization sequence for the assignment of patients to the different study arms
    (E) the bias of the experimenter is kept from influencing patient selection through blinding

Questions 68 Through 70

A 33-year-old woman (G2,P2002) presents with a history of menorrhagia, which has been worsening in the last 3 years. She has been advised to have a hysterectomy and consults you for a second opinion. Her work-up has included an endometrial biopsy that showed benign secretory endometrium. A pelvic ultrasound revealed an enlarged uterus measuring $18 \times 14 \times 10$ cm with multiple uterine fibroids, the largest measuring 5×5.6 cm. None of the fibroids appear to be submucosal.

68. The MOST likely cause of her hypermenorrhea is

    (A) coagulopathy
    (B) leiomyomata uteri
    (C) endometrial polyps
    (D) anorexia nervosa
    (E) spontaneous abortion

69. A laparotomy was performed in order to do multiple myomectomy. Laparotomy showed multiple small nodules over the surface of the pelvis and abdominal cavity. A biopsy of one of these nodules demonstrates benign-appearing fibrous whorls that resemble small myomas. The MOST likely diagnosis is

    (A) carneous infarction of a myoma
    (B) intravenous leiomyomatosis
    (C) leiomyomatosis peritonealis disseminata
    (D) malignant transformation of a myoma to adenocarcinoma
    (E) myxomatous degeneration of a myoma

70. Benign leiomyomas of the uterus carry a risk of malignant transformation in what percentage of cases?

    (A) 0.05%
    (B) 0.1%
    (C) 0.5%
    (D) 1%
    (E) 5%

Questions 71 Through 74

A 28-year-old African-American man has had a persistent marked erection of the penis, which is frequently painful. He has been hospitalized in the past for diffuse abdominal and bone pain. He has chronic pain in his back and lower legs.

71. Which of the following is depicted in Figure 4.8?

    (A) Peyronie's disease
    (B) priapism
    (C) satyriasis
    (D) balanitis
    (E) paraphimosis

72. Which of the following disorders is the patient MOST likely to have?

    (A) pulmonary fibrosis
    (B) nephrotic syndrome
    (C) sickle cell anemia
    (D) cirrhosis
    (E) congenital heart disease

73. Which of the following statements concerning the patient's underlying disease is true?

    (A) His risk of developing cholelithiasis is reduced.
    (B) He is at risk for deep venous thrombosis.

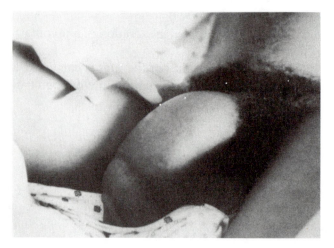

Figure 4.8

(C) Septicemia with encapsulated organisms is common.
(D) *Salmonella* is the most common cause of osteomyelitis in this group of patients.
(E) He has renal stones.

74. The number of his pain crises can be decreased by treatment with

    (A) more aggressive treatment with fluids, antibiotics, and pain medicine including narcotics as an outpatient
    (B) hydroxyurea
    (C) long-acting analgesics for his chronic pain
    (D) intermittent injections of meperidine (Demerol) and hydroxyzine (Vistaril)
    (E) morphine by a patient-controlled analgesia (PCA) device

Question 75

A 4$\frac{1}{2}$-year-old boy has a 4-month history of increasing neurologic disorders. The findings include paresis of conjugate gaze, hemiparesis and hyperreflexia, Babinski response, horizontal nystagmus, and truncal and extremity ataxia. The child does not exhibit sensory defects. Basal ganglia manifestations are not detected. Cerebrospinal fluid (CSF) pressure, cell count, protein, and sugar are normal. Plain x-rays of the skull are normal.

75. At this point, the diagnosis is probably

    (A) Sydenham's chorea
    (B) meningitis
    (C) pinealoma
    (D) agenesis of the corpus callosum
    (E) none of the above

Questions 76 and 77

A 70-year-old woman is being seen in the emergency department for abdominal discomfort in the right upper quadrant. She has a history of cholelithiasis. She is afebrile and her vital signs are stable. Her abdominal x-ray shows air in the billary tree.

76. A possible reason for the noted abnormality on the abdominal x-ray is

    (A) cholecystoenteric fistula
    (B) a nonobstructing colon cancer
    (C) gastritis
    (D) a left 3-cm adrenal mass
    (E) a rectal carcinoma

77. The MOST common site of intestinal obstruction due to this lesion is the

    (A) pylorus
    (B) duodenum
    (C) jejunum
    (D) ileum
    (E) sigmoid colon

Questions 78 Through 80

A 6-year-old boy with no significant past medical history appears at your office. He has recently recovered from an upper respiratory infection and since early this morning has had a number of episodes of vomiting. His mother states that he seems somewhat sleepy this morning as well. He has minimal fever and no obvious site of infection. He vomits after your exam, and you are concerned with his degree of lethargy. Bedside tests for meningitis are negative.

78. Important points to note in the history include

    (A) history of having taken aspirin lately
    (B) cases of Lyme disease in the community
    (C) history of bowel movements
    (D) history of asthma
    (E) history of renal infection

79. The MOST appropriate next step at this time would be to

    (A) perform an immediate spinal tap
    (B) admit for observation and obtain liver profile
    (C) take throat, urine, and blood cultures, and send home with instructions to keep you informed of the child's condition

    (D) start on pencillin for presumed strep throat after taking a throat culture
    (E) obtain a magnetic resonance imaging (MRI) scan and neurosurgical consult

80. Which of the following statements is true concerning Reye syndrome?

    (A) It will never result in coma or death because the disorder is "self-limited."
    (B) It is characterized by normal cerebrospinal fluid except for elevated pressure.
    (C) It is epidemiologically associated with medications, including actaminophen, laxatives, and caffeine.
    (D) A liver biopsy is necessary for correct diagnosis.
    (E) Deepening of coma is most likely when the serum ammonia level suddenly drops.

Questions 81 Through 83

A 74-year-old nulliparous woman, whose last menstrual period (LMP) was 25 years ago, presents with a 10-month history of vulvar itching not responsive to the topical ointments prescribed by her doctor. She recently noticed that the area is hard and bleeds easily. The lesion is 1 cm in diameter. It is located in the midportion of the right labia majus. The urethra and the anus are not involved. The inguinal lymph nodes are not palpable. She has otherwise been in good health. The vaginal wet smear is significant for yeast.

81. The next step should be to

    (A) treat with intravaginal and vulvar antifungal agents
    (B) perform a Papanicolaou (Pap) smear
    (C) refer her for colposcopy of the vulva
    (D) biopsy the lesion
    (E) schedule wide local excision

82. The tissue diagnosis of the lesion is invasive squamous (epidermoid) carcinoma with a depth of invasion of 1.5 mm. There is no lymphadenopathy. The following tests were performed and were negative: chest x-ray, intravenous pyelogram (IVP), cystoscopy, barium enema, and proctoscopy. Your treatment planning should be based on which diagnosis?

    (A) stage I vaginal carcinoma
    (B) stage I vulvar carcinoma
    (C) stage II vaginal carcinoma
    (D) stage II vulvar carcinoma
    (E) stage III vulvar carcinoma

83. The selected treatment plan is

    (A) chemotherapy
    (B) wide local excision
    (C) radical vulvectomy with internal iliac lymph nodes
    (D) radiation to the pelvis
    (E) topical chemotherapy

Questions 84 Through 88

A 55-year-old woman comes for a routine office visit and brings up her concerns about osteoporosis. Her menstrual periods have recently stopped, and her gynecologist is strongly encouraging her to begin hormone replacement therapy (HRT). You take a family history that reveals many family members with cardiac disease. The patient's mother suffered a hip fracture at the age of 64.

84. Which of the following statements concerning osteoporosis is true?

    (A) The main underlying cause of fractures in osteoporosis is trauma.
    (B) Initial bone density is unrelated to the risk of developing osteoporosis in later years.
    (C) Short women of Asian extraction tend to have an increased incidence of osteoporosis.

    (D) Postmenopausal HRT has no significant effect on the occurrence of fractures associated with osteoporosis.
    (E) Smoking and high alcohol intake increase the risk of developing osteoporosis twofold.

85. Which of the following drugs used in the treatment of osteoporosis is associated with significant gastrointestinal side effects?

    (A) vitamin D
    (B) calcium
    (C) estrogen
    (D) calcitonin
    (E) alendronate

86. Which of the following is associated with HRT?

    (A) an increased risk of endometrial cancer
    (B) a decreased risk of osteoporosis
    (C) an increased incidence of depression and memory loss
    (D) an increased risk of cardiovascular disease
    (E) an increase in incidence of urethral mucosa atrophy

87. The patient expresses concern about an increased risk of breast cancer in women receiving HRT. You tell her that

    (A) HRT does increase the risk of breast cancer, and you suggest that she should accept menopause and its symptoms as a natural part of life. You recommend that she follow up with her gynecologist in 1 or 2 years.
    (B) HRT does increase the risk of breast cancer, but with her family history, the benefits outweigh the risks. You recommend HRT with a mammogram every 6 months.

(C) HRT decreases the risk of breast cancer, and with her family history, she really should take it. You schedule her for a screening mammogram.

(D) HRT has no effect on breast cancer risk, and she should follow her gynecologist's recommendation. You schedule her for a screening mammogram.

(E) HRT and breast cancer studies are not conclusive. You recommend HRT because of her family history, a mammogram at least every 2 years, breast exam by a physician yearly, and pelvic exam as her gynecologist recommends.

88. Although she has been without a period for many months, she calls a few weeks after beginning her HRT to report vaginal bleeding lasting 5 days and quite heavy. You suggest that she

(A) go to the emergency department immediately

(B) call her gynecologist for an urgent appointment

(C) inform her gynecologist if bleeding beyond another few days, but that it is normal for women to have some irregular bleeding when starting HRT and, after not menstruating for months, normal for the flow to be quite heavy

(D) stop taking the HRT because vaginal bleeding is a sign of endometrial cancer

(E) come to your office for a pregnancy test

89. A 31-year-old multigravida had a cesarean section for cephalopelvic disproportion after a prolonged labor. On the second postoperative day, she has a temperature of 101.5°F, tachycardia, malodorous lochia, and uterine tenderness. A clinical diagnosis of postpartum endometritis was made, and she was started on appropriate antibiotic therapy. After 72 hours of therapy, the patient continues to demonstrate significant evening temperature elevations. The breasts show no engorgement. Her lungs are clear. The wound is clean and healing well. The next appropriate step is to

(A) obtain a CT scan of the abdomen and pelvis, looking for an intra-abdominal abscess

(B) perform an adequate pelvic examination to rule out a pelvic collection

(C) initiate anticoagulation therapy with intravenous heparin therapy

(D) initiate anticoagulation therapy with oral warfarin therapy

(E) discontinue the antibiotic therapy to rule out a drug fever

90. A patient presents to the emergency department at 12 weeks after the first day of her last normal menstrual period. Her chief complaint is cramping, bleeding, and passage of tissue that looks like hamburger. On examination, the cervix is open and tissue is present in the os. The diagnosis is

(A) incomplete abortion

(B) criminal abortion

(C) inevitable abortion

(D) missed abortion

(E) therapeutic abortion

91. Which of the following polyps of the colon and rectum is MOST likely to contain a malignancy?

(A) villous adenoma

(B) juvenile polyp

(C) tubular adenoma

(D) inflammatory polyp

(E) hyperplastic polyp

Questions 92 Through 94

A healthy 36-year-old man with a strong family history of cardiac disease presents to the preventive cardiology clinic for advice about how he can mitigate his risk of premature death. His father, two uncles, and one grandfather all died of heart attacks before they reached the age of 50. He has never had any specific testing related to heart disease risk. He eats a well-balanced vegetarian diet and does not smoke.

92. What further history is MOST important to assess possible avenues for prevention?

    (A) age of onset of puberty
    (B) family history of heart disease in female relatives
    (C) alcohol use
    (D) physical activity level
    (E) current symptoms of heart disease

93. Which of the following laboratory tests should be done as soon as possible?

    (A) 5-hour glucose tolerance test
    (B) fasting lipid panel (cholesterol, high-density lipoprotein [HDL], low-density lipoprotein [LDL], triglycerides)
    (C) nonfasting glucose and cholesterol levels
    (D) testosterone and GnRH levels
    (E) thyroid hormone levels

The following test results were obtained during the next week:

Glucose	103 mg/dL
Cholesterol	176 mg/dL
HDL	32 mg/dL
LDL	144 mg/dL
Triglycerides	128 mg/dL
Thyroxine	10 µg/dL

94. What advice would you give him?

    (A) Reduce intake of refined sugars.
    (B) Increase physical activity.
    (C) Eliminate eggs, cheese, and dairy products from the diet.
    (D) Switch from butter to stick margarine.
    (E) There is no need to change current habits.

95. A 23-year-old woman presents to her physician 2 days after completing final examinations at college. She has several complaints. On further questioning, the physician finds that the student had been drinking large quantities of coffee while studying for exams and has not consumed any coffee in the past 2 days. Which of the following statements is true regarding caffeine withdrawal?

    (A) Caffeine is a very strong reinforcer.
    (B) The most characteristic symptoms of caffeine withdrawal are headache and fatigue.
    (C) Caffeine withdrawal syndrome generally lasts less than a day.
    (D) Caffeine tolerance is rare in heavy users of caffeine-containing drinks.
    (E) Ten percent of adult Americans consume more than 500 mg of caffeine per day.

96. A 32-year-old man complains of headache pain in the area of his left eye, extending to the left side of his face. The pain began the day following his friend's bachelor party; it caused him to be awakened from his nap and has been present daily for the last 2 weeks. The MOST likely diagnosis is

    (A) migraine headache
    (B) hangover
    (C) tension headache
    (D) cluster headache
    (E) postconcussional disorder

97. A 76-year-old widow presents to her family physician stating that her skin has been infested by spiders. She points to numerous excoriations on all four extremities and states that these are the areas of infestation. She describes in great detail cleaning an oven, which was filled with spider eggs, and notes that her symptoms began after this event. She has tried numerous over-the-counter medicines and home remedies without success.

She now wonders if she might need to see a "skin doctor."

The patient is polite and cooperative during the examination. There is no evidence of hallucinations or disorganized thoughts. Mental status examination, neurologic studies, and laboratory screening fail to reveal evidence of any organic disorder. The MOST likely diagnosis of this patient is

(A) delusional disorder, somatic type

(B) schizophreniform disorder

(C) alcohol-induced psychotic disorder with delusions

(D) Münchhausen syndrome

(E) conversion disorder

Questions 98 Through 100

A slender 62-year-old woman with fair skin is being seen for her annual physical examination. She is postmenopausal and in good health, with no known medical problems. She is a nonsmoker. She works in an office setting as a school administrator. She is an avid table-tennis player, and her other main leisure-time activity is reading.

98. Which of the following conditions is she probably at lowest risk for?

(A) osteoporosis

(B) basal cell skin cancer

(C) coronary artery disease

(D) breast cancer

(E) peptic ulcer disease

99. Which of the following screening tests would be advisable following this visit?

(A) serum PSA level

(B) treadmill stress test

(C) endometrial biopsy

(D) serum lipid panel

(E) thyroid hormone levels

100. What preventive advice should you give her?

(A) Return semiannually for a Pap smear.

(B) Use sunscreen of sun protective factor (SPF) 8 or higher.

(C) Increase weight-bearing exercise.

(D) Reduce intake of dietary fats.

(E) Drink 1 to 2 glasses of red wine per day.

Questions 101 and 102

A 60-year-old man presents with a long-standing history of gastroesophageal reflux. He undergoes upper endoscopy, and an abnormality is present in the appearance of the mucosa 30 to 40 cm from the incisors. The final pathologic findings on the biopsy demonstrate Barrett's esophagus.

101. All of the following statements regarding Barrett's esophagus are true EXCEPT

(A) it is a metaplastic change in which the epithelium changes from columnar to squamous epithelium

(B) an esophagectomy is appropriate if severe dysplasia is present.

(C) patients can develop ulceration in this area of the metaplasia more similar to peptic ulceration of the stomach or duodenum

(D) in the absence of dysplasia, and with the failure of medical therapy alone, a Nissen fundoplication (an antireflux surgical procedure) is an appropriate surgical option

(E) a significant percentage of patients with benign esophageal stricture have Barrett's esophagus

102. All of the following are associated with an increased risk for esophageal cancer EXCEPT

(A) alcohol ingestion

(B) smoking

(C) chronic ingestion of hot beverages

(D) aflatoxin

(E) poor oral hygiene

Questions 103 Through 107

You are asked to consult on a case of failure to thrive in a 6-month-old girl. There is a history of bulky diarrheal stools and chronic cough. Your initial suspicion from the history alone is that cystic fibrosis (CF) is an important diagnostic consideration.

103. Which of the following is a true statement about CF?

    (A) Prognosis is steadily improving, with up to 90% cumulative survival beyond 20 years if diagnosis and treatment begin before lung damage occurs.
    (B) Renal infection causes most of the morbidity.
    (C) It is inherited as a sex-linked recessive disease.
    (D) Administration of influenza vaccine is not indicated in these patients.
    (E) The basic defect has not yet been identified.

104. Complications of the disease include

    (A) meconium ileus
    (B) hypoglycemic episodes
    (C) renal failure
    (D) hypotension
    (E) aplastic anemia

105. Which of the following statements is correct with respect to infections of the respiratory tract in patients with CF?

    (A) Pathogens include *Pseudomonas, Staphylococcus aureus,* and *Aspergillus.*
    (B) Respiratory infections are due to aspiration.
    (C) Hospitalization is indicated when a CF patient has symptoms of a respiratory tract infection.
    (D) *Pneumocystis carinii* is the most frequent pathogen.
    (E) With current treatments available, respiratory tract infections are uncommon.

106. Pulmonary complications of the disease include

    (A) pneumothorax
    (B) fibrosis
    (C) pulmonary dysplasia
    (D) reactive airway disease
    (E) anoxia

107. Important treatment steps in CF should include

    (A) genetic counseling for the parents
    (B) pancreatic enzyme supplements
    (C) chest physical therapy and postural drainage
    (D) inhalation therapy
    (E) all of the above

Questions 108 and 109

A 40-year-old man presents with a chief complaint of dysphagia. He has not had significant weight loss. You obtain a barium swallow, which demonstrates a dilated esophagus, absent primary peristalsis, and a narrow stricture at the cardioesophageal junction. Manometry confirms absence of primary peristalsis. On endoscopy, the endoscope is passed into the stomach without difficulty, but some retained food is present in the esophagus.

108. The MOST likely diagnosis is

    (A) esophageal cancer
    (B) benign esophageal stricture
    (C) achalasia
    (D) infiltrating intramural carcinoma of the cardia
    (E) biliary colic

109. The MOST definitive treatment choice would be

    (A) dilation
    (B) cholecystectomy
    (C) esophagectomy
    (D) myotomy of the esophagus distally extending through the gastroesophageal junction
    (E) right hemicolectomy

110. All of the following are nonsurgical causes of abdominal pain EXCEPT

    (A) pneumonia
    (B) diabetic ketoacidosis
    (C) acute salpingitis
    (D) head trauma
    (E) myocardial infarction

111. All of the following stimulate gastric acid secretion EXCEPT

    (A) sight of food
    (B) presence of food in the stomach
    (C) fat in the duodenum
    (D) gastrin
    (E) histamine

Questions 112 and 113

A 26-year-old woman who is 26 weeks pregnant presents with a swollen left leg. Evaluation reveals a deep venous thrombosis (DVT) involving the femoral vein. She has no personal or family history of thrombosis.

112. Which of the following statements is true?

    (A) Only pregnant women with protein C or S deficiency are at risk for thrombosis.
    (B) Protein C, protein S, antithrombin II level, lupus inhibitor, and APC resistance studies should be drawn once she is stabilized on her anticoagulant.
    (C) Heparin should be used to treat the thrombosis, and anticoagulation should continue until 4 to 6 weeks after delivery.
    (D) Coumadin can be started the day after she is started on heparin.
    (E) She will require anticoagulation for all subsequent pregnancies.

113. The most common predisposing factor to the development of a venous thrombosis is

    (A) protein C deficiency
    (B) protein S deficiency
    (C) antithrombin III deficiency
    (D) tobacco use
    (E) surgery

Questions 114 Through 116

114. A patient presents at 37 weeks with a known twin gestation. The presentation is cephalic/breech. The decision is made to allow this patient to attempt a vaginal delivery. After the delivery of baby A, baby B is still breech. The preferred route of delivery for baby B is

    (A) assisted breech delivery
    (B) total breech extraction
    (C) internal podalic version with extraction
    (D) external version followed by vaginal delivery
    (E) cesarean section

115. Which of the following factors is associated with the highest rate of twins?

    (A) race
    (B) heredity
    (C) maternal age
    (D) maternal size
    (E) infertility agents

116. If division of the zygote occurs on the second day after conception, the fetuses will have

    (A) two separate placentas, two amnions, and one chorion
    (B) two separate placentas, two amnions, and two chorions
    (C) one chorion and one amnion
    (D) two chorions and one amnion
    (E) one chorion and two amnions

Questions 117 and 118

A 55-year-old woman whose family are Ashkenazi Jews wants to know why you continue to recommend Pap smears for her every 2 to 3 years when she has heard that she is at low risk for developing cervical cancer.

117. You tell her which of the following?

(A) She is at lower risk of cervical cancer, but the risk is not zero, and she is still at risk for endometrial cancer, so an ongoing relationship with a gynecologist is important.

(B) She is right that cervical cancer is not seen in Jewish and Muslim women because their husbands are uniformly circumcised, so she does not need to see the gynecologist anymore.

(C) The peak incidence for cervical cancer is 28 to 30 years.

(D) Her obesity places her at increased risk for developing cervical cancer.

(E) Pap smears pick up endometrial and ovarian cancer too.

118. She goes on to tell you that her mother developed breast cancer at age 52 and that she has three aunts with breast cancer. She had heard about a drug, tamoxifen, that is supposed to decrease the risk of breast cancer but increase the risk of endometrial cancer. You tell her which of the following?

(A) Tamoxifen has been seen in retrospective studies to decrease the incidence of breast cancer by as much as 90%.

(B) It doubles the risk of uterine cancer.

(C) It increases the risk of arterial thrombosis.

(D) The benefits of taking it outweigh the risks for women under 55.

(E) It decreases the risk of coronary artery disease in postmenopausal women.

119. A 65-year-old Native American woman presents with a history of intermittent bouts of right upper quadrant abdominal pain associated with having eaten fatty meals. She cur-

rently has some mild right upper quadrant tenderness. Her vital signs are stable. She is afebrile. Her laboratory studies disclose only mildly elevated transaminases. You obtain an x-ray of her abdomen that shows a calcified gallbladder wall. Which of the following statements is correct?

(A) Sigmoidoscopy should be the next diagnostic test.

(B) A CT myelogram should be the next diagnostic test.

(C) She has a significantly increased risk of having carcinoma of the gallbladder.

(D) The x-ray and CT scan demonstrate evidence of cholelithiasis.

(E) Cholecystectomy is not indicated at this time.

120. Having an established infection with which of the following organisms increases the risk of acquiring HIV from an infected partner?

(A) human papillomavirus (HPV)

(B) *Mycobacterium tuberculosis*

(C) *Neisseria gonorrhoeae*

(D) *Pneumocystis carinii*

(E) herpes simplex virus-2

121. You are a county public health director in a region of the state that is experiencing an epizootic of rabies affecting the racoon population. The disease spread through the region south of you last year, killing approximately 80% of the racoon population in one year. (See Figure 4.9.) What should you do to prevent human rabies in your area?

(A) Immunize all susceptible individuals living in rural locations.

(B) Advise residents to avoid swimming in lakes where racoons may drink.

(C) Sponsor free rabies vaccination clinics for pets.

(D) Ask residents to report any sighting of a dead racoon to the animal control officer.

(E) Restrict access to public parks after dusk.

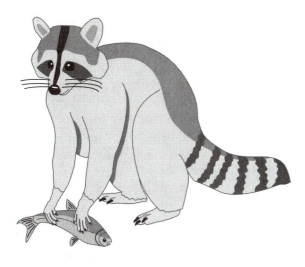

Figure 4.9

122. A 38-year-old patient (P2002) is admitted in active labor. She previously delivered a 4000-g fetus without difficulty. The fetus has an estimated weight of 4800 g. A protraction disorder of labor is diagnosed. The baby is in a right occiput posterior position. The patient has pushed for 3 hours. Heavy molding is present. The caput is at +1/5 station. Clinical pelvimetry performed early in labor was consistent with a clinically adequate android pelvis. The recommendation for the management of this patient should be

(A) expectant management with oxytocin augmentation
(B) outlet forceps delivery
(C) low forceps delivery
(D) midpelvic forceps delivery
(E) cesarean section

Questions 123 and 124

A 64-year-old woman presents to your office requesting a referral to a dermatologist because of some unsightly, brown, thickened skin in her axillae. She denies any other problems and is on no medication apart from a multivitamin and calcium, 1000 mg daily.

123. You recommend which of the following?

(A) no intervention at this time
(B) a corticosteroid cream
(C) an antifungal cream
(D) a plastic surgeon instead of a dermatologist
(E) mammogram; pelvic exam; blood studies; CT scan of chest, abdomen, and pelvis

124. On initial blood studies, you find that the patient has a mild elevation in her fasting blood sugar. She wants to know if additional studies are really necessary. You answer

(A) yes, because diabetes is not associated with this skin condition
(B) yes, because although diabetes can cause this, an underlying malignancy is more common
(C) yes, because she is overdue for her CT scan, which is recommended every 2 years for women over 50
(D) no, diabetes explains the whole problem
(E) no, because the CT contrast can cause renal failure in diabetics

125. The two MOST common complications of macrosomia are

(A) postpartum hemorrhage and shoulder dystocia
(B) cesarean section and neonatal hypoglycemia
(C) genital tract laceration and shoulder dystocia
(D) antepartum hemorrhage and shoulder dystocia
(E) lower uterine segment laceration and neonatal intracranial hemorrhage

Questions 126 and 127

A 42-year-old woman presents to her gynecologist with complaints of abdominal bloating and irregular menstrual periods. On physical examination, she has a bulky mass in her right pelvis, which is mobile. There is shifting dullness. Laboratory evaluation reveals an alpha-fetoprotein level of 2, beta-human chorionic gonadotropin of 10, and a CA 125 of 312.

126. Which of the following is true about this patient's disease?

    (A) Seventy percent of patients present with stage I disease.
    (B) There tends to be discomfort early on because of twisting of the infundibulo-pelvic ligament.
    (C) The CA 125 is the gold standard in evaluating pelvic masses.
    (D) The patient should have a laparoscopic evaluation of the pelvic mass.
    (E) Ultrasound is the preferred staging radiologic test because of its sensitivity in imaging the pelvic structures.

127. Which of the following is true regarding surgery in this patient?

    (A) With advanced stage disease, surgical evaluation only delays the institution of very effective chemotherapy.
    (B) Most explorations of this disease can be done by gynecologists with minimal experience.
    (C) Surgery increases the risk of blood-borne spread, but the advantages to debulking outweigh the complications.
    (D) Cytoreduction (debulking) of these patients improves survival.
    (E) CA 125 levels are useful for initial diagnosis but are not helpful in follow-up.

Questions 128 and 129

A 40-year-old man is taken to the operating room for an acute abdomen. On exploration, he is found to have a 3-cm mass involving the mesenteric border of the terminal ileum, with a desmoplastic reaction involving the surrounding mesentery. A small portion of the small bowel appears tethered and ischemic. No evidence exists of liver metastases. He undergoes a small bowel resection of the distal ileum and a right hemicolectomy. The final pathologic report demonstrates carcinoid tumor, with several positive lymph nodes.

128. All of the following statements are true regarding carcinoid tumor EXCEPT

    (A) this location of tumor can present a picture similar to Crohn's disease
    (B) the small bowel is the second most common location for carcinoid tumors
    (C) tumor growth is generally slow
    (D) the correct surgical management is to resect all tumor possible
    (E) obstruction secondary to luminal encroachment is common

129. All of the following statements are true regarding carcinoid syndrome EXCEPT

    (A) the major clinical manifestations are flushing and diarrhea
    (B) metastases are rare
    (C) serotonin levels and urinary 5-hydroxyindolacetic acid (5-HIAA) are abnormally elevated
    (D) treatment is directed at relief of symptoms
    (E) octreotide can be effective at suppressing some of the symptoms

Questions 130 and 131

130. In which of the following species is rabies endemic in the United States?

    (A) dogs
    (B) white-tailed deer
    (C) groundhogs
    (D) bats
    (E) red squirrels

131. Which of the following is a prominent feature of advanced rabies?

    (A) paralysis of the hind legs
    (B) photophobia, leading to avoidance of bright lights
    (C) bleeding from mucosal surfaces
    (D) convulsions
    (E) fetid odor

DIRECTIONS (Questions 132 through 142): Each group of items in this section consists of lettered headings followed by a set of numbered words or phrases. For each numbered word or phrase, select the ONE lettered heading that is most closely associated with it. Each lettered heading may be selected once, more than once, or not at all.

Questions 132 Through 136

Match the side effects with the medication.

    (A) alprazolam
    (B) dextroamphetamine
    (C) fluoxetine
    (D) haloperidol
    (E) lithium
    (F) nortriptyline
    (G) phenelzine
    (H) thioridazine
    (I) trazodone
    (J) valproic acid

132. Priapism

133. Sedation greater than risk of dystonia

134. Acute dystonia

135. Arrhythmias

136. Tyramine-induced hypertensive crisis

Questions 137 and 138

    (A) weight
    (B) bilirubin
    (C) both
    (D) neither

137. In the first 3 days of postnatal life, which could rise?

138. In the breast-fed infant, which could rise in the first 3 weeks?

Questions 139 Through 142

    (A) decreased fremitus, low diaphragms, prolonged expiration
    (B) absent fremitus, hyperresonance, absent breath sounds
    (C) decreased fremitus, tracheal shift away from the affected side, flat percussion, absent breath sounds
    (D) decreased fremitus, tracheal shift toward the affected side, dull or flat percussion, absent breath sounds
    (E) increased fremitus, dull to percussion, bronchophony

139. Atelectasis

140. Complete pneumothorax

141. Acute asthmatic attack

142. Lobar pneumonia

DIRECTIONS (Questions 143 through 145): The following set of matching questions in this section consists of a list of lettered options followed by several numbered items. For each numbered item, select the appropriate lettered options. Each lettered option may be selected once, more than once, or not at all.

(A) a true allergic reaction
(B) may be mediated by drug effect on kinin system
(C) skin rash is most likely manifestation
(D) predictive skin test available
(E) final mediator of symptoms are leukotrienes
(F) desensitization is feasible
(G) may be more common in women and African Americans
(H) never fatal

143. A 23-year-old man has a reaction after being given oral penicillin for a sore throat. (Select FOUR)

144. A 56-year-old woman is given an angiotensin-converting enzyme (ACE) inhibitor for control of hypertension and develops a reaction. (Select TWO)

145. A 23-year-old man has an exacerbation of asthma when he takes aspirin for a headache. (Select TWO)

DIRECTIONS (Questions 146 Through 150): Each group of items in this section consists of lettered headings followed by a set of numbered words or phrases. For each numbered word or phrase, select

A if the item is associated with (A) *only*,
B if the item is associated with (B) *only*,
C if the item is associated with *both* (A) *and* (B),
D if the item is associated with *neither* (A) *nor* (B).

(A) measles
(B) rubella
(C) both
(D) neither

146. A single attack confers lifelong immunity.

147. Complications may include keratoconjunctivitis, pneumonia, and encephalitis.

148. Transient polyarthritis is a common manifestation among children.

149. Infection during pregnancy may result in a newborn with deafness, congenital heart disease, cataracts, and retardation.

150. An enanthem may be present.

Answers and Explanations

1. **(C)** The x-ray findings in Figures 4.1 and 4.2 are consistent with a small bowel obstruction. Dilated loops of small bowel with air fluid levels are present on the upright films. In addition, colonic gas is absent. If a colonic obstruction is present, there should be colonic distention. No evidence exists of a pneumoperitoneum, which would be evident on the upright films and would indicate a perforated viscus. If the obstruction does not resolve, the patient will require exploratory laparotomy.

2. **(C)** Bowel stimulants are contraindicated in obstruction and usually of no use in cases of ileus. Distention and dilated loops of bowel are common to both ileus and bowel obstruction. Bowel obstruction is treated by operation if it does not resolve spontaneously; ileus is not usually treated operatively. Tinkling bowel sounds are characteristic of early bowel obstruction before the onset of ischemia. Rushes may also be heard and coincide with crampy pain. As ischemia and infarction progress, bowel sounds decrease. Periods of pain, interspersed with relatively pain-free times, is the definition of colic and characteristic of obstruction.

3. **(E)** A small bowel obstruction is most commonly secondary to adhesions from previous abdominal surgery. An incarcerated external hernia is the next most likely cause, followed by neoplasm. Volvulus and intussusception are less common causes of a small bowel obstruction.

4. **(B)** More than 2 days after fetal death, brain liquefaction occurs and the fetal skull bones overlap (Spalding sign). Exaggerated fetal spine curvature is often demonstrable. Gas in the great vessels, a very specific sign, occurs rarely. Movements of the fetus secondary to maternal movement must be distinguished from fetal spontaneous movements. The amniotic fluid eventually becomes a turbid reddish-brown color.

5. **(C)** The risk of DIC for this patient, who does have not any other DIC risk factors, is very low but never zero. Most patients with an IUFD will go into spontaneous labor 2 to 3 weeks after fetal death. Only 6% of all patients with IUFD will develop a coagulopathy (1 to 2% will be severe). The vast majority of these develop after the fourth week.

6. **(D)** Erythema chronicum migrans is the unique clinical marker for Lyme disease, a tick-borne spirochetal illness. The rash (when it occurs, which is not all the time) begins as a red macule or papule at the site of the tick bite. As the area of redness expands, there is often central clearing. Dermatophytosis of the trunk (tinea corporis) can be caused by several species of *Trichophyton* and result in annular, inflamed patches with elevated scaling and, at times, vesicular borders with a tendency for central clearing. Nummular eczema does not have a definitive cause, although dry skin or underlying infections may play a role. It manifests by coin-shaped patches on the extensor areas of the extremities or trunk. The most common cutaneous

manifestations of a drug reaction are hives or morbiliform rashes, although lesions similar in appearance to erythema migrans can occur. Sporotrichosis occurs at a site of inoculation, usually on the foot, hand, or arm. The most common form begins as a hard, nontender, subcutaneous nodule.

7. **(D)** Each of the listed illnesses are tick-borne except for pediculosis, which is a louse-borne disease.

8. **(D)** Acrodermatitis chronica atrophicans is a chronic skin lesion associated with late (years later) Lyme disease. It is rare in the United States, though common in Europe. It appears as violaceous, infiltrated plaques or nodules that eventually atrophy. It is most common on extensor surfaces. The typical rash is not a diffuse, maculopapular rash but multiple annular lesions. Vasculitis and hematuria are not seen.

9. **(B)** Doxycycline and amoxicillin are considered by most physicians to be the drugs of choice for the treatment of Lyme disease. Trimethoprim–sulfamethoxazole is ineffective in the treatment of Lyme disease. Ibuprofen may help the joint aches but does nothing for the infection. Prednisone also fails to treat the underlying problem, although it may appear to make the rash better.

10–12. **(10-E, 11-A, 12-A)** All of the conditions listed would be considered in the differential in this case, except chronic, nonspecific diarrhea of infancy, which does not cause failure to thrive. Decreased appetite is more a feature of the disease than increased appetite. It is essential in this condition that the diagnosis be confirmed by biopsy, because the treatment (proper diet) is lifelong. Wheat, rye, oats, and barley should be eliminated. These patients are allowed to have corn in their diet. Steroids have no place in the treatment of this disorder. Fat-soluble vitamins K and D may be needed. Symptoms should improve within weeks, with improvement in ir-

ritability within days. Normal weight may be reached within 6 months.

13. **(E)** The patient's symptoms are consistent with those caused by compression of the median nerve. Up to 25% of pregnant women will have at least occasional symptoms of median nerve compression. In a large study of 2400 patients, diagnoses were verified in 2.3%. It is more common closer to term. The symptoms improve with simple wrist splinting at night as well as decreased inciting activity (keyboard operation). Approximately 80% of patients will have bilateral involvement. If the symptoms persist, further evaluation is appropriate.

14. **(D)** Terbutaline and ritodrine are beta-2-adrenergic receptor agonists. The stimulation of the beta-2 receptor, which is dominant in the myometrium, blood vessels, and bronchi, results in relaxation of the affected muscle. Ritodrine is approved by the Food and Drug Administration (FDA) for use in preterm labor. Uterine tocolysis appears to be transient because of beta-adrenergic receptor desensitization. Magnesium sulfate is commonly used for tocolysis.

15. **(D)** A patient with a significant postoperative ileus is generally disinterested in food. Hypokalemia, hypomagnesemia, sigificant intraperitoneal inflammation, and opioid medications are predisposing factors to the development of a postoperative ileus.

16. **(C)** Ileus is usually a reflection of the postoperative state or a metabolic abnormality. Correction of the underlying cause will result in its resolution. Bowel stimulants are usually ineffective in cases of ileus.

17. **(E)** The standard treatment of ileus is to stop all oral intake, give intravenous fluid, institute nasogastric suction, and correct any electrolyte imbalances. Operative therapy is usually not necessary.

18. **(A)** Linear streaks are very typical of poison ivy, and the recent hike in the woods assists

in the diagnosis as well. Chickenpox, or varicella, begins on the body and spreads to the extremities. It is also not linear. Lyme disease begins with a circular rash (erythema marginatum).

19. **(D)** Type IV cell-mediated reaction is also known as delayed-type hypersensitivity reaction. Contact allergies are the prototype of these reactions (poison ivy, graft–host reaction, tuberculosis reactivity). This reaction results from antigen interaction with sensitized thymus-derived lymphocytes.

20. **(C)** Anti-Sm detects a protein complexed to six species of small nuclear ribonucleic acid (RNA). It is felt to be very specific for systemic lupus erythematous (SLE). However, only 30% of patients have a positive test. In the case presented, there are enough clinical criteria to confirm the diagnosis of SLE with 98% specificity. The most sensitive test is the ANA, which is positive in 98% of patients with SLE.

21. **(C)** About 95% of patients will develop musculoskeletal symptoms during the course of SLE. Arthralgias and myalgias predominate, but arthritis, hand deformities, myopathy, and avascular necrosis of bone can occur. About 85% of patients will have hematologic disease, and 80% will have skin manifestations.

22. **(A)** Pericarditis, sometimes leading to tamponade, is the most common manifestation of cardiac disease. Myocarditis does occur and can cause arrhythmias, sudden death, or heart failure. Libman–Sachs endocarditis is associated with thrombotic events or, less commonly, valvular regurgitation. Myocardial infarction is more commonly a result of atherosclerotic heart disease than vasculitis.

23. **(B)** Cytoid bodies are a diagnostically helpful ophthalmic finding in SLE. Cytoid bodies are white exudates in the retina. As they indicate a retinal vasculitis that can lead to blindness, aggressive immunosuppression should be instituted.

24. **(D)** Renal damage is generally secondary to deposition of circulating immune complexes. The presence of high titer anti-ds deoxyribonucleic acid (DNA), persistently abnormal urinalysis, and low complement increases the risk of severe nephritis. Although most patients have immunoglobulin deposition in the glomeruli, only half develop clinical nephritis. Some patterns of involvement, mesangial or mild focal proliferative nephritis, have a good prognosis. Rapidly deteriorating renal function with an abnormal urine sediment mandates urgent treatment, but not necessarily urgent biopsy.

25. **(E)** If a statistically significant difference is not found between two treatments, there has been a failure to reject the null hypothesis. It should be noted that failing to reject the null hypothesis is not the same as accepting the null hypothesis. In statistical science, it is never possible to accept the null hypothesis.

26. **(D)** Most patients with acute, severe lung injury have multiple causes. This patient has sepsis, fluid overload, and preeclampsia as potential etiologies. Additionally, other etiologies include shock, trauma, and aspiration. A PO_2 of less than 50 with an FiO_2 greater than 0.60 and decreased respiratory compliance with shunting are commonly found in the presence of ARDS. Management is directed at oxygenation and correcting the inciting causes—in this case, sepsis and fluid overload. Mechanical ventilation with varying manipulations may be necessary.

27. **(D)** The x-ray shows bilateral hilar adenopathy. The x-ray picture and spontaneous resolution of the abnormalities are most consistent with a diagnosis of sarcoidosis. Sarcoidosis has been reported to occur in African Americans with a higher frequency than Caucasians. Organ involvement is usually asymptomatic, and the disease most frequently regresses spontaneously, although progression to debilitating disease can occur. The etiology is unknown.

28. (C) Erythema nodosum may be associated with sarcoidosis as a secondary vasculitic reaction. Sarcoid granulomas also occur directly in the skin to produce a variety of small, asymptomatic macular and papular lesions that are present either superficially or more deeply in the dermis. Lupus pernio, consisting of violaceous plaques over the nose, cheeks, and ears, is the most commonly described skin lesion and may be disfiguring.

29. (A) Sarcoid is treated with corticosteroids if spontaneous regression does not occur or if the symptoms are significant. The minimum amount is used. Chloroquine is useful in treating chronic mucocutaneous sarcoidosis. When patients develop chronic fibrocystic sarcoidosis, they can get colonization of the cyst with *Aspergillus.* Hemoptysis is a significant problem. It can be treated with antibiotics to control the bacterial infection of the cysts, which can precipitate the bleeding. Occasionally, embolization of the dilated bronchial arteries, which supply the inflamed areas of the lung, is necessary to control the bleeding. Surgery is reserved for only the most difficult situations.

30. (A) The edema of caput succedaneum usually disappears within the first few days of life and requires no specific therapy. It may extend across the midline or across suture lines. The scalp may show mild bruising.

31. (C) The constellation of complaints and physical findings is most consistent with the diagnosis of infectious mononucleosis. In most cases, this is caused by primary Epstein–Barr virus (EBV) infection. Although this infection occurs during the first decade of life in less developed countries, among middle and higher socioeconomic groups in industrialized countries, primary infection occurs in the adolescent and postadolescent groups, usually as a result of close contact. Rashes occur significantly more often if ampicillin is given to a patient with acute EBV infection, but they are not usually vesicular in nature, as is the rash of varicella infection. Recurrent strep infection of the throat

is not usually accompanied by hepatosplenomegaly and does not give a highly positive heterophile test (which is 95% specific and 95% sensitive in the adolescent population). Acute HIV infection can certainly cause a mono-like syndrome and should always be part of your differential. However, it should be suspected if the heterophile is negative, or positive only at a low level. The incubation period for hepatitis B (assuming the patient has an illness similar to his girlfriend's) is too long to be the cause of his complaints.

32. (A) Specific serologic testing for EBV infection involves measuring antibodies to latently infected (anti-EBNA), early replication cycle (anti-EA), or late replication cycle (anti-VCA) viral proteins, usually by enzyme-linked immunoassay or indirect immunofluorescence microscopy. With acute primary infection, EA and IgM VCA titers are high, and EBNA and IgG VCA titers are low. Patients recovering from recent primary infection have lower IgM VCA or EA titers, a low EBNA tier, and a higher IgG VCA titer. After several months, IgM VCA and EA titers are low or negative, but EBNA and IgG VCA titers are high.

33. (C) No treatment is necessary for most cases of infectious mononucleosis. Rest during the acute symptomatic period and gradual return to normal activities as tolerated are advised. Patients with splenomegaly should restrict their involvement in sports until the spleen returns to normal size, as they run the risk of traumatic rupture. The patient's signs and symptoms are consistent with intra-abdominal bleeding, and his spleen must be removed immediately.

34. (A) Trisomy 18 is one of the more frequent chromosomal abnormalities associated with a single umbilical artery. About one third of these infants are found to have congenital abnormalities that may involve the genitourinary tract. The rate of twins is 35 per 1000.

35. **(D)** Breast cancer occurs in approximately 1 of 4000 pregnancies. Pregnancy does not significantly influence the natural history of breast cancer. Survival in both the pregnant and nonpregnant populations is stage dependent. Any suspicious mass in the breast should be promptly evaluated with mammography and fine-needle aspiration. Others will recommend open biopsy. The value of mammography is diminished because of the increased density of the breast. The radiation associated with the mammography is not in a teratogenic range. Fine-needle aspiration is both sensitive and specific. If breast cancer is diagnosed, surgical therapy should not be delayed. Chemotherapy in selected cases may be given during pregnancy.

36. **(B)** *Chlamydia trachomatis* is the most common sexually transmitted pathogen. In men, it typically presents with odorless penile discharge and in women is often asymptomatic. Gonorrhea's presentation is similar, but it is less common. In trichomoniasis, the discharge is apt to be malodorous, and the female partners would probably have had symptomatic vaginitis. The other infections listed present with skin lesions, rather than discharge. (See Figures 4.10 and 4.11.)

37. **(D)** *Chlamydia* can be treated with doxycycline, tetracycline, erythromycin, or azithromycin. Penicillin is the drug of choice for syphilis and gonorrhea (though drug resistance is a problem). Acyclovir is an antiviral drug used to treat herpes. Metronidazole and tinidazole are both used in treating trichomoniasis.

38. **(E)** Female infertility secondary to fallopian tube scarring from chronic salpingitis is a serious sequela of chlamydial infections. If a neonate is exposed to *Chlamydia* during birth, visual impairment can result from conjunctivitis, not uveitis. Neurologic and cardiac complications are seen in late-stage syphilis. Chronic persistent hepatitis can be caused by hepatitis B, another sexually transmitted infection.

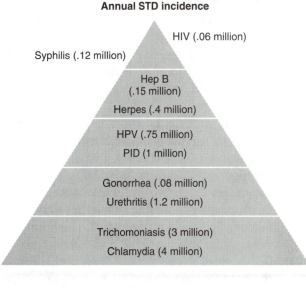

Figure 4.10

39. **(A)** Koro is a nonpsychotic hysterical reaction that occurs in Southeast Asia in epidemic form. Men may complain that their penises are retracting into their abdomens. It is a good example of a culture-bound psychiatric disorder. Antisocial personality disorder is characterized by a pervasive pattern of disregard for and violation of the rights of others, beginning by age 15. Alcohol intoxication and amphetamine intoxication cause multiple

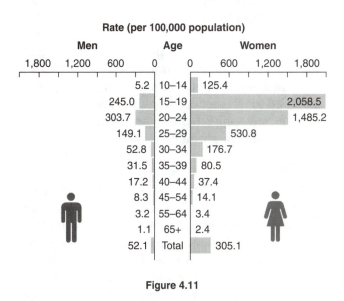

Figure 4.11

symptoms rather than a single, well-defined delusion. This man does not have an amphetamine-induced psychotic disorder, with delusions, or paranoid schizophrenia, which present similarly, because he has a single discrete delusion with no other symptoms.

40. **(D)** It is important for the psychiatric interviewer to establish rapport with the patient and to give the patient a chance to answer open-ended questions. Also, it is important not to feel defensive while interviewing or to insult a patient, causing him or her to become defensive.

41. **(B)** A smear will show a predominance of eosinophils, and a good history and physical will elicit many of the characteristic signs.

42. **(A)** Failure rates from lowest to highest: injectable progestins, combination birth control pills, progestin-only pills, IUD, condom, diaphragm, spermicide, withdrawal, periodic rhythmic abstinence, douche, chance.

43. **(D)** The major advantages of injectable progestins are effectiveness and convenience. Disadvantages are prolonged irregular bleeding and anovulation after discontinuation; thus, they would not be a good choice for this 39-year-old who hopes to achieve pregnancy in the near future. The risk of thromboembolism is equal to that for oral combination contraceptives.

44. **(E)** Heavy smoking, particularly over age 35, is an absolute contraindication. Additional contraindications include pregnancy, suspected breast cancer, hepatic neoplasm, thrombophlebitis, and so forth. The others are relative contraindications.

45. **(D)** This patient is exhibiting many of the signs of major depressive disorder: subjective depressed mood, inability to sleep, loss of appetite, diminished concentration, feelings of self-worthlessness, and guilt. However, because there is an identifiable life just before the onset of symptoms, the Diagnostic and Statistical Manual, 4th edition (DSM-IV) sug-

gests a diagnosis of adjustment disorder. For such a diagnosis, symptoms must appear within 3 months of the stressor and subside within 6 months of the event. However, this patient is only 4 months from the event, so the most appropriate diagnosis is adjustment disorder, depressive type. She is not exhibiting a manic symptomatology, and a diagnosis of bipolar disorder would be inappropriate without such a history. Similarly, while she is potentially abusing benzodiazepines, and this is an issue which should be discussed during the session, DSM-IV allows the diagnosis of benzodiazepine dependence only in the absence of another mental disorder that could better explain the symptoms.

46. **(D)** Studies of psychopharmacological or biological intervention in adjustment disorder have provided disappointing results. Supportive psychotherapy has been shown to help a large number of patients.

47. **(A)** Now that the patient's symptoms have lasted more than 6 months after her stressor, and have actually worsened, she should now be diagnosed with major depression and treated accordingly.

48. **(E)** Although administration of a selective serotonin reuptake inhibitor (SSRI) such as fluoxetine might be beneficial, the most important first step is determination of the patient's suicidal ideation and potential planning. Patients must always be asked if they have thought of hurting themselves, especially in the setting of depression. Until such an assessment is made, hospitalization cannot be entertained. Electroconvulsive therapy is usually reserved for those patients who fail trials of antidepressant medications and psychotherapy. Haloperidol is not indicated, because the patient has no obvious psychotic symptoms.

49. **(A)** The AIDS epidemic in New York and many other urban centers in the United States is intimately linked to intravenous drug use. The primary routes of disease

transmission are sharing of contaminated "works" (syringes, needles, etc.) *and* sexual contact between intravenous drug users and others, often in exchange for drugs or to earn money to buy drugs. In San Francisco, the epidemic is more closely associated with homosexual transmission among men who have sex with men. In third world cities, such as Kampala and Manila, heterosexual transmission is the primary mode of spread. (See Figure 4.12.)

50. **(B)** AIDS Clinical Trial Group Study 076 demonstrated the effectiveness of zidovudine therapy during pregnancy, delivery, and the neonatal period, to prevent mother-to-child HIV transmission. Prevention of blood-product transmission depends on donor screening and testing the blood supply. Breast milk transmission is best prevented by using artificial baby milk ("formula") rather than breast feeding. Prevention of transmission following occupational exposure involves use of multiple drugs, including protease inhibitors.

51. **(D)** The patient's mildly elevated total T_4 and low T_3 resin uptake are consistent with the increased quantity of thyroid-binding globulin in pregnancy. The patient's free T_4, or calculated free thyroxin index, is within the normal range. Her sensitive TSH is also within normal range. The patient should be observed for the development of signs or symptoms of thyrotoxicosis. Propylthiouracil is the medication of choice for the treatment of active thyrotoxicosis during pregnancy.

52. **(B)** The most likely kinds of foods to harbor high concentrations of bacteria are those that are high in protein and are inadequately cooked or left at room temperature prior to serving. The iced tea meets neither of those criteria. The omelets were cooked immediately prior to being served, and cooking kills bacteria; however, they may have been undercooked. The fruit compote, sorbet, and coffee cake are low-protein foods, relatively unlikely to promote bacterial growth. (See Figure 4.13 on page 158.)

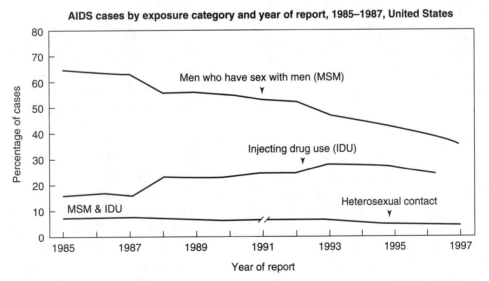

Figure 4.12

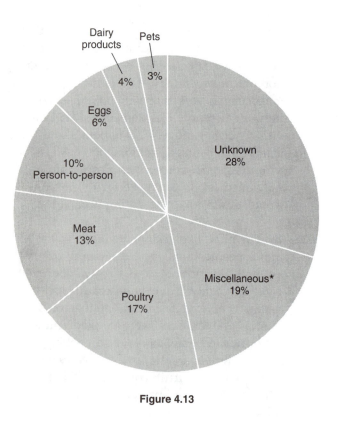

Dairy
products   Pets

4%   3%

Eggs
6%

Unknown
28%

10%
Person-to-person

Meat
13%

Miscellaneous*
19%

Poultry
17%

Figure 4.13

53. **(C)** *Salmonella* strains are frequent causes of food-borne gastroenteritis, and eggs are frequently infected with *Salmonella* despite heavy use of antibiotics in the poultry industry. *V. cholerae* is generally water-borne and leads to profuse, watery diarrhea. *V. parahaemolyticus* is most often associated with seafood contamination. *Shigella* causes bloody diarrhea. *Giardia lamblia* is associated with chronic diarrhea and is typically transmitted by person-to-person contact or through contaminated water.

54. **(E)** Staphylococcal food poisoning is caused by heat-stable enterotoxins, and the clinical course is characterized by abrupt onset of severe gastrointestinal symptoms soon after eating: nausea, crampy abdomial pain, vomiting, and diarrhea. The attack rate is generally high, but we have no information about food-specific attack rates in this case.

55. **(B)** This is a typical presentation of meningococcal meningitis, with meningococcemia leading to the purpuric rash. Children and

young adults are more susceptible than older people. Outbreaks are relatively common in groups of young adults living in close proximity (eg, in college dormitories or military bases). Pneumococcal and *H. influenzae* meningitis are uncommon in young adults, the former occurring primarily in infants and the elderly and the latter in young children. Coxsackievirus is a frequent cause of aseptic meningitis, often associated with a maculopapular or vesicular rash. Purpuric lesions are not typical of coxsackievirus infections. Cryptococcal meningitis presents less acutely than the case described, and it most frequently affects immunocompromised individuals.

56. **(D)** Rifampin prophylaxis is indicated for close contacts of the index case, and the college and local health care providers should be vigilant for additional cases. After only one case, however, more extreme outbreak control measures are not yet warranted. If there were a more widespread outbreak on campus, group travel to other campuses should be restricted to avoid broadening the epidemic, and all susceptible individuals should be immunized if the strain of meningitis is one covered by the meningococcal vaccine (primarily serogroups A and C). Screening for carriers is not worthwhile, because nasopharyngeal colonization with *N. meningitidis* is very widespread (often greater than 25%) and does not indicate risk of infection. Extra chlorination in the college swimming pool is unlikely to affect the course of an infection that is spread by person-to-person respiratory contact.

57. **(B)** The nitrazine test is a pH test only. It is not specific for amniotic fluid. If the pH of the vaginal pool is greater than 6.5, there is a presumption that the membranes are ruptured. Other bodily fluids, including blood, semen, and infected urine, are associated with a pH above 6.5. Soaps are also associated with a very alkaline pH. If the patient has not had a cervical examination in the preceding 48 hours, bloody show or the passage of a few drops of blood or blood-tinged mu-

cus predictably precedes the onset of labor by up to a few days. Patients who have had a cervical examination performed may pass their mucous plug or have bloody show and not go promptly into labor.

58. **(A)** Braxton–Hicks contractions commonly occur late in pregnancy. The greatest significance of these is that a patient may confuse early preterm labor with Braxton–Hicks contractions and discount the preterm labor. The Braxton–Hicks contractions represent a normal transient contractility of the uterus. They are neither rhythmic nor progressive. The uterus begins contracting as early as the first trimester. These incoordinate contractions do not result in any cervical change. The contractions of active labor are regular, increasing in strength and duration, with progressive cervical dilatation.

59. **(A)** The combination of an African-American woman and iron-resistant microcytic anemia should make alpha-thalassemia come to mind. Single alpha gene deletions are very prevalent in this population. While compliance with oral iron is notoriously low, the fact that she has a normal RDW (usually elevated in iron deficiency), combined with a very low MCV, makes iron deficiency less likely, although certainly a ferritin should be performed to evaluate the possibility. Beta-thalassemia minor will have an abnormal hemoglobin electrophoresis.

60. **(A)** Single gene deletions are very common and may approach 80% in some populations. Double gene deletions are not unusual and are of two types in the sense that patients can have two genes deleted with very different implications for reproduction. The single gene deletion is more common in African patients, whereas the doubly deleted gene is more often seen in Asians. This makes hemoglobin H or hydrops fetalis rare in Africans. Cord blood testing is available, and hemoglobin Bart's is elevated even in alpha-thalassemia–trait patients in the perinatal period. All menstruating women are prone to iron deficiency, and with the complicating

presence of the thalassemia, one cannot rely on the MCV or hemoglobin to make the diagnosis. Therefore, periodic ferritin levels are probably indicated, especially now that recent studies suggest detrimental effects of iron deficiency on the body before anemia develops.

61. **(D)** Life stressors that may affect treatment and outcome are axis IV, and the GAF is axis V.

62. **(A)** Alcohol hallucinosis is defined as a condition of vivid auditory or visual hallucinations that develop within a few days of reduction or cessation of drinking in a physiologically dependent person. Delusions are not a prominent feature of the disorder.

63. **(A)** Amphetamine-induced psychotic disorder with delusions develops following recent use of a sympathomimetic drug. It apparently does not develop following a single large dose unless such a dose is preceded by chronic use. The syndrome develops rapidly, and persecutory delusions are the most common feature.

64. **(B)** The patient is severely disturbed, agitated, delusional, and has already proven himself a danger to others. Admission is crucial; treatment including antipsychotic medication should be instituted promptly.

65. **(E)** In general, to be found not responsible for criminal activity, it must be determined that at the time of such conduct, as a result of mental disease or defect, the patient lacked substantial capacity either to appreciate the wrongfulness of the conduct or to conform such conduct to the requirement of the law. Usually, states do not recognize substance-induced disorders as mental disease or defect. Competency to stand trial is an issue separate from criminal responsibility.

66. **(C)** Autosomal dominant inheritance indicates that the trait is not sex-linked. In a mating in which a parent passes either a normal or a mutant gene to the offspring and the cor-

responding genes derived from the other parent are normal, 50% of the children will be normal and 50% (male or female) will exhibit the trait.

67. **(B)** When a trial is controlled, the therapy studied is being compared to a different therapy that has a well-known effect on an illness. A trial that uses a negative control (frequently called a placebo-controlled trial) uses a control technique with no effect on the illness. A trial that compares the therapy being studied to an active therapy, usually the gold standard, is using a control technique with a positive effect on the illness and thus uses a positive control.

68. **(D)** Uterine fibroids most commonly present as increased menstrual bleeding (menorrhagia, more than 80 mL menstrual blood). Hypermenorrhea or menorrhagia can be caused by a variety of conditions. Spontaneous abortion should be ruled out, as a surgical treatment may be necessary. Coagulation factor deficiencies can cause significant menorrhagia, leading to severe anemia, particularly in a young woman. Anorexia nervosa leads to a premenarchal pattern of gonadotropin-releasing hormone (GnRH) release and amenorrhea.

69. **(C)** Leiomyomatosis peritonealis disseminata (LPD) is a rare but fortunately benign condition in which multiple small myomatous nodules are found over the surface of the pelvis and abdominal peritoneum. Grossly, thenodules mimic disseminated carcinoma but are histologically benign appearing. Intravenous leiomyomatosis is also another rare condition in which benign smooth muscle fibers invade the venous channels of the pelvis and even involve the vena cava and right heart.

70. **(C)** Malignant degeneration of a benign uterine fibroid to a sarcoma occurs in 0.3 to 0.7% of cases. Leiomyosarcoma is diagnosed in 3% of uterine malignancies. The number of mitotic figures per high-power field correlates to its severity.

71. **(B)** Priapism refers to a persistent erection of the penis, which is not associated with sexual desire. It results fom vaso-occlusion within the corpus cavernosum.

72. **(C)** The patient has sickle cell anemia, which is a common cause of priapism. It results from vaso-occlusion within the corpus cavernosum. Other vaso-occlusive clinical syndromes that may be associated with sickle cell anemia include cerebrovascular accidents, hepatic crises, acute chest syndrome, and acute renal papillary infarction.

73. **(C)** Common vaso-occlusive clinical syndromes include cerebrovascular accidents caused by involvement of the cerebral vasculature. There is no increase in the number of venous thromboses. Although not directly related to the sickling phenomenon, patients are at increased risk of developing infections and cholelithiasis (caused by chronic hemolysis leading to increased bilirubin production), but not renal stones. Childhood infections with encapsulated organisms, such as *Haemophilus influenzae* and *Streptococcus pneumoniae*, are common. Although *Salmonella* occurs almost exclusively in this population, *Staphylococcus aureus* remains the most common cause of bone infections. Although there may be no overt sign of renal dysfunction, when studied, all patients with an S gene, even if only the trait, will have a concentration defect.

74. **(B)** Hydroxyurea increases the amount of hemoglobin F in some patients, which has been associated with a milder course and fewer painful crises. Its effects are also seen without a demonstrable increase in hemoglobin F, but the etiology of this is unclear. Beginning treatment of painful crises at inception with oral fluids, antibiotics if indicated, and oral analgesics including narcotics can significantly decrease hospitalizations for pain crises but does not decrease their frequency. Control of chronic pain may decrease hospitalizations and will certainly improve the quality of his life. Demerol has been used in the past to manage sickle crisis pain, but mul-

tiple studies have shown the use of morphine, especially by PCA device, to be superior in control of pain, incidence of side effects, and duration of hospital stay.

75. (E) The signs and symptoms described are characteristic of none of the items noted. The neurologic findings are most suggestive of brain stem pathology. There is evidence of pyramidal tract and cerebral pathway involvement, as well as cranial nerve involvement. A computed tomography (CT) scan is performed, revealing a brain stem glioma, a tumor constituting about 10% of intracranial childhood tumors.

76. (A) The abdominal x-ray demonstrates pneumobilia. A cholecystoenteric fistula has direct communication between the biliary tract and the bowel lumen; therefore, it would not be unusual to see air in the biliary tree. The other choices listed do not explain why air would be in the biliary tree.

77. (D) The ileum is the narrowest portion of the intestines and, thus, the most frequent site of gallstone ileus.

78–80. (78-A, 79-B, 80-B) The case presented is that of a child with Reye syndrome, which is associated with outbreaks of influenza, especially B; varicella; and use of aspirin. It is important to have a high index of suspicion for the disease. Diagnosis can be made through clinical observations of level of consciousness, and an abnormal liver profile and serum ammonia levels will be found early in the process. A liver biopsy is helpful but not essential. Early support, including administration of vitamin K, treating intracranial pressure, and avoidance of hypoglycemia, can be lifesaving. The disorder can result in coma or death and is not "self-limited."

81. (D) Postmenopausal patients with vulvar lesions self-medicate or are treated with topical agents by physicians prior to the determination of a diagnosis. A simple office biopsy will under most circumstances be diagnostic. A wide local excision is not wrong but does

introduce delay. The magnification of the colposcope may facilitate the biopsy, but it is not necessary. A Pap smear may be performed in addition to the biopsy. Although this patient has a concurrent yeast infection, an alternative diagnosis for the vulvar lesion must be sought. Preinvasive lesions occur in the sixth decade and invasion is diagnosed in the seventh. Most vulvar carcinomas are found by the patient because of mass, pruritus, or bleeding.

82. (B) Excision of the lesion and involved nodes is performed, as well as assessment of local and distant areas of spread. The International Federation of Gynecology and Obstetrics (FIGO) system uses T, M, and N levels to describe the lesions and assign the stage. Approximately 50% of patients present with stage I or II disease. Advanced disease is diagnosed with chest x-ray, IVP, cystoscopy, barium enema, or proctosigmoidoscopy.

83. (B) Surgery is the primary therapy; however, the extent of surgery is individualized to optimize survival against the morbidity of radical surgery. Stage I–II carcinoma of the vulva is typically treated with either radical hemivulvectomy with ipsilateral node dissection or radical vulvectomy with bilateral superficial and deep inguinal node dissection. Preoperative radiation to the vulva and regional lymph nodes is used for locally advanced disease prior to excision of residual disease. Adjuvant chemotherapy is used for advanced metastatic disease with limited success.

84. (E) Insufficient accumulation of bone mass during skeletal growth predisposes to fractures later in life as age-related bone loss ensues. Although trauma can certainly cause fractures, it is the increased bone fragility that increases the risk of fracture in patients with osteoporosis. Height, weight, genetics, calcium intake during skeletal growth, exercise, and hormonal factors are all important in determining bone mass. Short women of Northern European descent tend to be at higher risk because their peak bone density is less. HRT significantly decreases the risk of fracture.

85. **(E)** Estrogen effectively reduces bone resorption, as do calcitonin and alendronate. Calcitonin therapy, now available as a nasal spray, must be accompanied by calcium therapy in order to prevent secondary hyperparathyroidism. Alendronate is a bisposphonate with once-a-day dosing but is contraindicated in patients with esophageal strictures and must be used with care in patients with reflux, gastritis, or peptic ulcers. Calcium, which may act by decreasing parathyroid hormone secretion, is a safe, well-tolerated, and inexpensive therapy. Vitamin D should be reserved for patients who show impairment of calcium absorption. The dose that increases calcium absorption is not much smaller than the dose that increases bone resorption.

86. **(B)** Initially, unopposed estrogen was used in the treatment of peri- and postmenopausal symptoms. This was associated with an increased risk of endometrial cancer. Currently, the use of combined estrogen and progesterone therapy appears to have eliminated the risk. HRT decreases the risk of osteoporosis, mitigates the psychological changes that accompany ovarian failure, decreases the risk of cardiovascular disease by 50%, and maintains the function of all estrogen-sensitive tissue such as the urethra.

87. **(E)** Studies looking at HRT and breast cancer are not conclusive. Some suggest an increased risk and some suggest no effect. Many earlier studies showing the risk used much higher doses of estrogen and progesterone than are commonly used now. However, with her family history, she is at high risk of cardiovascular disease and osteoporosis. Most clinicians would agree that the benefits for this patient outweigh the risks. Mammogram recommendations are in flux, but for patients over 50, a minimum of every other year is acceptable, while some people still recommend yearly. Doing screening mammograms more often than yearly is not recommended. A yearly breast exam by a physician and instruction in breast self-exam should be standard for all women.

88. **(C)** Her gynecologist should be alerted to the issue, but it is not an emergency. Especially in a woman who has recently ceased menstruating, the endometrium is still able to respond to the hormonal stimulation and begin cycling again, a sign that it is returning to its pre–ovarian failure function. Vaginal bleeding *is* a sign of endometrial cancer but does not occur at increased frequency in patients taking combined therapy. When it does occur in patients on unopposed estrogen, it takes more than a few weeks to develop. Although pregnancy is possible, it is unlikely at this point; however, most physicians do perform a pregnancy test prior to starting sexually active women on HRT.

89. **(B)** An adequate pelvic examination should be performed before option A, C, or E is chosen. The differential diagnosis for persistent fever after antibiotic therapy includes pelvic collection or abscess, drug fever, and septic pelvic thrombophlebitis. In the last case, the patients have a spiking, picket fence temperature pattern, and intravenous anticoagulation with heparin is a common treatment.

90. **(A)** An incomplete abortion is spontaneous partial expulsion of the uterine contents. The cervical os is typically open and bleeding is present. Frequently, surgical evacuation of the remaining contents is necessary to stop the bleeding. Spontaneous abortions are frequently complete prior to 10 weeks' gestation. An inevitable abortion means that there is gross rupture of the membranes and/or cervical dilatation without passage of tissue. A missed abortion is diagnosed when the embryo or fetus has died but the products remain in utero for an extended period of time. The use of an arbitrary time period was dropped by most because it does not serve a clinically useful purpose. Recurrent spontaneous abortion refers to three or more consecutive spontaneous abortions. Criminal abortion is an induced abortion that does not

conform to the state statutes. More than 10% of abortions are associated with fetal to maternal hemorrhage. Rh immune globulin is recommended for Rh-negative patients. Sepsis following abortion is much more frequently associated with criminal abortions than with legal abortions. Prompt, aggressive treatment, including evacuation of the uterus and antibiotic therapy, is necessary.

91. (A) Approximately 40% of villous adenomas show malignant change. Adenomas have a 5% chance of showing malignant change, whereas the other polyps have little or no increase in malignant potential.

92. (D) Physical activity is one of the most important modifiable risk factors for cardiac disease. Family history, age, and gender are important but nonmodifiable risk factors. Alcohol use is a weaker risk/protective factor. Age at puberty is not strongly associated with cardiac risk. Current symptoms may influence specific advice related to physical activity, but they do not preclude increasing activity.

93. (B) Fasting lipid levels are a key biochemical indicator of cardiac risk. They can help guide preventive advice regarding both diet and exercise. A glucose tolerance test would diagnose diabetes, an important cardiac risk factor, but it is not indicated in this asymptomatic man. Nonfasting tests vary too greatly to be useful for guiding prevention plans, and the hormone levels listed are not useful in assessing cardiac risk except possibly in special circumstances.

94. (B) All of the results are within normal limits except that the HDL cholesterol level is somewhat low. Exercise can significantly increase HDL levels, which in turn helps the body prevent deposition of cholesterol in atherosclerotic plaques. Refined sugar intake and even dietary cholesterol do not influence cholesterol levels. Reducing the amount of fat, particularly saturated fat, is the most important dietary intervention for lowering cholesterol (total and LDL) levels. Butter and stick margarine are roughly equal in fat and saturated fat content.

95. (B) Caffeine withdrawal syndrome causes headaches and decreased alertness, which generally reach peak intensity 24 to 48 hours after the last dose of caffeine. Caffeine is a weak reinforcer in laboratory studies. Tolerance occurs to caffeine intake. Twenty to thirty percent of adult Americans consume more than 500 mg of caffeine per day.

96. (D) Cluster headaches generally begin between the ages of 20 and 40. Men are affected more commonly than women. Pain typically is in the area of the orbit but may affect adjacent areas. Cluster headaches typically awaken the patient during rapid eye movement (REM) sleep; alcohol is a common precipitant. Migraine headaches are often associated with visual symptoms or exacerbated by light and relieved by darkness. In general, migraines do not awaken a person from sleep. A "hangover" headache does not awaken a person from sleep and does not last for an extended period of time. Tension headaches occur when a person is awake, are not usually located in a specific single location, and typically are not present every day for an extended period of time. Postconcussional disorder can occur after head trauma that caused significant cerebral concussion. Criteria for postconsussional disorder include the presence of at least three of several possible symptoms for at least 3 months.

97. (A) The patient best meets criteria for a diagnosis of delusional disorder, somatic type. She demonstrates nonbizarre delusions, with normal behavior apart from the delusions. The patient does not have schizophreniform disorder because she has nonbizarre delusions only; she does not have hallucinations, disorganized speech, disorganized or catatonic behavior, or negative symptoms. It is unlikely that she has alcohol-induced psychotic disorder with delusions because there is no evidence that she has recently consumed a large quantity of alcohol. The patient does not have Münchhausen syndrome,

also known as factitious disorder, because she does not seem to be intentionally creating her complaints and wanting to be considered sick. This patient does not have conversion disorder because she does not have symptoms suggesting a neurologic or other medical condition, and her complaints were not precipitated by a conflict or other stressor.

98. **(B)** All of the activities mentioned are indoor pursuits, so the woman is probably at low risk for excessive sun exposure, the major risk factor for skin cancer. Because she is slender and postmenopausal, osteoporosis is a significant risk for her. Coronary artery disease is the number one killer of postmenopausal women. Other than her age, no specific risk factors for breast cancer were mentioned, but it is one of the most common forms of cancer in women. Her job as a school administrator is probably a high-stress position, which could put her at risk for ulcer disease.

99. **(D)** Because coronary artery disease is such a common and preventable cause of death in older Americans, assessment of lipid levels is advisable. Because she has no cardiac symptoms, nor even any specific risk factors, a treadmill test is not necessary. Similarly, endometrial biopsy and thyroid hormone levels are not indicated in asymptomatic individuals. Serum PSA (prostate-specific antigen) is a test that may be useful for detecting prostate cancer, a condition that does not affect women.

100. **(C)** Weight-bearing exercise is an important preventive measure for osteoporosis, a condition for which she is at significant risk. She does not need to have a Pap smear more than once a year unless her Pap is abnormal. Because she does not spend a significant amount of time outdoors, sunscreen is not necessary. She is already thin, and without knowing her lipid levels, there is no reason to believe that she needs to cut back on fat. Drinking moderate amounts of alcohol, particularly red wine, seems to lower the risk of heart disease, but without further informa-

tion (eg, about personal or family history of alcoholism), it may be unwise to recommend alcohol intake. (See Figure 4.14.)

101. **(A)** Barrett's esophagus is a metaplastic change in the epithelium in which the epithelium changes from squamous to columnar epithelium. Barrett's esophagus is considered a premalignant lesion. The principles of therapy are directed at lifestyle changes and medical therapy. If the reflux is severe and the patient does not have dysplasia, an antireflux procedure is done. An esophagectomy in a patient with significant dysplasia is appropriate. As many as 45% of patients with esophageal stricture have changes consistent with Barrett's esophagus.

102. **(D)** Factors that increase the risk of esophageal cancer include alcohol ingestion, smoking, zinc, nitrosamines, malnutrition, anemia, poor oral hygiene, previous gastric surgery, and chronic ingestion of hot foods or beverages. Aflatoxin increases the risk of hepatocellular carcinoma.

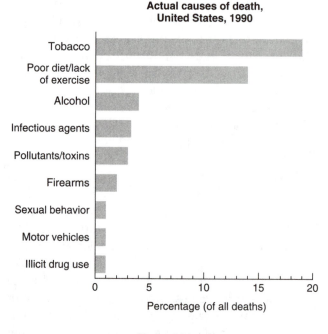

Figure 4.14

103–107.   (103-A, 104-A, 105-A, 106-A, 107-E)
Cystic fibrosis is an autosomal recessive disease. Pulmonary infection results in most of the morbidity. Influenza vaccination is indicated. The most common gene mutation has been identified as AF508. It is not hypoglycemia but hyperglycemia that is seen as the condition affects the pancreas. Most of the morbidity comes from pulmonary involvement, with a wide variety of chronic infections and complications possible. Meconium ileus, the most common cause of intestinal obstruction in the newborn, allows immediate diagnosis in about 10% of patients. Rectal prolapse, nasal polyps, and biliary cirrhosis may be associated features of the disease. Atelectasis, hemoptysis, and acute respiratory failure may be found. Renal failure, hypotension, and aplastic anemia are not typical. All of the treatments are effective in improving the survival rate.

108.   (C) Achalasia is a neuromuscular disorder of the esophagus, characterized by dilation and thickening, absent peristalsis, and no true stricture. The manometric criteria of achalasia are failure of the lower esophageal sphincter to relax reflexively when swallowing and lack of progressive peristalsis through the length of the esophagus. Dysphasia, weight loss, and aspiration pneumonia with secondary lung abscesses are also possible complications of achalasia. The fact that an endoscope was passed through the area of narrowing without difficulty would make a true stricture unlikely. Esophageal cancer is unlikely because no lesion was seen on endoscopy. Infiltrating intramural carcinoma at the cardia is relatively rare. Biliary colic is characterized by right upper quadrant pain radiating to the back and is unrelated to the current scenario.

109.   (D) Myotomy provides the best long-term benefit. Forceful dilation is an option, but the results are not as good as myotomy. Esophagectomy is not an appropriate, given that this is a benign condition. Cholecystectomy and hemicolectomy do not address the appropriate diagnosis.

110.   (D) Common causes of abdominal pain not requiring operation for treatment include: myocardial infarction, pneumonia, pulmonary infarction, pancreatitis, gastroenteritis, hepatitis, diabetic ketoacidosis, hyperlipidemia, rectus muscle hematoma, peripheral neuralgia, pyelonephritis, acute salpingitis, and sickle cell crisis. Head trauma may have associated abdominal trauma but is not, in itself, a cause of abdominal pain.

111.   (C) The sight or smell of food results in a vagus-mediated increase in gastric secretion (cephalic phase). Food in the stomach (gastric phase) results in gastrin release and increased gastric secretions. In the proper neurohormonal milieu, histamine is released from stores within the gastric mucosa and stimulates acid secretion. Gastric acid secretion is inhibited by the presence of acid, fat, or hyperosmotic solutions in the duodenum.

112.   (C) Pregnancy is a naturally occurring hypercoagulable state. The incidence of DVT during pregnancy is increased when compared to women with similar risk factors (ie, tobacco use, obesity, and exercise level). This is probably secondary to the hormonal changes occurring. Heparin is the drug of choice because it does not cross the placenta. Coumadin is probably safe in the third trimester and postpartum, but the possible risk is usually avoided and the patients are maintained on heparin by subcutaneous or intavenous infusion through delivery. Women remain hypercoagulable for several weeks after delivery. All of the studies listed in option B are of limited use in the setting of an acute thrombosis. They will often be low secondary to consumption. A better approach is to treat the acute problem and then follow the delivery and return of the woman's system to the nonpregnant state to perform the studies. If an abnormality is found then, most patients do receive anticoagulation for subsequent pregnancies. The majority of women will have normal studies, and anticoagulation is not routinely recommended for those women.

113. **(E)** All of the options are predisposing factors for venous thrombosis usually in combination with other factors such as pregnancy, inactivity, or use of birth control pills. Evaluation of patients immediately postoperatively demonstrates that nearly 100% have evidence of venous thrombosis. The majority are not clinically significant, and efforts to decrease the incidence, including compression boots, are ongoing. The fact remains that surgery is the single most common predisposing factor to the development of a venous thrombosis.

114. **(A)** The method for delivery of the second twin presents a challenge. An attempted vaginal breech delivery is used if the requirements for a vaginal breech birth are present. These include anesthesia, average fetal weight, adequate pelvic diameters, flexed head, and experienced operator. If these are not available, external version during the period of uterine quiescence is appropriate. A cesarean section is also an alternative. Approximately 40% of all twin gestations present as cephalic/cephalic, with another 25% being cephalic/breech. The second twin should be monitored by a continuous technique to maximize the chances for a good outcome.

115. **(E)** The incidence of multiple births is approximately 30% when ovulation-inducing agents are used. All of the factors mentioned are associated with an increased rate of twinning. The incidence of dizygotic twinning is commonly approximately 1 in 80 for African-American women and 1 in 100 for Caucasian women. A woman who is a dizygotic twin has a twin birth rate of 1 in 60. Larger and older women are more likely to have twins. The frequency of monozygotic twinning is constant, at approximately 1 in 250 births. Monozygotic twinning is independent of external factors. Twin gestation is associated with a very high incidence of admission for evaluation and management of problems during the pregnancy. Hypertension and preterm labor are extremely common. Approximately 25% (18 to 35%) of all twin gestations are associated with pregnancy-induced hypertension. The perinatal mortality rate for twin gestations is approximately 54 per thousand births compared to the 10 per thousand in singleton births.

116. **(E)** Division of the zygote prior to the fourth day results in two amnions, two chorions, and two placentas that may be fused. Division between the fourth and the eighth days results in one chorion, two amnions, and one placenta. Division between the eighth and twelfth days postconception results in a monoamniotic, monochorionic gestation. Division after the thirteenth day results in conjoined twins. The incidence is approximately 1 in 60,000 births.

117. **(A)** Jewish and Muslim women do seem to have a lower incidence of cervical cancer, and it is postulated that this is related to the circumcision rate among their partners, but the risk is not zero. The peak incidence for cervical cancer is 48 to 55 years and for endometrial cancer 55 to 60, so she should continue her regular visits to her gynecologist. Obesity, nulliparity, and diabetes all increase the risk of developing endometrial cancer but not cervical cancer. Pap smears are useful only for detecting abnormalities in the cervix. The review of systems, speculum exam, and bimanual exam are important in detecting other malignancies of the female reproductive system.

118. **(B)** As of this moment, only retrospective studies have been published regarding the benefits of tamoxifen in preventing breast cancer; therefore, an assessment of risk versus benefit is not yet available. In retrospect, it does appear to decrease the incidence of new breast cancers for women with a history of breast cancer, but only by 40 to 50%. It increases the incidence of endometrial cancer from .0005 to .001. These cancers are typically low grade and cured by hysterectomy. It increases the risk of *venous* thrombosis, especially in women with other risk factors such as tobacco use and obesity. No effect on coronary artery disease has been consistently demonstrated.

119. **(C)** This patient has calcification of the wall of the gallbladder, known as a porcelain gallbladder, which is associated with a 25 to 60% increased risk for carcinoma of the gallbladder. Unless some form of contraindication exists for other medical issues, a cholecystectomy should be performed. Sigmoidoscopy and CT myelogram are inappropriate for this evaluation.

120. **(E)** Herpes simplex virus-2 is the leading cause of genital ulceration in the United States. Sexually transmitted diseases (STDs) that cause genital ulcers increase the risk of HIV infection by disrupting the body's physical barriers against infection. Gonorrhea and HPV are both sexually transmitted infections but do not lead to ulcerative lesions. Tuberculosis and *Pneumocystis carinii* are both common infections in individuals with HIV, but they do not increase the risk of acquiring the disease.

121. **(C)** Most human rabies exposure is indirect, through pets getting into fights with rabid wildlife. Vaccinating all pets reduces the risk to humans significantly. Rabies vaccine is recommended only for individuals at high risk, such as veterinarians, or for postexposure prophylaxis. Avoiding swimming in lakes is unnecessary, because rabid animals avoid drinking or even being near water due to painful throat spasms. It is not necessary to test all dead animals for rabies, only ones where human exposure is a possibility. Rabid animals are as likely to be out in the middle of the day as after dusk, so restricting use of parks in the evening is unnecessary.

122. **(E)** The use of oxytocics increases the risk of uterine rupture. This patient has several characteristics consistent with cephalopelvic disproportion (CPD). The combination of the arrest with suspected CPD is best treated by a cesarean section. Although the caput is at +1 station, this fetal head is probably not engaged. The use of forceps would most likely result in a high application, which is contraindicated. The outcome would most likely be fetal and maternal trauma. The midpelvic forceps delivery of a macrosomic fetus places the mother and baby at significant risk for birth trauma, including shoulder dystocia

123. **(E)** Acanthosis nigricans is a skin change seen in association with adenocarcinoma and insulin resistance. Recognition of the lesion warrants a thorough evaluation for underlying malignancy as well as diabetes. The skin is gray-brown or sometimes black. It is thickened with small papillomatous elevations that feel almost velvety.

124. **(B)** Diabetes (insulin resistance) is associated with acanthosis nigricans but is also commonly seen in patients with underlying adenocarcinomas. CT scans are not a recommended routine screening test. The use of contrast is problematic in patients with renal insufficiency but is not a problem for a diabetic with normal renal function studies.

125. **(A)** Approximately 1% of vaginal deliveries are associated with shoulder dystocia; however, 3% of deliveries of babies weighing between 4100 and 4500 g, and 8% of those weighing greater than 4500 g, are associated with shoulder dystocia. Approximately one half of shoulder dystocia occurs, however, in the baby that weighs less than 4000 g. Management decisions based solely on the estimated weight of the baby as determined by ultrasound are discouraged because of the high degree of error involved in the estimation of weight. The increased risk of postpartum hemorrhage is caused by uterine atony related to oxytocics, prolonged labor, and genital tract laceration.

126. **(C)** The presentation of a relatively asymptomatic woman with abdominal bloating and vaginal bleeding with an elevated CA 125 is ovarian cancer unless proven otherwise. The CA 125 is the gold standard, a very sensitive test for epithelial tumors of the ovary. Unfortunately, 70% of these women present with advanced-stage disease because there is not as much of an effect on the infundibulopelvic ligament as with germ cell tumors. The patients should next have a CT or MRI of the

pelvis, followed by a surgical evaluation; generally, this is not laparoscopic if the picture is as clear-cut as this. Laparoscopic evaluations are useful in patients with unexplained pelvic pain.

127. **(D)** Cytoreduction is considered standard for all patients with stage III and IV disease, although there are some patients for whom it is clear from the staging radiographs that optimal reduction is not possible, and those patients are usually treated first with chemotherapy. Adequate cytoreduction requires meticulous attention to surgical technique and a thorough knowledge of abdominal and pelvic anatomy. Physicians with minimal experience or who do the procedure infrequently tend to have fewer complications because they are less aggressive but have poorer outcomes. Patients with stage III disease who have optimal cytoreduction have an improved survival from about 20 months to 40 months. Surgery does not increase the incidence of blood-borne metastases, and most patients die of abdominal disease. CA 125 levels are useful both in the initial diagnosis and in follow-up.

128. **(E)** Patients can have an obstruction, but the most common reason for the obstruction is a tethering or kinking of the small bowel.

129. **(B)** Most patients with carcinoid tumor are asymptomatic, with relatively small tumor burden. Patients with carcinoid syndrome manifest as late-stage disease with metastatic disease to the liver. The major symptoms are flushing and diarrhea. High serotonin levels are present in patients with significant disease. A major metabolite of serotonin is 5-HIAA, which is excreted in the urine and is a common way to evaluate a patient for carcinoid. Treatment is directed at relief of symptoms and oetreotide, a naturally occurring inhibitory peptide of somatostatin, is used for management of symptoms.

130. **(D)** Rabies is endemic in bats in North America, affecting roughly 1% of the population. Bats are the source of most cases of hu-

man rabies in this country. In some parts of the world, where there are large populations of feral dogs, rabies is endemic in that species. In this country, most dogs are pets and by law must be vaccinated. Deer and groundhogs may occasionally be infected with rabies. Small animals such as squirrels rarely survive an encounter with a rabid animal: They die acutely of injuries inflicted by the rabid animal and do not live long enough to develop rabies.

131. **(A)** Hind limb paralysis is a late manifestation of the disease. Photophobia does not seem to be a symptom; in fact, a common sign of rabies among normally nocturnal animals is that they wander around in broad daylight. Rabies used to be called "hydrophobia"; affected humans and animals avoid water because the mere thought of swallowing can induce painful spasms of the throat muscles. Bleeding, seizures, and odor are not characteristic of rabies.

132. **(I)** Priapism is often reported as a side effect of trazodone, a tricyclic antidepressant.

133. **(H)** Although sedation is a side effect of many psychoactive drugs, it is especialy important to recognize the differing side effect profiles of the low-potency (eg, thioridazine) and high-potency (eg, haloperidol; see question 134) antipsychotics.

134. **(D)** See answer to question 133.

135. **(F)** Because of their chemical similarities to antiarrhythmic medications, the tricyclic antidepressants, including nortriptyline, can cause arrhythmias.

136. **(G)** Tyramine-induced hypertensive crisis is a common adverse reaction to the monoamine oxidase inhibitor (MAOI) class of antidepressants. Patients should be warned not to eat foods rich in tyramine, such as cheeses and red wines.

137. **(B)** Weight loss occurs during the first 3 to 4 days of life. Jaundice may be present at birth

or arise at any time in the neonatal period depending on the condition producing the elevation in bilirubin level.

138. **(C)** The course of breast-feeding jaundice can have prolonged elevation of bilirubin levels through the third week of life. Breast-fed infants should regain their birth weight by 14 days of life compared to 10 in the formula-fed infant.

139. **(D)** Atelectasis and large pulmonary effusions both can present with decreased fremitus, dullness or flatness to percussion, and absent breath sounds. In atelectasis, tracheal shift, if present, is toward the affected side, and the opposite for a large pleural effusion.

140. **(B)** A complete pneumothorax results in absent fremitus, hyperresonance or tympany, and absent breath sounds.

141. **(A)** Asthma's most typical manifestations are prolonged expiration and diffuse wheezing. However, impaired expansion, decreased fremitus, hyperresonance, and low diaphragms can also be found.

142. **(E)** Lobar pneumonia is characterized by consolidation with increased fremitus, dullness, and auscultatory findings of bronchial breathing, bronchophony, pectoriloquy, and crackles.

143. **(A, C, D, F)** Penicillin can cause numerous allergic reactions, including anaphylaxis, interstitial nephritis, rashes (the most common manifestation), urticara, fever, pneumonitis, dermatitis, and even asthma in workers exposed to airborne penicillin. Hemolytic anemia in often IgG-mediated. Skin tests are reliable in predicting low risk (similar to the general population) for those claiming previous penicillin reactions, and desensitization is feasible. The frequency of reactions to cephalosporins in penicillin-allergic patients is not definitely known.

144. **(B, G)** ACE inhibitors can cause angioedema of the face and oropharyngeal structures. This is felt to be a pseudoallergic reaction, possibly due to the drug's effect on the kinin system. It is thought that reactions may be more common in women, African Americans, and those with idiopathic angioedema. If this occurs, therapy with alternate ACE inhibitors should NOT be attempted.

145. **(E, F)** Aspirin frequently can precipitate asthma in susceptible individuals. At highest risk are asthmatics with chronic rhinosinusitis and nasal polyps. This is probably a pseudoallergic reaction related to inhibition of cyclo-oxygenase, with a resultant enhancement of leukotriene synthesis or effect. Desensitization regimens have been developed.

146–150. **(146-C, 147-A, 148-D, 149-B, 150-C)** A single attack of either rubella or measles confers lifelong immunity. Both diseases are vaccine preventable. Both may have an enanthem that appears before the rash. In measles, Koplik's spots appear on the buccal mucosa. In rubella, there may be punctate or larger red spots on the soft palate. Rare complications of rubella include encephalitis and thrombocytopenia purpura. Polyarthritis is more common in women and is uncommon in children. The congenital rubella syndrome is where prevention efforts are placed. Measles' complications include keratoconjunctivitis, myocarditis, pneumonia, secondary bacterial infections, encephalitis, and subacute sclerosing panencephalitis.

Practice Test 5
Questions

DIRECTIONS (Question 1 through 128): Each of the numbered items or incomplete statements in this section is followed by answers or by completions of the statement. Select the ONE lettered answer or completion that is BEST in each case.

Questions 1 Through 5

You are called to the nursery to examine an infant whose father has a history of intravenous drug abuse. The mother denies any drug use and was discovered to be positive for human immunodeficiency virus (HIV) antibody in her third trimester. The infant appears healthy, and his HIV antibody status is pending. His white blood cell (WBC) count is normal, as are his other baseline laboratory tests. At a follow-up visit 2 weeks later, you inform the mother that his HIV antibody test is positive.

1. Without treatment, what percentage of infants born to HIV-infected mothers will be infected?

   (A) 10%
   (B) 20%
   (C) 40%
   (D) 60%
   (E) 80%

2. Clinical manifestations of acquired immune deficiency syndrome (AIDS) in infants and young children may include

   (A) periorbital ecchymosis
   (B) failure to thrive
   (C) cardiac arrhythmia
   (D) rhinitis
   (E) Kaposi's sarcoma

3. "Safe sex" will help prevent the spread of the HIV virus. Which of the following procedures is also considered "safe"?

   (A) blood transfusion
   (B) history of receiving gamma globulin
   (C) intravenous drug use
   (D) history of receiving factor VIII concentrate
   (E) breast feeding by an HIV-infected mother

4. Laboratory findings in pediatric AIDS may include

   (A) elevated levels of immunoglobulin G, M, and D (IgG, IgM, IgD)
   (B) unaltered helper–suppressor T-cell ratio
   (C) increase in absolute number of T cells
   (D) high levels of interferon
   (E) normal monocyte chemotaxis

5. Which of the following vaccines is contraindicated in a pediatric AIDS patient?

   (A) measles, mumps, rubella (MMR)
   (B) diphtheria, pertussis, tetanus (DPT)
   (C) *Hemophilus influenzae b* (HIB)
   (D) influenza vaccine
   (E) oral polio vaccine

6. A 34-year-old woman (P1011) at 41⁵/₇ weeks' gestation presents in labor. Her prenatal course was totally unremarkable. She was 5 cm on admission. The electronic fetal monitoring strip was interpreted as completely reassuring. Approximately 2 hours later, the patient was reexamined and was found to be 5 cm, 80% effaced, with the vertex at 0 station in a left occiput anterior position. The fetal monitoring strip (Figure 5.1) is shown. The MOST reasonable diagnosis and plan is

(A) reassuring electronic fetal monitoring; arrested dilatation; oxytocin augmentation

(B) reassuring electronic fetal monitoring; normal labor progress; continued observation

(C) nonreassuring fetal monitoring; late deceleration; in utero resuscitation

(D) reassuring electronic fetal monitoring; arrested dilatation; if cephalopelvic disproportion is ruled out, begin oxytocin augmentation

(E) nonreassuring electronic fetal monitoring; arrested dilatation; oxytocin augmentation

7. A 55-year-old chronic schizophrenic patient who has been involuntarily hospitalized sues

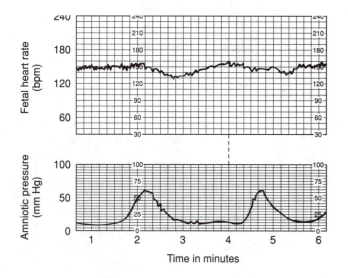

Figure 5.1

the hospital on the grounds that he is receiving no therapy. He has not had a documented physical examination or psychiatric evaluation for over a year. His attorney is likely to base his case on

(A) the constitutional right to refuse treatment

(B) the importance of informed consent prior to treatment

(C) the right to treatment in return for confinement

(D) testamentary capacity

(E) competency to stand trial

8. A 62-year-old woman was diagnosed with major depressive disorder 10 years ago. She has been on several antidepressant medications, with minimal improvement. Her psychiatrist is considering treating her with electroconvulsive therapy (ECT). An absolute contraindication to ECT is

(A) brain tumor

(B) increased intracerebral pressure

(C) hypertension

(D) myocardial disease

(E) none of the above

9. Postpartum blues is another name for mild transient depression that occurs typically within 1 to 2 weeks of delivery. Its incidence in postpartum women is

(A) 10%

(B) 25%

(C) 50%

(D) 75%

(E) 90%

Questions 10 and 11

A 35-year-old otherwise healthy man presents with a 24-hour history of increasing umbilical pain. You elicit from the history that he has had intermittent tenderness and a mass in his umbilical area on coughing or straining. On physical examination, he has a soft abdomen, with a focal, 3-cm, erythematous, firm, tender mass in the region of his umbilicus. His temperature is 100.8°F, and the vital signs are stable. His serum laboratory findings disclose a WBC count of 13,000/mm³.

10. The MOST likely diagnosis is

   (A) Sister Joseph's node
   (B) a benign tumor of the umbilicus
   (C) incarcerated umbilical hernia
   (D) abdominal wall abscess
   (E) a malignant tumor of the umbilicus

11. The MOST appropriate treatment choice is

   (A) antibiotics alone
   (B) incision and drainage
   (C) resection of the tumor
   (D) umbilical herniorrhaphy with examination of the contents in the hernia sac
   (E) chemotherapy

Questions 12 and 13

A 42-year-old man is found to have a high ferritin level during evaluation for elevated liver enzymes. He remembers that other members of his family have died of complications of diabetes and cardiovascular disease. It is a family joke about how they all get darker as they age.

12. The MOST common finding in this disease is

   (A) insulin-dependent diabetes
   (B) impaired renal function
   (C) arthropathy
   (D) hypogonadism
   (E) skin pigment changes

13. Which of the following is true of this disease?

   (A) No specific genetic abnormality has been identified in this disorder.
   (B) Symptomatic treatment is recommended as complications develop.
   (C) Therapeutic phlebotomies begun early in the disease may prevent end-organ damage.
   (D) Screening of asymptomatic family members with ferritin levels is not helpful.
   (E) Women never develop evidence of disease until after menopause.

14. Which of the following is a feature of constitutional growth delay?

   (A) Puberty usually begins at the usual time.
   (B) Osseous maturation (bone age) is not delayed.
   (C) Growth rate (velocity) is normal after age 18.
   (D) Final adult height is within normal limits.
   (E) A parent with a similar pattern of growth is rare.

Question 15 and 16

15. A 72-year-old woman presents with vaginal bleeding. Her last mentrual period was 20 years ago. A speculum examination reveals a friable, necrotic lesion in the left vaginal fornix. The cervix does not appear to be involved. Bimanual and rectovaginal examination demonstrates that there is extension into the soft tissues on the left posterior fornix, but the pelvic sidewall is not involved. Biopsy of the lesion demonstrates invasive squamous carcinoma. The following tests were next performed: chest x-ray, cystoscopy, intravenous pyelogram (IVP), proctoscopy, and barium enema. All were negative. The correct diagnosis is

   (A) stage I vaginal carcinoma
   (B) stage IIB cervical carcinoma
   (C) stage II vaginal carcinoma
   (D) stage II cervical carcinoma
   (E) stage III vaginal carcinoma

16. The MOST appropriate treatment would be

   (A) chemotherapy
   (B) whole pelvis radiation therapy
   (C) intracavitary radiation to the uterus, cervix, and vagina
   (D) total abdominal hysterectomy with appropriate vaginal cuff excision
   (E) radical hysterectomy and pelvic lymphadenectomy

Questions 17 and 18

A 21-year-old man who has just moved into your area presents with a neck mass that has been gradually growing over the past 5 or 6 years. It is painless but becoming unsightly. You examine him and find a midline tracheal mass, which is smooth, firm, and relatively symmetric.

17. The MOST likely cause of this growth is

(A) goiter
(B) thyroid carcinoma
(C) laryngeal carcinoma
(D) branchial cleft cyst
(E) parathyroid adenoma

18. The principal cause of this disorder worldwide is

(A) poor dietary habits
(B) drug toxicity
(C) genetic predisposition
(D) deficiency of iodine in soil and water
(E) thyroid carcinoma

19. A 30-year-old athlete had sudden shortness of breath when jogging. He complains of right-sided chest and shoulder pain. His breath sounds are decreased on the right. His chest x-ray is shown in Figure 5.2. Fifteen minutes after obtaining a chest x-ray, he becomes hemodynamically unstable. The MOST important intervention is

(A) administration of oxygen
(B) antibiotics for pneumonia
(C) bronchoscopy
(D) nebulizer treatment
(E) chest tube thoracostomy

Questions 20 Through 22

A 42-year-old journalist is leaving in several weeks to go to Central America, sub-Saharan Africa, and Southeast Asia on assignment to write about overpopulation. He is concerned about illnesses he may encounter while traveling and wants information about what he can do to stay healthy.

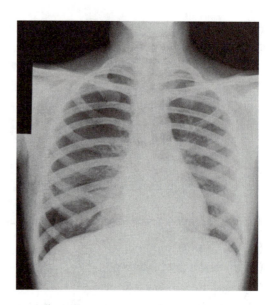

Figure 5.2. Spontaneous pneumothorax on right side.

20. Which of the following illnesses is he MOST likely to contract?

(A) plague
(B) cholera
(C) schistosomiasis
(D) typhoid fever
(E) *Escherichia coli* enteritis

21. What sort of chemoprophylaxis would be effective to prevent this condition?

(A) norfloxacin
(B) penicillin
(C) erythromycin
(D) metronidazole
(E) iodochlorhydroxyquin (Entero-Vioform)

22. Which of the following vaccines is required for travel in endemic areas?

(A) yellow fever vaccine
(B) smallpox vaccine
(C) meningococcal vaccine
(D) Japanese encephalitis vaccine
(E) African trypanosomiasis vaccine

23. A patient with sudden, rapid, recurrent movements that involve multiple muscle groups would MOST likely have

   (A) Huntington's disease
   (B) Tourette's disorder
   (C) Parkinson's disease
   (D) Alzheimer's disease
   (E) Sydenham's chorea

24. Clincal features of respiratory syncytial virus (RSV) may be described by which of the following?

   (A) RSV bronchiolitis usually manifests itself by wheezing and reaches its peak severity in 48 to 72 hours.
   (B) CO_2 retention may be presumed to begin when the respiratory rate surpasses 20/min.
   (C) Distinction between RSV bronchiolitis and RSV penumonia is usually easily made.
   (D) RSV disease in younger infants is generally milder than in older children.
   (E) RSV pneumonia generally will not resolve spontaneously over several weeks.

25. The MOST common complication of preterm premature rupture of membranes at 28 weeks is

   (A) fetal compression anomalies
   (B) pulmonary hypoplasia
   (C) intrauterine infection
   (D) limb contractions
   (E) abruptio placentae

Questions 26 Through 30

A 35-year-old obese woman complains of recent weight loss in spite of a large appetite, vulvar pruritus, waking frequently at night to urinate, and the leg lesions seen in Figure 5.3.

26. What is the MOST likely diagnosis?

   (A) diabetes mellitus
   (B) diabetes insipidus

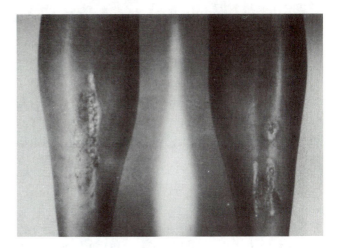

Figure 5.3

   (C) vaginitis and cystitis
   (D) myxedema
   (E) pheochromocytoma

27. What is the MOST likely diagnosis of the leg lesions?

   (A) eruptive xanthomas
   (B) necrobiosis lipoidica diabeticorum
   (C) gangrene
   (D) staphylococcal infection
   (E) erythema nodosum

28. The diagnosis is generally established by

   (A) a urine glucose
   (B) an insulin tolerance test
   (C) a fasting blood sugar
   (D) a glucose tolerance test
   (E) an intravenous glucose tolerance test

29. The metabolic effects of insulin on adipose tissue are MOST likely to include

   (A) decrease of glucose transport
   (B) decrease in glucose phosphorylation
   (C) decrease in cyclic adenosine monophosphate (AMP)
   (D) decrease in lipoprotein lipase
   (E) enhancement of glucagon effect

30. Which of the following renal diseases is this patient MOST likely to develop?

    (A) acute glomerulonephritis
    (B) obstructive uropathy
    (C) polycystic kidneys
    (D) renal infarction
    (E) glomerulosclerosis with mesangial thickening

Questions 31 Through 33

A 30-year-old woman presents with a 12-year history of ulcerative colitis. She has had persistent problems with malnutrition and arthritis in addition to abdominal discomfort and bloody diarrhea. At this point, she has an exacerbation of her disease every time the steroids are tapered. She has been reluctant to have a definitive surgical procedure until now. On her last colonoscopy, she had dysplastic changes in her colon, with her entire colon and rectum involved with ulcerative colitis.

31. What would be the procedure of choice in this patient?

    (A) proctocolectomy with an ileal pouch–anal anastomosis
    (B) right hemicolectomy
    (C) proctocolectomy with permanent ileostomy
    (D) total colectomy and ileoproctostomy
    (E) small bowel resection

32. Which of the following is a complication of ulcerative colitis?

    (A) pyoderma gangrenosum
    (B) toxic megacolon
    (C) uveitis
    (D) colon and rectal cancer
    (E) all of the above

33. All of the following statements are true regarding Crohn's (granulomatous) colitis EXCEPT

    (A) the rectum is often not involved
    (B) the bowel wall is thickened
    (C) chronic inflammation involves all layers of the bowel wall
    (D) the colonic lesions are generally confluent and diffuse
    (E) internal fistulas are relatively common

Questions 34 Through 36

A patient who presented with signs and symptoms of labor and ruptured membranes is 5 cm dilated. She is now in active labor. The fetal assessment is reassuring. She is requesting analgesia. She chose to have parenteral analgesia with perineal anesthesia provided, if necessary, by either local infiltration or a pudendal block. Her husband asks the following questions:

34. The use of parenteral analgesics in labor is associated with which of the following?

    (A) maternal respiratory stimulation
    (B) fetal agitation
    (C) late decelerations
    (D) diminished beat-to-beat variability
    (E) increased neonatal appetite

35. Select the two correct responses that are commonly associated with pudendal anesthesia.

    (A) sensory nerve block from the ventricle branch of the second, third, and fourth sacral nerves
    (B) sensory block of the sensory portions of the tenth, eleventh, and twelfth thoracic and first lumbar nerves
    (C) residual paralysis
    (D) paraspinal abscess
    (E) paravaginal abscess

36. One hour later, she is 6 to 7 cm dilated and the meperidine is wearing off. An epidural analgesic is administered, and 15 minutes later, late decelerations begin. Appropriate management measures include

(A) immediate cesarean section for cord prolapse

(B) no change as the problem will resolve spontaneously

(C) immediate administration of ephedrine and discontinue epidural

(D) fluid resuscitation and repositioning to correct maternal hypotension

(E) cesarean section for fetal distress

Questions 37 Through 39

A 2-year-old girl is seen for a well-child check-up. She is a healthy child, and her development is appropriate for her age.

37. Which of the following is a leading potential cause of death for this child for which a preventive measure is available that should be discussed with the child's parents?

(A) motor vehicle accident

(B) lead poisoning

(C) HIV

(D) acute lymphoblastic leukemia

(E) Wilms' tumor

38. Assuming that she is caught up on her immunizations, which of the following diseases is she now fully protected against without further boosters after this visit?

(A) measles

(B) diphtheria

(C) tetanus

(D) HIB

(E) polio

39. If this girl had been HIV positive, what change would you have made in her childhood immunization schedule?

(A) Use dT instead of DPT.

(B) Omit MMR vaccination.

(C) Substitute inactivated polio vaccine (IPV) for oral polio vaccine (OPV).

(D) Delay all immunizations by 6 months.

(E) Use split doses of all live attenuated vaccines.

40. In the use of the multiaxial system for evaluation of patients with suspected psychiatric disorders, which of the following refers to the physical condition?

(A) axis I

(B) axis II

(C) axis III

(D) axis IV

(E) axis V

41. You decide to prescribe a benzodiazepine to an 84-year-old woman. You recognize the importance of choosing a benzodiazepine with a short half-life. Which of the following would you prescribe for this patient?

(A) chlordiazepoxide

(B) diazepam

(C) clorazepate

(D) oxazepam

(E) phenobarbital

42. Posttransfusion hepatitis is MOST often due to

(A) hepatitis A

(B) hepatitis B

(C) hepatitis C

(D) delta-associated virus

(E) Epstein–Barr virus

Questions 43 and 44

43. A fetal heart rate pattern described as a slowing of the heart rate for more than 60 to 90 seconds and less than 15 minutes is best classified as a

    (A) prolonged bradycardia
    (B) prolonged deceleration
    (C) bradycardia
    (D) late deceleration
    (E) variable deceleration

44. The ideal management for the patient whose fetus demonstrates a prolonged deceleration is

    (A) cesarean section
    (B) operative vaginal delivery
    (C) continued observation
    (D) individualized management based on the clinical situation
    (E) amino infusion

Questions 45 Through 50

A 29-year-old woman develops painful swelling of both hands. She is also very stiff in the morning. Physical examination reveals involvement of the proximal interphalangeal joints and the metacarpophalangeal joints.

45. The rheumatoid factor is

    (A) positive in 10 to 20% of juvenile rheumatoid arthritis (JRA) patients
    (B) positive in almost 100% of "classical" rheumatoid arthritis patients
    (C) seen only in rheumatoid arthritis
    (D) an immunoglobulin that attaches to the Fc fragment of an IgM molecule
    (E) frequently present in osteoarthritis

46. The MOST likely cause of the inflammation in her joints is

    (A) activated T cells
    (B) activated B cells

    (C) microvascular injury
    (D) interleukin-4
    (E) precipitated rheumatoid factor

47. The MOST likely place for her to develop vasculitis is

    (A) kidneys
    (B) heart
    (C) lungs
    (D) bowel
    (E) skin

48. The MOST likely drug to relieve the signs and symptoms of disease is

    (A) D-penicillamine
    (B) an antimalarial
    (C) methotrexate
    (D) aspirin
    (E) gold

49. The MOST frequently used drug to prevent the progression of disease is

    (A) D-penilillamine
    (B) an antimalarial
    (C) methotrexate
    (D) aspirin
    (E) gold

50. After having this disease for a number of years, she is started on gold therapy. Which of the following toxic reactions is she MOST likely to experience?

    (A) nausea and vomiting
    (B) agranulocytosis
    (C) dermatitis and stomatitis
    (D) thrombophlebitis
    (E) alopecia

Questions 51 and 52

A 42-year-old woman has a painless solitary thyroid nodule on the right side of her neck. Her medical history is that of lymphoma with neck irradiation in the remote past.

51. The single MOST important diagnostic study to be performed in this patient is

   (A) computed tomography (CT) scan
   (B) fine-needle aspiration
   (C) open biopsy
   (D) radioiodine scan
   (E) ultrasound

52. The MOST frequent variety of thyroid cancer is

   (A) follicular carcinoma
   (B) papillary carcinoma
   (C) anaplastic carcinoma
   (D) Hashimoto's associated lymphoma
   (E) medullary carcinoma

Questions 53 Through 56

A 23-year-old female patient, whom you have seen in your office several times, telephones with a complaint of progressive vulvar itching and burning for 4 days. She has tried an over-the-counter (OTC) antifungal preparation, which caused increased burning. On further questioning, she tells you that she had sexual relations with a new partner 1 week earlier and used a condom. She also takes oral contraceptives.

53. From this history, you are concerned that she has an infection due to

   (A) bacterial vaginosis
   (B) *Chlamydia*
   (C) herpes simplex virus (HSV)
   (D) *Monilia*
   (E) *Trichomonas*

54. You ask her additional questions and particularly want to know whether

   (A) there is a discharge with a fishy odor
   (B) she has any pelvic cramping
   (C) she has swollen inguinal lymph nodes, fever, or malaise
   (D) there is a discharge with a milky or cheesy consistency
   (E) there is a bubbly or blood-tinged discharge

55. Upon learning the answer, you advise her that

   (A) she has a bacterial infection and you telephone the pharmacy with a prescription for metronidazole gel 0.75%, per vagina hs for 5 days
   (B) she should come to the office that day
   (C) she has a herpes infection and you telephone the pharmacy with a prescription for famciclovir, 125 mg bid for 5 days
   (D) some women are allergic to vaginal yeast preparations and you telephone the pharmacy with a prescription for fluconazole, 150 mg PO single dose
   (E) yeast infections are resistant to some OTC preparations and you telephone the pharmacy with a prescription for terconazole, 80 mg suppository per vagina hs for 3 days

56. The patient is extremely anxious that she might have contracted a sexually transmitted disease (STD) and insists on coming to the office for a definitive diagnosis. Upon seeing her you observe bilateral vulvar vesicles and ulcerations, increased but otherwise normal-appearing leukorrhea with a pH of 4.0, and swollen inguinal nodes. You give this patient an appropriate prescription and reassure her that

   (A) the symptoms should resolve in 3 to 5 days
   (B) condoms are effective protection, and this is not an STD
   (C) there is no effective treatment and symptoms will continue to recur monthly
   (D) she may be advised to have a cesarean section but only if she has active lesions around the time of obstetric delivery
   (E) there is no need to discuss this infection with her current or future sexual partners

Questions 57 Through 59

You have been asked to advise a nearby rural school district about measures they should take to stem the alarming rise in teen pregnancy in their district. The number of pregnancies among girls in the high school has risen by 30% in the past 10 years, and there have even been a few pregnancies among girls in the middle school (6th through 8th grades).

57. Which of the following educational approaches during the middle school years has been shown to delay the onset of sexual activity and reduce the risk of teen pregnancy?

   (A) abstinence education stressing the dangers of premarital sexual activity

   (B) general health education focusing on health promotion

   (C) sexuality education that includes information about contraception

   (D) family life education focusing on family roles and interpersonal communication

58. What is the highest-risk time during the week for teen pregnancies to occur?

   (A) weekday afternoons

   (B) Saturday mornings

   (C) Friday and Saturday nights

   (D) Sunday afternoons

   (E) after 9:00 P.M. daily

59. Which of the following interventions should you recommend to the school administrators as a first step?

   (A) Meet with the director of the local Planned Parenthood clinic to arrange for their staff to provide individual contraceptive counseling in the school nurse's office.

   (B) Survey the middle school and high school students about their health practices, using the Centers for Disease Control and Prevention's (CDC's) Youth Risk Behavior Survey as an instrument.

   (C) Revise the health education curriculum to address pregnancy prevention and STDs earlier than 11th grade.

   (D) Expand the after-school intramural athletic program.

60. True statements concerning grief and bereavement include

   (A) the initial physical symptoms may be indistinguishable from depression

   (B) widowers and widows have an increased death rate in the first year following the death of a spouse

   (C) identification phenomenon may occur

   (D) grief may extend from 1 to 2 years

   (E) all of the above

61. Puerperal endomyometritis is

   (A) a polymicrobial infection

   (B) primarily limited to anaerobic gram-positive cocci

   (C) an aerobic gram-positive cocci

   (D) an anaerobic gram-negative bacilli

   (E) an aerobic gram-negative bacilli

Questions 62 and 63

A 71-year-old man is seen for a routine check-up. He complains of a slight decrease in his energy level so a complete blood count (CBC) is ordered. It demonstrates a WBC count of 27,000, with a differential of 31% segs, 63% lymphs, 2% bands, 1% eos, and 3% monos. His hemoglobin is 12.4 g/dL and platelet count 231,000. A review of the peripheral smear shows the lymphocytes to be small lymphs with densely packed nuclei. He has no abnormalities on physical examination.

62. Which of the following statements is true regarding this man's diagnosis?

   (A) A bone marrow biopsy is necessary to make the diagnosis.

   (B) The lymphocytes will be polyclonal.

   (C) He is likely to experience progression of his disease in the next 5 years.

(D) He is likely to require treatment in the next year.

(E) He may develop a large cell lymphoma.

63. At the advice of a hematologist, you repeat the patient's CBC at 3-month intervals to develop an understanding of the doubling time of his disease process. Eighteen months later, you note a dramatic drop in his hemoglobin to 8.2 g/dL, and he complains of worsening fatigue and shortness of breath. His WBC count is now 32,000 with a similar differential. The platelets are still in the normal range. On physical examination, he is pale with a resting pulse of 92 beats per minute. Neither his spleen nor any lymph nodes are palpable. Which of the following tests would be diagnostic?

(A) CT scan

(B) blood culture

(C) creatinine

(D) reticulocyte count

(E) serum iron

64. A woman initially presents with a complaint of nipple discharge. All of the following statements concerning nipple discharges are true EXCEPT

(A) a yellow or greenish discharge is consistent with fibrocystic changes

(B) when bloody, the discharge is due to a malignancy 70% of the time

(C) a milky discharge may be due to a pituitary adenoma

(D) benign duct papillomas are the most common cause of bloody discharges

(E) excision of the involved duct may be necessary to determine the cause

65. During an asthma attack, which of the following is expected?

(A) lung volumes increase

(B) residual volumes increase

(C) expiratory flow rates increase

(D) bronchial hyperreactivity decreases

(E) mediastinal air decreases

66. The MOST common benign solid tumor of the vulva is a

(A) lipoma

(B) hidradenoma

(C) fibroma

(D) syringoma

(E) endometrioma

Questions 67 and 68

A 42-year-old severely depressed woman was found unconscious, with an empty bottle of propoxyphene hydrochloride (Darvon) at her side. She was promptly taken to the emergency department, where she was noted to be comatose.

67. Which of the following would be MOST likely to be found in this patient?

(A) respiratory alkalosis

(B) apnea

(C) increase in blood pressure

(D) vomiting

(E) hypervigilant state

68. After a patent airway has been ensured and artificial respiration instituted, which of the following would be most helpful in treating the patient's respiratory depression?

(A) physostigmine

(B) naloxone (Narcan)

(C) atropine

(D) propranolol (Inderal)

(E) none of the above

Questions 69 and 70

A 48-year-old man presents to the hospital outpatient clinic complaining of numbness and pain in his hands on exposure to cold. The physician diagnoses his problem as Raynaud's phenomenon.

69. Which of the following occupations may have led to this condition?

    (A) jackhammer operator
    (B) data-processing keyboard specialist
    (C) meat-packing plant freezer-room technician
    (D) anesthetist
    (E) dairy farmer

70. What other occupational risk is likely in a person in this occupation?

    (A) repetitive motion injury
    (B) chemical burns
    (C) hearing loss
    (D) visual impairment
    (E) torn rotator cuff

Questions 71 and 72

A 71-year-old woman complains of recent onset pneumaturia. A CT scan is consistent with, but not diagnostic of, a vesicoenteric fistula.

71. The MOST common cause of vesicoenteric fistulas is

    (A) colorectal malignancy
    (B) iatrogenic
    (C) inflammatory bowel disease
    (D) bladder malignancy
    (E) sigmoid diverticulitis

72. All of the following statements are true regarding fistulas EXCEPT

    (A) barium enema, ultrasound, CT scan, and cystoscopy are used for diagnosis
    (B) the presence of a colovesical fistula is a surgical emergency

(C) the fistula may close spontaneously in patients with diverticular disease
(D) if surgical resection is required, the bladder is separated from the colon and the segment of bowel is resected
(E) some patients present with a refractory urinary tract infection

Questions 73 Through 75

A 42-year-old woman comes for frequent office visits over a 6-month period. She has numerous somatic complaints, including diffuse aches and pains. On physical examination, she has gained 20 pounds in 6 months and her voice has become somewhat hoarse. She also reports menorrhagia and dryness of her skin.

73. Which of the following is the MOST likely diagnosis in this patient?

    (A) Addison's disease
    (B) Cushing's disease
    (C) primary hypothyroidism
    (D) thyrotoxicosis
    (E) acromegaly

74. The MOST common cause of this disorder is

    (A) drug induced
    (B) congenital
    (C) iatrogenic
    (D) autoimmune destruction
    (E) trauma

75. Which of the following laboratory abnormalities is seen in this disorder?

    (A) elevated creatinine
    (B) normal thyroid-stimulating hormone (TSH)
    (C) low folate levels
    (D) elevated alkaline phosphatase
    (E) microcytic anemia

TABLE 5.1 STAGES OF PUBIC HAIR AND PUBERTAL GENITAL DEVELOPMENT IN MALES

Stage	Characteristics
1	No pubic hair
2	A little soft, thin hair; testes enlarging
3	Some darker, curlier hair; skin over testicles thinner; testicles larger
4	More dark, thick, curly hair but not on upper legs; testes getting larger
5	Upper line of hair is straight across; hair has spread to upper legs

Questions 76 Through 78

76. During the process of normal adolescent growth and development (see Table 5.1), which of the following statements is correct regarding male gynecomastia?

    (A) It occurs at midpuberty in about 50% of boys.
    (B) It always involves both breasts.
    (C) It usually resolves with hormonal treatment.
    (D) It is usually effectively treated with corticosteroids.
    (E) Surgical consultation is prudent to confirm the diagnosis.

77. Which of the following is true of puberty in a normal female?

    (A) begins with menarche
    (B) occurs at Tanner 1 or 2
    (C) begins with the thelarche
    (D) occurs between 14 and 16 years
    (E) growth spurt occurs at Tanner 1 or 2

78. The first sign of puberty in a normal male is usually the

    (A) increase in size of the testes
    (B) appearance of facial hair
    (C) appearance of axillary hair
    (D) appearance of pubic hair
    (E) appearance of "girl watching"

Questions 79 Through 81

A 29-year-old nulliparous woman at 36 weeks' gestation with a previously uncomplicated pregnancy has an incidental finding of a consistently elevated blood pressure of 190/110 and 4+ proteinuria. She thinks she has some increased "water weight." Otherwise, she is without complaint.

79. The patient's diagnosis is

    (A) essential hypertension
    (B) nephrotic syndrome
    (C) mild preeclampsia
    (D) severe preeclampsia
    (E) HELLP (hemolysis, elevated liver enzymes, and low platelet count) syndrome

80. The next step in her management is to

    (A) perform a pelvic exam to plan for delivery
    (B) draw platelet count and liver enzymes and start a 24-hour urine collection for protein
    (C) admit the patient for hospital bedrest
    (D) perform a cesarean section
    (E) perform a nonstress test

81. The cornerstone of the medical management of a preeclamptic patient is the administration of $Mg\ SO_4, 7H_2O$, which

    (A) decreases maternal mean arterial pressure
    (B) increases uterine blood flow
    (C) stops uterine contractions
    (D) prevents neonatal intraventricular hemorrhage
    (E) prevents eclamptic seizures

Questions 82 Through 85

A 45-year-old divorced woman is self-referred for psychiatric services. She complains of a depressed mood for 4 to 5 months, accompanied by anger, irritability, poor appetite and weight loss, social isolation, tearfulness, poor concentration, impaired sleep, and suicidal ideation. Past psychiatric history is significant for a 6-month course of marital therapy. Current psychosocial stressors include financial pressures and conflicts in her relationship with a significant other.

82. Which of the following BEST describes this patient's DSM-IV diagnosis?

    (A) major depression, single episode
    (B) major depression, chronic
    (C) benzodiazepine dependence
    (D) adjustment disorder, depressive type
    (E) bipolar disorder, depressive episode

83. Which of the following medications would MOST appropriately treat the symptoms of this patient?

    (A) fluoxetine
    (B) carbamazepine
    (C) diphenhydramine
    (D) fluphenazine
    (E) risperidone

84. After 4 weeks of treatment with the medication chosen above, the patient reports improvement in all of her symptoms. She adds that she and her significant other are getting along much better. She is concerned, however, because she has experienced some decreased interest in sex and anorgasmia. What is the MOST likely etiology of her new complaint?

    (A) a previously undiagnosed sexual dysfunction disorder
    (B) severe interpersonal conflict with her significant other
    (C) a manifestation of her underlying personality disorder

    (D) a side effect of the medication chosen
    (E) a factitious complaint in keeping with her attention-seeking behavior pattern

85. What is the MOST appropriate treatment at this point?

    (A) Decrease the medication dosage and schedule a follow-up appointment.
    (B) Refer the patient for couples counseling.
    (C) Refer the patient to a sexual disorders clinic.
    (D) Confront the patient regarding her attention-seeking behavior.
    (E) Refer the patient for ECT.

Questions 86 Through 88

You are present at the delivery of an infant suspected of being postdates. There was some evidence of fetal distress with the passage of terminal meconium. After the delivery, the baby is dried and assigned Apgar scores of 4 at 1 minute and 8 at 5 minutes. The baby's birth weight was 8 pounds. The mother expresses her choice to breast feed the baby.

86. Which of the following is a true statement about breast feeding?

    (A) Intubation for suctioning meconium can inhibit attachment to the breast.
    (B) A postdates baby always needs stabilization before breast feeding.
    (C) Newborns will not root immediately after birth for the mother's nipple.
    (D) Studies have demonstrated that longevity of the breast-feeding experience is unaffected by early attachment after birth.
    (E) Mothers should not put their babies to breast before delivery of the placenta and repair of the perineum.

87. After the mother and baby leave the delivery area, routine assessment of the baby with a Dextrostix finds evidence of a low glucose. The baby has meconium staining but does not appear jittery or cyanotic. The next treatment step in management of this baby is to

(A) obtain a serum glucose level, place a feeding tube into the baby's stomach, and give 15 cc glucose water

(B) obtain a serum glucose level and give the baby a bottle of glucose water

(C) feed the baby a bottle of glucose water and then repeat the Dextrostix in 30 minutes

(D) administer intravenous glucose as a bolus of 200 mg/kg

(E) send a serum glucose level, allow the baby to return to the mother's breast, observe for symptoms, and recheck a Dextrostix in 30 minutes

88. Several days after discharge, you receive a call from a home health care nurse regarding the mother. The nurse informs you that the mother wants to know if the medications she took home from the hospital will pass into her breast milk. Which of the following is contraindicated for breast feeding?

(A) acetaminophen

(B) codeine

(C) metronidazole

(D) low-estrogen–containing oral contraceptive pills

(E) erythromycin

89. Under which of the following circumstances does the law require reporting of suspected child abuse by a psychiatrist who evaluates a child?

(A) in all cases

(B) only when the psychiatrist believes it is in the child's best interest

(C) only when consent of a parent or guardian is obtained

(D) only in cases in which the child shows behavioral manifestations of abuse

(E) only when the psychiatrist has examined all members of the family

Questions 90 Through 92

During a periodic health evaluation, a 67-year-old man is noted to have microhematuria. The patient complains that he gets up six to eight times each night to urinate. He has been treated for a urinary tract infection three times in the past 6 months. An intravenous pyelogram (IVP) and cystogram are performed. On rectal examination, his prostate is noted to be enlarged, but no masses are present. His prostate-specific antigen (PSA) is normal.

90. All of the following conditions show radiologic features of benign prostatic hypertrophy (BPH) EXCEPT

(A) filling defect at base of the bladder

(B) calcification of the prostate

(C) diverticula of the bladder

(D) bladder stones

(E) ureteric dilation

91. All of the following are indications to undergo prostatectomy for BPH EXCEPT

(A) poor stream

(B) annoying frequency and nocturia

(C) large amount of infected residual urine

(D) obstructive uropathy

(E) enlarged prostate

92. Advantages of transurethral prostatectomy over open prostatectomy include all of the following EXCEPT

(A) lower mortality and morbidity

(B) bladder diverticula can be removed

(C) less risk of wound healing or urinary fistula

(D) shorter period of catheterization

(E) fewer bleeding problems

93. The MOST rapid acquisition of a behavior is found in

    (A) partial reinforcement
    (B) positive reinforcement
    (C) negative reinforcement
    (D) continuous reinforcement
    (E) Pavlovian conditioning

94. The following are different levels of intelligence quotient (IQ) scores. Patients falling within which range would be reported as having "moderate mental retardation"?

    (A) IQ level below 20 or 25
    (B) IQ level 20–25 to 35–40
    (C) IQ level 35–40 to 50–55
    (D) IQ level 50–55 to approximately 70
    (E) IQ level 71–85

95. A 24-year-old sexually active patient presents with a maculopapular rash mostly involving her palms and soles. She admits to having developed, several months prior to this rash, a solitary, painless, ulcerative lesion in the right labia majus along with painless inguinal lymphadenopathy. A serum test for syphilis using the rapid plasma reagin test (RPR) was nonreactive at the time the ulcer was present. This patient should be treated with which antibiotic regiment?

    (A) benzathine penicillin G, 2.4 million units IM
    (B) benzathine penicillin G, 2.4 million units IM given weekly for 3 consecutive weeks
    (C) aqueous procaine penicillin G, 4.8 million units IM, and probenecid 1 g PO just before the injection, plus doxycycline, 100 mg PO bid for 7 days
    (D) cefixime, 400 mg PO, plus doxycycline, 100 mg PO bid for 7 days
    (E) amoxicillin, 500 mg PO tid for 7 to 10 days

96. A 95-year-old nursing home resident arrives at the emergency department after being found on the floor next to her bed. She is unable to provide a history, but transfer records from an outside hospital indicate she has a displaced hip fracture. They do not indicate which side, but this is clinically apparent because the affected limb is

    (A) shortened
    (B) externally rotated
    (C) shortened and externally rotated
    (D) flexed, abducted, and internally rotated
    (E) flexed, abducted, and externally rotated

Questions 97 Through 99

A sexually active 18-year-old man complains of a painful urethral discharge.

97. Which of the following organisms is responsible for up to 50% of all cases of acute urethral syndrome?

    (A) *Escherichia coli*
    (B) *Pseudomonas aeruginosa*
    (C) *Staphylococcus aureus*
    (D) *Candida albicans*
    (E) *Chlamydia trachomatis*

98. After appropriate studies, a diagnosis of gonorrhea is made. Which of the following would MOST likely be found on a smear of his discharge?

    (A) gram-positive rods
    (B) gram-negative rods
    (C) gram-positive cocci
    (D) gram-negative cocci
    (E) acid-fast bacilli

99. Treatment options could include which of the following?

    (A) ceftriaxone, 125 mg IM daily for 2 days
    (B) amoxicillin, 500 mg PO qid for 10 days
    (C) ciprofloxacin, 500 mg PO once
    (D) cefixime, 400 mg PO tid for 10 days
    (E) spectinomycin, 1 g IM daily for 7 days

Questions 100 Through 102

A 3-week-old, first-born male infant presents with projectile vomiting void of bile. He appears to be hungry all the time and has lost weight since his 2-week check-up.

100. The MOST likely diagnosis is

(A) duodenal stenosis
(B) adrenogenital syndrome
(C) aminoaciduria
(D) gastroesophageal reflux
(E) pyloric stenosis

101. The diagnostic physical finding in the above condition is

(A) abdominal tenderness
(B) peristaltic waves in lower abdomen
(C) hyperactive bowel sounds
(D) olive-shaped mass in upper abdomen
(E) abdominal distention

102. If the physical examination is NOT diagnostic, which of the following tests should be obtained?

(A) sweat chloride
(B) esophageal pH probe
(C) abdominal ultrasound
(D) urine metabolic screen
(E) abdominal films

103. The MOST common etiology of asymmetric intrauterine growth retardation (IUGR) is

(A) aneuploidy
(B) maternal smoking
(C) maternal vascular disease
(D) congenital malformation
(E) maternal drug ingestion

Questions 104 Through 106

A 69-year-old woman changes insurance and can no longer see her old physician. She comes to you for the first time with a long-standing history of pruritus treated prn with Benadryl and emollient lotions. She also suffers from recurrent superficial phlebitis. Her CBC is shown in Figure 5.4. On physical examination she has an enlarged spleen and has a slightly erythematous face.

104. The MOST likely diagnosis is

(A) acute myelogenous leukemia
(B) polycythemia rubra vera
(C) thrombocytopenic purpura
(D) leukemoid reaction
(E) metastatic carcinoma

Tech:
Date reported:
Time reported:

□ Routine □ Today □ STAT
□ CBC □ WBC □ DIFF □ RBC □ HBG □ HCT
□ RETIC □ PLAT. CT □ ESR □ PT □ PTT □ SICKLE CELL
Name:
Date requested:
Doctor:
Chart no.:

Results	Test	Normal values
24.8□	WBC $\times 100^6$	M 4.3–10 F 4.3–10
□□7.48□	RBC $\times 1012^6$	M 4.4–6.0 F 4.2–5.4
15.0□	HGB g/dL	M 14–18 F 12–16
48.5□	HCT m^2/dL	M 41–51 F 37–47
65□	MCV m	80–96
20□	MCH Pg	20–32
31	MCHC gm/dL	31–36

Differential		Relative nor. value
Sef	89□	34.6–71.4
Band	1□	
Lymph	7□	19.6–32.7
Alyphed Lymph	□□□	
MONO	2□	2.4–11.8
EOSIN	□	0–7.8
Baso		0–1.8
Meta-Myelo		0
Myelo		0
Pre-Myelo		0

Test	Result
RETIC count	
Platelet count	□581,□000
SED plate	
PROTH time	
PT control	
PTT	
Platelet EST	↑

RBC morph:
Microcytic□
Normochromic□
Slight Poikilocytosis□
Slight Basophilia

Figure 5.4

105. This patient's splenomegaly is MOST probably caused by

    (A) recurrent infection
    (B) increased adipose tissue
    (C) extramedullary hematopoiesis
    (D) portal hypertension
    (E) none of the above

106. Which of the following would be MOST
likely in this patient?

    (A) elevated copper level
    (B) low leukocyte alkaline phosphatase
    (C) normal 24-hour urine uric acid
    (D) normal arterial blood gas
    (E) increased marrow iron stores

Questions 107 and 108

A 34-year-old woman (G4,P3) at 34 weeks' gestation is admitted with significant vaginal bleeding
and a blood pressure of 140/90. Ultrasound shows
no placenta previa. Her platelet count is 57,000, and
the fibrinogen is 150 mg/dL.

107. Which of the following statements is true regarding this patient?

    (A) This patient has HELLP syndrome and
    should be given betamethasone and de-
    livered in 48 hours.
    (B) This patient has disseminated intravas-
    cular coagulation (DIC) and should be
    treated with heparin.
    (C) This patient has a consumptive coagu-
    lopathy and should be treated with re-
    placement of blood and clotting factors.
    (D) This patient has an abruption, resulting
    in a consumptive coagulopathy, and
    should be delivered promptly.
    (E) This patient has an abruption, but thera-
    peutic intervention is *not* required if the
    fetal monitor tracing is normal.

108. Risk factors for placental abruption include

    (A) increasing maternal age and parity, dia-
    betes, and hypertension
    (B) increasing maternal parity and age,
    IUGR, and Rh isoimmunization

    (C) hypertension, diabetes, and IUGR
    (D) increasing maternal age, parity, hyper-
    tension, cocaine use, and cigarette smok-
    ing
    (E) IUGR, diabetes, and Rh isoimmunization

Questions 109 Through 111

The infant mortality rate (IMR) is a major indicator
of a population's overall health status.

109. Which of the following statements is true
about infant mortality in the United States?

    (A) The U.S. IMR has dropped precipitously
    since the turn of the century and contin-
    ues to fall.
    (B) The IMR among African-American in-
    fants is nearly four times the IMR among
    Caucasian infants.
    (C) The U.S. IMR is among the lowest rates
    in the industrialized world.
    (D) It shows significant regional and small
    area variation, due primarily to variation
    in access to specialized health care ser-
    vices.
    (E) It is composed in roughly equal propor-
    tions of neonatal (0 to 28 days) and post-
    neonatal (29 to 365 days) mortality.

110. To have the greatest positive impact on infant mortality in the United States, we should
increase access to and utilization of

    (A) neonatal intensive care for babies born
    prematurely
    (B) prenatal ultrasound screening to detect
    treatable anomalies
    (C) preconceptional genetic testing of
    prospective parents
    (D) family planning counseling and contra-
    ceptive services
    (E) screening for and treatment of toxemia

111. Birth defects are a major cause of infant mortality as well as long-term morbidity and disability during childhood. The causes of most
defects are multifactorial, involving environmental, genetic, nutritional, and other con-

tributors. Primary prevention is effective on a population level for which of the following major malformations?

(A) renal agenesis

(B) tetralogy of Fallot

(C) anencephaly

(D) achondroplastic dwarfism

(E) hypertrophic pyloric stenosis

112. Your associate delivered a very anxious patient approximately 8 hours ago. Meperidine was used for analgesia. The Apgar scores were 3 at 1 minute and 8 at 5 minutes. Although your associate discussed the Apgar score and the pH with her after the delivery, she is still concerned. She is a third-year medical student and has not yet had an obstetrics rotation. She is worried about the low 1-minute Apgar score. A low Apgar score at 1 minute

(A) is highly correlated with late neurologic sequelae

(B) indicates an acidemic newborn

(C) has the same significance in premature and term infants

(D) is of minimal prognostic value

(E) is a useful index of resuscitative efforts

Questions 113 Through 115

A 3-year-old boy is found on routine screening to have a blood lead level of 23. His mother reports that the family lives in an apartment building that was built in 1926 and that is not well maintained by the landlord. There is peeling paint around several window frames. The apartment is on a busy street, and there is no yard or playground nearby, so the children play inside or out on the sidewalk.

113. Which of the following is the MOST likely source of this boy's lead poisoning?

(A) paint chips

(B) dust in the apartment

(C) dirt from the sidewalk outside

(D) tap water

(E) all of the above

114. What should the parents do to reduce their son's lead exposure?

(A) Use a power sander to sand smooth any peeling pain in the apartment.

(B) Help the boy to wash his hands before eating.

(C) Sweep up all visible paint chips and paint dust.

(D) Increase the amount of vitamin B_6 in the boy's diet.

(E) Administer oral chelation therapy under physician supervision.

115. Which of the following can result from long-term, low-level exposure to lead?

(A) reduced IQ and behavioral problems

(B) chronic fatigue syndrome

(C) hepatocellular carcinoma

(D) saturnine gout

(E) osteoporosis

116. Which of the following is the MOST common indication for cesarean section in the United States?

(A) breech presentation

(B) fetal distress

(C) dystocia/failure to progress

(D) repeat cesarean section

(E) all other indications

Questions 117 Through 119

A 54-year old woman has come to see you for help with quitting smoking. She says she has already tried twelve times to quit, but each time she starts again after a few days. Her husband, who quit 15 years ago on his first try, has told her that she has no will power. (See Figure 5.5.)

117. What do her past failures to quit smoking tell you about how to increase the likelihood of success this time?

   (A) She is not sufficiently motivated; she would benefit from information about the ways smoking is harmful to her, physically and financially.
   (B) She has never gotten beyond nicotine withdrawal; nicotine replacement therapy would probably be helpful.
   (C) She has no social support system; she should join a support group.
   (D) She has reached a point of diminishing returns in her effort to quit; you should inform her that if she does not quit permanently this time, success is unlikely.

118. Which of the following population-based tobacco control efforts is most useful in encouraging current smokers to quit?

   (A) prohibiting outdoor advertising
   (B) increasing cigarette taxes by 25 cents per pack
   (C) restricting smoking in public places
   (D) conducting "sting operations" in places where cigarettes are sold
   (E) prohibiting sale of cigarettes in vending machines

119. Which of the following female cancers is most strongly associated with cigarette smoking?

   (A) breast
   (B) cervical
   (C) ovarian
   (D) endometrial
   (E) vaginal clear cell

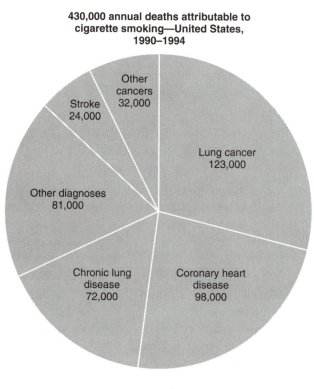

430,000 annual deaths attributable to cigarette smoking—United States, 1990–1994

Other cancers 32,000
Stroke 24,000
Lung cancer 123,000
Other diagnoses 81,000
Chronic lung disease 72,000
Coronary heart disease 98,000

Figure 5.5

120. Of the following psychotropic drugs, which is the MOST likely to produce pigmentary retinopathy?

   (A) lithium
   (B) thioridazine
   (C) maprotiline hydrochloride
   (D) haloperidol
   (E) amitriptyline

121. In negligence,

   (A) a standard of care must exist
   (B) a duty must be owed by the defendant or someone for whose conduct he or she is answerable
   (C) the duty must be owed the plaintiff
   (D) there must be a breach of duty
   (E) all of the above

122. Which of the following sets of laboratory results would be MOST consistent with a diagnosis of alcohol dependence?

(A) elevated bilirubin; microcytic anemia

(B) elevated serum glutamic oxaloacetic transaminase (SGOT); folate toxicity

(C) elevated gamma-glutamyl transpeptidase (GGT); macrocytosis

(D) elevated serum glutamic pyruvic transaminase (SGPT); vitamin B_{12} deficiency

(E) blood alcohol level; iron deficiency

123. Information learned from the National Institute of Mental Health Epidemiologic Catchment Area Program includes

(A) as a group, anxiety disorders were the most prevalent, with a lifetime prevalence rate of 14.6%

(B) substance abuse was found to be more prevalent in older age groups

(C) prevalence of affective disorders was equal to that of schizophrenia

(D) men were found to have higher overall rates of mental disorders than women

(E) women had higher prevalence rates of alcoholism than men

124. Infants and children are vertically infected with HIV

(A) in utero

(B) at delivery

(C) after delivery

(D) in utero, at delivery, and after delivery

(E) none of the above

125. Among people who have attempted suicide, which of the following groups would be at the HIGHEST risk for completed suicide?

(A) women

(B) those under the age of 45

(C) the employed

(D) those living with relatives

(E) those with previous attempts by violent methods

126. Which of the following statements is true of patients with amnestic syndrome?

(A) They may be oriented and alert but cannot remember what happened a few hours earlier.

(B) They are able to remember recent events.

(C) They have delusional psychoses.

(D) Alcohol abuse and deficiency of niacin combine to cause the clinical picture.

(E) Tactile hallucinations are often found in the syndrome.

127. The largest diagnostic group among suicide completers is

(A) depression

(B) alcoholism

(C) schizophrenia

(D) anxiety disorders

(E) drug dependence

128. A 53-year-old man with no significant medical history arrived at the emergency department with complaints of cataclysmic headache while engaging in sexual intercourse, accompanied by nausea, vomiting, nuchal rigidity with meningismus, and diffuse occipital headache. A CT scan confirmed subarachnoid hemorrhage. All of the following are true about subarachnoid hemorrhage EXCEPT

(A) it rarely occurs in sleep

(B) it can be precipitated by physical activity

(C) patients are frequently hypertensive following hemorrhage

(D) it causes retinal hemorrhages

(E) it causes changes in the electrocardiogram (ECG)

DIRECTIONS (Questions 129 through 150): Each group of items in this section consists of lettered headings followed by a set of numbered words or phrases. For each numbered word or phrase, select the ONE lettered heading that is most closely associated with it. Each lettered heading may be selected once, more than once, or not at all.

Questions 129 Through 135

The following group of questions pertains to patients who have AIDS.

(A) pneumocystis carinii pneumonia (PCP)
(B) *Mycobacterium avium-intracellulare* complex (MAC)
(C) cytomegalovirus
(D) herpes simplex
(E) *Cryptosporidium*
(F) *Cryptococcus neoformans*
(G) *Mycobacterium tuberculosis*
(H) *Toxoplasma gondii*
(I) non-Hodgkin's lymphoma
(J) Kaposi's sarcoma

129. A 22-year-old man has brain lesions. Biopsy shows an obligate intracellular protozoan.

130. A 34-year-old woman has retinitis.

131. A 15-year-old boy with hemophilia A has meningitis.

132. A 62-year-old man has intractable diarrhea.

133. You recommend prophylaxis when your patient's CD4 counts fall below 200.

134. A 26-year-old woman has weight loss, fever, and liver function abnormalities.

135. A 50-year-old man is found to have the most common neoplasm seen in HIV infection.

Questions 136 Through 139

The following group of questions pertains to "milestones."

(A) 18 months
(B) 30 months
(C) 3 years
(D) 40 months
(E) 5 years
(F) 4 months
(G) 6 months

136. Can name four colors and count 10 pennies

137. Expected to know age and sex

138. First one-word utterances

139. Uses two- and three-word phrases

Questions 140 Through 144

(A) simple partial seizures
(B) complex partial seizures
(C) tonic–clonic (grand mal) seizures
(D) absence (petit mal) seizures
(E) myoclonic seizures
(F) status epilepticus

140. A 55-year-old man, recently arrived from Great Britain, has a long history of beef consumption. He has now developed a rapidly progressive dementia.

141. A 27-year-old woman's magnetic resonance imaging (MRI) reveals temporal lobe sclerosis.

142. A teenager has a long history of "daydreaming" in school. Electroencephalogram (EEG) reveals evidence of a generalized seizure disorder, but there has never been a history of convulsive muscular activity.

143. A 23-year-old woman has a history of repetitive involuntary movements of her right hand associated with abnormal facial movements. At times, the movements spread to involve the entire arm.

144. This form of epilepsy almost always starts in childhood.

Questions 145 Through 150

    (A) esophageal atresia
    (B) pyloric stenosis
    (C) chalasia
    (D) duodenal atresia
    (E) intussusception

145. It has a high incidence in Down syndrome.

146. Bloody stool may be seen.

147. Surgery is usually not indicated.

148. Passage of a radiopaque catheter is usually diagnostic.

149. It is more frequent in male infants.

150. Barium enema is indicated if there is no intestinal perforation.

Answers and Explanations

1–5. (1-B, 2-B, 3-B, 4-A, 5-E) Pediatricians are being faced daily with the reality of caring for infants with AIDS. The fastest growing segment of patients with pediatric AIDS is described in this patient. Perinatal transmission from a drug-abusing, HIV-positive mother accounts for the greatest number of children with AIDS. Twenty to thirty-five percent of infants who test positive at birth will go on to develop full-blown AIDS. Receiving gamma globulin is not a risk factor for AIDS. In contrast to adult AIDS, Kaposi's sarcoma is rare in children. Clinical manifestations may include hepatosplenomegaly, chronic interstitial pneumonia, and chronic parotid swelling. HIV-positive children need immunizations to protect them against childhood diseases. Oral polio vaccine, however, as a live virus vaccine, is contraindicated. (MMR is also a live virus vaccine but is recommended unless the patient is severely immunocompromised.) (See Table 5.2 and Figure 5.6.)

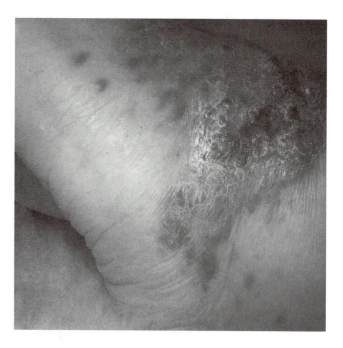

Figure 5.6. Crusted, violaceous papules and nodules on the lower leg and foot with classic Kaposi's sarcoma.

6. (C) The electronic fetal monitor demonstrates a baseline heart rate of 160 bpm, decreased to absent variability, and repetitive late decelerations. The interpretation is nonreassuring. The patient's labor graph shows an arrest of dilatation pattern. The nonreassuring electronic fetal monitor precludes augmentation and further attempts at a vaginal delivery. Oxytocin is contraindicated in the presence of late decelerations. In utero resuscitation should be performed while preparing for a cesarean delivery, since this patient is unlikely to deliver vaginally within a reasonable period of time.

7. (D) The right to treatment has been formulated as an important legal question in all categories of noncriminal confinement. To fulfill this treatment right, a state must provide a humane physical and psychological environment, qualified staff in sufficient numbers, and individual treatment or rehabilitation plans for each patient. Refusal of treatment and informed consent are not applicable because the man has been hospitalied involuntarily and thus must have been determined to not have capacity. Without capacity, a person is generally not competent to stand trial, but capacity is determined by a psychiatrist and competence is determined by a judge.

TABLE 5.2 COMMON PRESENTING SYMPTOMS AND SIGNS OF HIV INFECTION IN CHILDREN

General
Growth delay or failure to thrive
Weight loss
Recurrent fever
Generalized lymphadenopathy
Hepatomegaly
Splenomegaly

Neurologic Conditions
Progressive encephalopathy
Delayed development
Loss of developmental milestones
Acquired microcephaly
Hypertonicity and spasticity, especially of the lower extremities

Pulmonary Conditions
Pneumocystis carinii pneumonia (PCP)
Lymphoid interstitial pneumonitis (LIP)
Cytomegalovirus (CMV) pneumonia
Recurrent bacterial pneumonia

Oral Conditions
Thrush (chronic, recurrent, or difficult to eradicate)
Parotitis or enlarged parotid glands

Gastrointestinal Tract Conditions
Recurrent or chronic diarrhea

Hepatic Conditions
Hepatitis

Hematologic Conditions
Anemia
Leukopenia
Lymphopenia
Thrombocytopenia (immune thrombocytopenic purura)

Dermatologic Conditions
Atopic dermatitis
Seborrhea
Candida diaper dermatitis

Opportunistic Infections
Recurrent otitis media
Serious bacterial infections (sepsis, pneumonia, meningitis, osteomyelitis)
Tuberculosis
Mycobacterim avium complex infection
Candida esophagitis
Toxoplasmosis (older than 1 month of age)
CMV, disseminated or organ-specific
DIsseminated herpes simplex virus infection
PCP

Other Conditions
Cardiomyopathy
Chronic or recurrent otitis media
Chronic rhinorrhea

Tumors
Lymphoma (non-Hodgkin's or primary central nervous system)
Leiomyosarcoma

8. **(E)** There are almost no absolute contraindications for ECT, given under modern anesthesia and with a modern machine. All the conditions listed can increase the risk of complications of ECT, but, in many cases, measures can be taken to reduce the risk. With modern methods, ECT is safer than the use of tricyclic medication.

9. **(A)** Approximately 7 to 10% of women will show signs and symptoms of a transient depression postpartum. This is commonly associated with an emotional letdown within the immediate postpartum period. The patient's discomforts and lifestyle changes associated with anxiety over her ability to care for the newborn and concern over becoming less attractive to her mate contribute significantly. In most cases, it lasts less than 2 weeks. Underlying chronic depression is also a factor. Persistent blues and severe depression are not variations of normal.

10. **(C)** By the history elicited, the patient describes an intermittent mass in the umbilical area present on straining, which is most consistent with an umbilical hernia. This patient had an incarcerated umbilical hernia containing a piece of strangulated omentum. The other choices would be much less common. Sister Joseph's node is a metastatic gastric tumor to the umbilical area.

11. **(D)** The correct diagnosis is an incarcerated umbilical hernia; therefore, the correct answer is to repair the hernia and examine the contents incarcerated in the hernia sac. In this case, a piece of strangulated omentum was resected before the herniorrhaphy. None of the other treatment options address the correct diagnosis.

12. **(E)** In hemochromatosis, arthropathy usually involves the second and third metacarpophalangeal joints, then knees, hips, and shoul-

ders. It occurs in one quarter to one half of patients. Diabetes occurs in 65% of patients and is more common in those with a family history of diabetes. Cardiac disease is the presenting symptom in 15% of patients, with heart failure being the usual manifestation. Hypogonadism may manifest as loss of libido, impotence, amenorrhea, testicular atrophy, and sparse body hair. Skin pigmentation is present in 90% of symptomatic patients at presentation, but renal involvement is not characteristic of the disease.

13. **(C)** A specific genetic abnormality has been localized to the sixth chromosome near the human lymphocyte antigen (HLA) complex. Screening relatives with ferritin levels and starting therapeutic phlebotomy early may indeed prevent or delay end-organ damage. The level to keep the ferritin is not yet established, but most hematologists aim for low normal. Although the regular blood and iron loss that occurs in menstruating and childbearing women balances the increased absorption of iron, some women still develop overt signs prior to menopause.

14. **(D)** Children with constitutional growth delay have a delayed puberty; therefore, they have more time to grow. They usually attain a normal adult height. Bone age is delayed, but growth rate (velocity) is normal after age 4. It is common for these children to have a parent with a similar growth pattern. See Table 5.3 for causes of limb length inequality.

15–16. **(15-B [or E with B], 16-C)** Vaginal carcinoma causes 1 to 2% of cancers in women. It is most common in the sixth or seventh decade. This disease is diagnosed and staged by clinical examination. If the cervix is involved, cervical cancer is diagnosed, not vaginal cancer. The most common histopathology is epidermoid. Clear cell adenocarcinoma is rare. Spread of the disease is by local extension and lymphatics. Upper vaginal lesions spread in a fashion similar to cervical cancer. Lower vaginal lesions may extend in a manner similar to vulvar carcinoma. The International Federation of Gynecology and

TABLE 5.3 CAUSES OF LIMB LENGTH INEQUALITY

Infectious causes
  Osteomyelitis
  Septic arthritis
Neoplastic causes
  Arteriovenous malformations
  Hemangioma
Neuromuscular causes
  Cerebral palsy
  Isolated limb paralysis
  Poliomyelitis
Traumatic causes
  Malunion of long bones
  Physeal injury
Other causes
  Avascular necrosis of femoral head (and physis)
  Congenital amputations
  Legg–Calvé–Perthes disease

Obstetrics (FIGO) staging is similar to cervical cancer but less detailed. The primary treatment for disease confined to the pelvis is similar to cervical cancer but less detailed. The primary treatment for disease confined to the pelvis is whole pelvis radiation therapy. If the lesion is at an early stage and confined to the upper vagina, in certain specific instances, radical hysterectomy, partial vaginectomy, and pelvic lymphadenectomy may be offered. Chemotherapy may be offered in the case of distant metastatic disease. The response of the tumor is usually poor when this treatment is employed.

17. **(A)** Autoimmune thyroiditis is a common cause of goiter attributable to lymphocytic infiltration of the gland. Enlargement of the thyroid is also seen in Graves' disease. Another cause of goiter is dietary iodine deficiency; although it is uncommon in North America and Europe, it still affects 100 million people around the world. Thyroid carcinoma is less common in younger patients and generally presents as a distinct nodule. Branchial cleft cysts and parathyroid adenomas, while found in this area, are usually distinct nodules and not symmetric. Laryngeal carcinoma would have to be very far advanced to be palpable externally and would have significant other symptoms.

18. **(D)** Iodine deficiency is the most common cause of thyroid disease in the world population, although iodination of salt has eliminated this problem in North America and Europe. Areas in which iodine intake remains low include mountainous regions such as the Andes and Himalayas, as well as some areas of Central Africa, New Guinea, and Indonesia. Iodine prophylaxis in the form of foodstuffs or the administration of iodinized oil injections has helped the situation in many areas.

19. **(E)** A pneumothorax is a collection of air or gas occupying the pleural space. A tension pneumothorax, in which the mediastinum shifts to the contralateral side, is an emergency because the patient can go into shock and die. Figure 5.3 demonstrates a right pneumothorax. This patient had a spontaneous pneumothorax that subsequently developed into a tension pneumothorax. The correct treatment for a tension pneumothorax is placement of a thoracostomy tube and re-expansion of the lung.

20. **(E)** Toxigenic *E. coli* is a major cause of "travelers' diarrhea," the most common illness among individuals from the United States and other industrialized countries traveling in the third world. The other illnesses are all endemic in areas of the world the journalist is planning to visit, but they are far less common than simple travelers' diarrhea.

21. **(A)** Norfloxacin, 400 mg daily, can prevent travelers' diarrhea; however, sanitary precautions (eg, handwashing, careful food preparation, use of bottled drinking water) are the most important means of prevention. The other drugs listed are not effective against *E. coli* enteritis.

22. **(A)** Many of these illnesses are endemic in the regions of the world this man is planning to visit. Yellow fever vaccination is the only mandatory one of the vaccines listed; it is required for travel to tropical Africa and to Central and South America. Vaccination for smallpox is no longer necessary since its worldwide eradication in October 1977. Meningococcal vaccination is recommended for travel in endemic areas (eg, Saudi Arabia, Nepal) during high-incidence seasons. Japanese encephalitis vaccination is recommended for travel in rural areas in Asia. There is no vaccine against trypanosomiasis, also known as sleeping sickness.

23. **(B)** Tourette's disorder is a syndrome that involves tics produced by multiple muscle groups. Additionally, at some point, there must be at least one vocal tic, such as hiccuping, sighing, whistling, belching, throat clearing, yawning, sniffing, or lip smacking. Criteria for diagnosis include the presence of symptoms for at least 1 year and onset of symptoms before age 18. Patients with Huntington's disease or Sydenham's chorea have choreiform movements, patients with Parkinson's disease have a resting tremor, and patients with Alzheimer's disease do not demonstrate a specific abnormal movement pattern.

24. **(A)** Rales and wheezing are found in both conditions, so the distinction is often arbitrary. CO_2 retention is presumed with a respiratory rate of over 60/min. The disorder is more severe in younger infants but will often resolve spontaneously over several weeks.

25. **(C)** Preterm premature rupture of membranes is a major cause of prematurity as well as perinatal morbidity and mortality. Infection of both the mother and the fetus is the most common and significant complication of preterm premature rupture of membranes except for the premature delivery itself. Approximately 13% of patients managed expectantly will develop chorioamnionitis. In some studies, amniotic fluid infection with intact membranes may cause 25 to 33% of cases of preterm labor. Evidence of infection requires delivery. The infants have a three- to fourfold increase in major morbidity and mortality. The fetal compression anomalies, limb contractions, and pulmonary hypoplasia seldom occur after 26 weeks.

26. **(A)** Diabetes mellitus is a syndrome consisting of hyperglycemia, large vessel disease, microvascular disease, and neuropathy. The classic presenting symptoms are increased thirst, polyuria, polyphagia, and weight loss. In type II (often called non–insulin-dependent diabetes), the presentation can be more subtle and is often made when the patient is less symptomatic.

27. **(B)** This lesion is more frequent in females and may antedate other clinical signs and symptoms of diabetes. The plaques are round, firm, and reddish-brown to yellow in color. They most commonly involve the legs but can also involve hands, arms, abdomen, and head.

28. **(C)** An insulin tolerance test does not establish the diagnosis of diabetes mellitus. Urine testing is not sensitive enough for diagnostic purposes and is no longer used to monitor treatment either. With typical symptoms, an elevated random sugar is diagnostic. The gold standard is still a fasting plasma glucose greater than 140 mg/dL on two separate occasions. Glucose tolerance tests are rarely required.

29. **(C)** Insulin lowers cyclic AMP, probably via an increase in phosphodiesterase activity. This probably inactivates cyclic AMP–dependent protein kinase. This promotes glycogen formation, stimulates glycolysis, and inhibits gluconeogenesis. Pyruvate becomes available for lipogenesis, ketone formation slows, and fatty acid synthesis increases. In the presence of glucose, insulin enhances the activity of lipoprotein lipase.

30. **(E)** The patient is most likely to develop glomerulosclerosis. This can be diffuse or nodular (Kimmelstiel–Wilson nodules). Poor metabolic control is probably a major factor in the progression of diabetic nephropathy.

31. **(A)** A patient who has had ulcerative colitis for more than 10 years is at a significantly increased risk for developing carcinoma of the colon and rectum. The surgical treatment of ulcerative colitis requires removal of the colon and rectal mucosa to obtain a definitive cure. Proctocolectomy with an ileal pouch–anal anastomosis is the procedure of choice. Total proctocolectomy and permanent ileostomy is also curative but is used for patients who are not candidates for the ileoanal procedure. Surgical treatment with total colectomy and ileoproctostomy is usually not indicated because the risk for proctitis and development of carcinoma remains. Small bowel resection does not address the disease process and is inappropriate, and a right hemicolectomy would be an inadequate operation.

32. **(E)** All of the diagnoses listed are complications of ulcerative colitis.

33. **(D)** The lesions generally have segmental involvement with or without skip areas. The rest of the statements are correct for Crohn's (granulomatous) colitis.

34. **(D)** Pain relief in labor is infrequently associated with several undesirable effects. The mother may experience respiratory depression if excessive quantities are given. Fetal respiratory depression may occur if the interval between administration and delivery is too close. Electronic fetal monitoring interpretation is also affected because of the decrease in variability. Late decelerations are not related to parenteral analgesics. The neonate's appetite and activity may be decreased because of the residual effect of the analgesic.

35. **(A)** Pudendal anesthesia is an effective form of regional nerve block affecting the ventral branches of the second, third, and fourth sacral nerves which form the pudendal nerve. Occasionally, the patient will have a unilaterally ineffective block resulting from inadequate distribution of local anesthetic around the nerve. Paravaginal abscess or hematoma occur infrequently. The hematomas are more common in patients with co-

agulation disorder. Convulsions secondary to a direct intervascular injection occur infrequently when proper technique is used.

36. **(D)** Under proper circumstances, epidural anesthesia provides excellent safe pain relief. Epidural anesthesia may cause late decelerations because of a decrease in maternal cardiac output due to peripheral pooling and decreased preload and hypotension. Repositioning and fluids are the first steps in resuscitation. Medications such as ephedrine are used only if the fetal heart rate abnormality does not resolve with hydration and position change.

37. **(A)** Motor vehicle accidents are among the top causes of death in young children. Many of these deaths can be prevented by use of car

safety seats, seating children in the back seat, and careful driving by parents and other caregivers. Lead poisoning is also common and preventable, but almost never fatal. HIV infection in childhood is almost always perinatally acquired and therefore not preventable at the age of 2. Leukemia and Wilms' tumor are relatively common cancers in childhood, but they are extremely rare compared with motor vehicle accidents. (See Figure 5.7.)

38. **(D)** The final booster dose of HIB vaccine is given at 12 to 15 months. The MMR vaccine requires a booster at the time of school entrance (4 to 6 years) or later in childhood (11 to 12 years) to prevent measles in adolescence or adulthood. Diphtheria and tetanus boosters should be taken at age 4 to 6 in the DPT vaccine, and lifelong every 10 years as diphthe-

10 Leading causes of deaths by age group—1995

Rank	<1	1–4	5–9	10–14	15–24	25–34	35–44	45–54	55–64	65+	Total
Age groups											
1	Congenital anomalies 6,554	Unintentional injuries 2,260	Unintentional injuries 1,612	Unintentional injuries 1,932	Unintentional injuries 13,642	Unintentional injuries 13,435	HIV 18,860	Malignant neoplasms 44,186	Malignant neoplasms 87,896	Heart disease 615,426	Heart disease 737,563
2	Short gestation 3,933	Congenital anomalies 695	Malignant neoplasms 523	Malignant neoplasms 503	Homicide 7,284	HIV 11,894	Malignant neoplasms 17,110	Heart disease 34,496	Heart disease 68,240	Malignant neoplasms 381,142	Malignant neoplasms 538,455
3	SIDS 3,397	Malignant neoplasms 488	Congenital anomalies 242	Homicide 405	Suicide 4,784	Suicide 6,292	Unintentional injuries 14,225	Unintentional injuries 9,261	Bronchitis Emphysema Asthma 9,988	Cerebro-vascular 138,762	Cerebro-vascular 157,991
4	Respiratory distress synd. 1,454	Homicide 452	Homicide 157	Suicide 330	Malignant neoplasms 1,642	Homicide 6,162	Heart disease 13,603	HIV 8,179	Cerebro-vascular 9,735	Bronchitis Emphysema Asthma 86,478	Bronchitis Emphysema Asthma 102,899
5	Maternal complications 1,309	Heart disease 251	Heart disease 130	Congenital anomalies 207	Heart disease 1,039	Malignant neoplasms 4,875	Suicide 6,467	Cerebro-vascular 5,473	Diabetes 8,188	Pneumonia & influenza 74,297	Unintentional injuries 93,320
6	Placenta cord membranes 962	HIV 210	HIV 123	Heart disease 164	HIV 629	Heart disease 3,461	Homicide 4,118	Liver disease 5,247	Unintentional injuries 6,743	Diabetes 44,452	Pneumonia & influenza 82,923
7	Perinatal infections 788	Pneumonia & influenza 156	Pneumonia & influenza 73	Bronchitis Emphysema Asthma 105	Congenital anomalies 452	Cerebro-vascular 720	Liver disease 3,705	Suicide 4,532	Liver disease 5,356	Unintentional injuries 29,099	Diabetes 59,254
8	Unintentional injuries 767	Perinatal period 87	Benign neoplasms 50	HIV 68	Bronchitis Emphysema Asthma 246	Pneumonia & influenza 622	Cerebro-vascular 2,772	Diabetes 3,996	Pneumonia & influenza 3,458	Alzheimer's disease 20,230	HIV 43,115
9	Pneumonia & influenza 492	Septicemia 80	Bronchitis Emphysema Asthma 38	Benign neoplasms 55	Pneumonia & influenza 207	Diabetes 614	Diabetes 1,844	Bronchitis Emphysema Asthma 2,756	Suicide 2,804	Nephritis 20,182	Suicide 31,284
10	Intrauterine hypoxia 475	Cerebro-vascular 57	Anemias 31	Pneumonia & influenza 55	Cerebro-vascular 172	Liver disease 604	Pneumonia & influenza 1,480	Pneumonia & influenza 2,079	HIV 2,320	Septicemia 16,899	Liver disease 25,222

Figure 5.7

ria–tetanus (dT) vaccine. The final polio booster is given at 4 to 6 years. (See Figure 5.8.)

39.   **(C)** Immunosuppressed individuals should not be given the live polio vaccine. A killed vaccine (IPV) is available and effective, and it does not pose the risk that the child could develop polio. All of the other vaccinations should be given at the usual doses and times. There is no reason for omitting vaccines or for using split doses, an unwarranted practice followed by some providers in hopes that it might reduce the risk of adverse reactions, particularly to the pertussis vaccine.

40.   **(C)** In the Diagnostic and Statistical Manual, 4th edition (DSM-IV), mental disorders are included in axes I and II. Axis I includes all mental disorders except personality disorders and mental retardation, which are included in axis II. General medical conditions, or physical disorders, are classified as axis III. Psychosocial and environmental problems are classified as axis IV. Axis V registers the clinician's global assessment of the functioning of the patient.

41.   **(D)** Oxazepam (Serax) has a half-life of about 8 hours. This short half-life may benefit elderly patients who are more vulnerable to the cumulative effects of agents such as hypnotics or sedatives. Chlordiazepoxide (Librium) has a half-life of about 24 hours. The half-life of diazepam (Valium) may be roughly estimated by adding 20 hours to the number of years the patient is above the age of 30. Clorazepate (Tranxene) has a half-life of about 50 hours. Phenobarbital is an anticonvulsant, not a benzodiazepine.

42.   **(C)** Posttransfusion hepatitis is most often due to hepatitis C. Hepatitis B and delta hepatitis are also principally transmitted by the parenteral route. Hepatitis A is usually transmitted by the fecal–oral route, and parenteral transmission is unusual.

43.   **(B)** Prolonged decelerations are isolated decelerations. If the deceleration lasts more than 10 to 15 minutes, it is referred to as a

baseline change. The common etiologies include examination, supine hypotension, cord accidents, uteroplacental insufficiency for a variety of reasons, complications of anesthesia, and second-stage labor. The significance of these is challenging. Their management should take into consideration their etiology, frequency, severity, fetal/placental reserve, and stage of labor.

44.   **(D)** Most fetuses with a normal placenta will be resuscitated spontaneously after the prolonged deceleration has recovered. Individualized management is necessary because of the wide variety of clinical situations in which this occurs. Amino infusion is used if oligohydramnios is considered to be the etiology.

45.   **(A)** The rheumatoid factor is positive in 10 to 20% of JRA cases. About 75% of classical rheumatoid arthritis patients have elevated titers. One third of patients have monarticular arthritis, most often in a knee or an ankle. The rheumatoid factor is frequently present in asymptomatic elderly patients and has little diagnostic efficacy in that group and is unrelated to the presence or absence of osteoarthritis. It is an immunoglobulin that attaches to the Fc fragment of IgG molecules.

46.   **(A)** Numerous mediators of inflammation are found in the synovium of patients with rheumatoid arthritis. The evidence favoring activated T cells as the initiators of the inflammation include the predominance of CD4 T cells in the synovium, the increase in soluble interleukin-2 receptors (a product of T-cell activation), and amelioration of symptoms by T-cell removal.

47.   **(E)** Although widespread vasculitis resembling polyarteritis nodosa can occur, most often the skin is involved. This presents as crops of small brown spots in the nail beds, nail folds, and digital pulp. Mononeuropathy is another relatively common presentation of rheumatoid vasculitis.

Vaccine	Birth	1 mo	2 mos	4 mos	6 mos	12 mos	15 mos	18 mos	4–6 yrs	11–12 yrs	14–16 yrs
Hepatitis B†	Hep B	Hep B									
		Hep B	Hep B		Hep B	Hep B	Hep B			Hep B	
Diphtheria, Tetanus, Pertussiss§			DTaP	DTaP	DTaP		DTaP	DTaP	DTaP	Td	
H. influenzae type b¶			Hib	Hib	Hib	Hib					
Poliovirus**			IPV	IPV	Polio	Polio	Polio		Polio		
Rotavirus††			*RV*	*RV*	*RV*						
Measles-Mumps-Rubella§§						MMR			MMR	MMR	
Varicella¶¶						Var	Var			Var	

Range of acceptable ages for vaccination

Vaccines to be assessed and administered if necessary

Incorporation of this new vaccine into clinical practice may require additional time and resources from health-care providers

* This schedule indicates the recommended ages for routine administration of currently licensed childhood vaccines. Any dose not given at the recommended age should be given as a "catch-up" vaccination at any subsequent visit when indicated and feasible. Combination vaccines may be used whenever any components of the combination are indicated and its other components are not contraindicated. Providers should consult the manufacturers' package inserts for detailed recommendations.

† **Infants born to hepatitis B surgace antigen (HBsAg)-negative mothers** should receive the second dose of hepatitis B (Hep B) vaccine at least 1 month after the first dose. The third dose should be administered at least 4 months after the first dose and at least 2 months after the second dose, but not before age 6 months. **Infants born to HBsAg-positive mothers** should receive Hep B vaccine and 0.5 mL hepatitis B immune globulin (HBIG) within 12 hours of birth at separate injection sites. The second dose is recommended at age 1–2 months and the third dose at age 6 months. **Infants born to mothers whose HBsAg status is unknown** should receive Hep B vaccine within 12 hours of birth. Maternal blood should be drawn at the time of delivery to determine the mother's HBsAg status; if the HBsAg test is positive, the infant should receive HBIG as soon as possible (no later than age 1 week). All children and adolescents (through age 18 years) who have not been vaccinated against hepatitis B may begin the series during any visit. Special efforts should be made to vaccinate children who were born in or whose parents were born in areas of the world where hepatitis B virus infection is moderately or highly endemic.

§ Diphtheria and tetanus toxoids and acellular pertussis vaccine (DTaP) is the preferred vaccine for all doses in the vaccination series, including completion of the series in children who have received one or more doses of whole-cell diphtheria and tetanus toxoids and pertussis vaccine (DTP). Whole-cell DTP is an acceptable alternative to DTaP. The fourth dose (DTP or DTaP) may be administered as early as age 12 months, provided 6 months have elapsed since the third dose and if the child is unlikely to return at age 15–18 months. Tetanus and diphtheria toxoids (Td) is recommended at age 11–12 years if at least 5 years have elapsed since the last dose of DTP, DTaP, or DT. Subsequent routine Td boosters are recommended every 10 years.

¶Three *Haemophilus influenzae* type b (Hib) conjugate vaccines are licensed for infant use. If Hib conjugate vaccine (PRP-OMP) (PEDvax HIB® or ComVax® [Merck]) is administered at ages 2 and 4 months, a dose at age 6 months is not required. Because clinical studies in infants have demonstrated that using some combination products may induce a lower immune response to the Hib vaccine component DTaP/Hib combination products should not be used for primary vaccination in infants at ages 2, 4, or 6 months unless approved by the Food and Drug Administration for these ages.

** Two poliovirus vaccines are licensed in the United States: inactivated poliovirus vaccine (IPV) and oral poliovirus vaccine (OPV). The ACIP, AAFP, and AAP recommend that the first two doses of poliovirus vaccine should be IPV. The ACIP continues to recommend a sequential schedule of two doses of IPV administered at ages 2 and 4 months followed by two doses of OPV at age 12–18 months and age 4–6 years. Use of IPV for all doses also is acceptable and is recommended for immunocompromised persons and their household contacts. OPV is no longer recommended for the first two doses of the schedule and is acceptable only for special circumstances (e.g., children of parents who do not accept the recommended number of injections, late initiation of vaccination that would require an unacceptable number of injections, and imminent travel to areas where poliomyelitis is endemic. OPV remains the vaccine of choice for mass vaccination campaigns to control outbreaks of wild poliovirus.

†† The first dose of Rv vaccine should not be administered before age 6 weeks, and the minimum interval between doses is 3 weeks. The Rv vaccine series should not be initiated at age 7 months, and all doses should be completed by the first birthday. The AAFP opinion is that the decision to use rotavirus (Rv) vaccine should be made by the parent or guardian in consultation with the physician or other health-care provider.

§§ The second dose of measles, mumps, and rubella vaccine (MMR) is recommended routinely at age 4–6 years but may be administered during any visit provided at least 4 weeks have elapsed since receipt of the first dose and that both doses are administered beginning at or after age 12 months. Those who have not previously received the second dose should complete the schedule no later than the routine visit to a health-care provider at age 11–12 years.

¶¶ Varicella (Var) vaccine is recommended at any visit on or after the first birthday for susceptible children (i.e., those who lack a reliable history or chickenpox [as judged by a health-care provider] and who have not been vaccinated). Susceptible persons aged ≥ 13 years should receive two doses given at least two weeks apart.

Use of trade names and commercial sources is for identification only and does not imply endorsement by CDC or the U.S. Department of Health and Human Services.

Source: Advisory Committee on Immunization Practices (ACIP), American Academy of Family Physicians (AAFP), and American Academy of Pediatrics (AAP).

Figure 5.8 Recommended childhood immunization schedule*—United States, January–December 1999

48. **(D)** Aspirin, or other nonsteroidal anti-inflammatory drugs (NSAIDs), are effective medications for relieving the signs and symptoms of disease. They do little to modify the course of the disease, however. A new generation of NSAIDs that are more specific inhibitors of cyclo-oxygenase-2 provide promise for less toxicity with therapy. Glucocorticoids are very powerful at suppressing signs and symptoms of disease and may alter disease progression.

49. **(C)** Methotrexate, 7.5 to 20 mg once a week, is the most commonly recommended disease-modifying drug, because its effect is more rapid and patients are able to tolerate it for longer periods of time. Maximum improvement with methotrexate occurs after 6 months of therapy. Toxicity includes gastrointestinal (GI) upset, oral ulceration, and liver function abnormalities. The GI upset in particular may be ameliorated by concurrent folic acid administration. Pneumonitis has also been reported.

50. **(C)** If salicylates and NSAIDs fail to control the inflammation or are not tolerated, alternative therapies such as gold can be tried. Because of the potential toxicity to kidneys and bone marrow, frequent urinalysis and blood counts must be done. The most common side effects include pruritic skin rashes and painful mouth ulcers.

51. **(B)** Fine-needle aspiration of the thyroid nodule is the single most important diagnostic test listed. An open biopsy is unnecessary. A radioiodine scan showing a "cold" nodule is suggestive but not diagnostic for carcinoma. Ultrasound can characterize the appearance of the lesion, but it is not definitive.

52. **(B)** Papillary carcinoma (pure and papillary–follicular mixed) accounts for 60 to 70% of all thyroid cancers. The patient's history of neck irradiation in the remote past increases her risk for a malignant nodule.

53. **(C)** HSV is endemic to the United States, with the highest incidence in young, sexually active women. The incubation period is 6 to 7 days, and male condoms and oral contraceptives are not protective due to direct contact of the unprotected vulva. The patient often confuses the initial symptoms with those of a yeast infection.

54. **(C)** Initial infection is often accompanied by fever, headache, malaise, and tender adenopathy.

55. **(B)** Presumptive diagnosis is made by clinical and cytologic findings. Culture is definitive if positive, but is more likely to be negative if done on older drying lesions.

56. **(D)** Recurrences are extremely variable in frequency, intensity, and duration. Patients will frequently be extremely distraught at the diagnosis and need to be counseled about the significance. Because neonatal herpes is life threatening, cesarean section may be performed, but only if there is suspicion of viral shed at the time of delivery.

57. **(C)** Carefully designed studies of sexuality education have demonstrated that a comprehensive approach, teaching young people about sex and birth control, prevents pregnancies by increasing effective use of contraceptives by those who are sexually active *and* by postponing the onset of sexual activity. The other approaches to health education have not shown similar results. Abstinence education, information about contraception and STD prevention, and communication skills are all important parts of comprehensive sexuality education.

58. **(A)** The hours between 3:00 and 6:00 on weekday afternoons have been shown to be the riskiest times for adolescent pregnancy. Teens are out of school in the late afternoon and are often unsupervised because their parents are at work. At the other times listed, there are more likely to be responsible adults nearby.

59. (D) Adolescent pregnancy prevention is a controversial issue that many communities have difficulty with. Interventions that involve addressing adolescent sexuality directly often engender significant opposition from parents and others in the community. Providing alternative activities for students who would otherwise be at risk for premature sexual experimentation is a noncontroversial way of *beginning* a teen pregnancy prevention program, though it should not be the only effort.

60. (E) Grieving is a dynamic state, with its symptoms lasting until the person has had the opportunity to experience the entire calendar year at least once without the lost person. The bereaved person may take on the qualities, mannerisms, or characteristics of the deceased to perpetuate that person in some way. Early in the grieving process, grief may be indistinguishable from depression and should be considered if an individual has recently suffered the loss of a spouse or other close family member. During the first year following the death of a spouse, both widowers and widows have an increased death rate.

61. (A) Endomyometritis is caused by a polymicrobial organism including members of all four groups. Infection typically makes a transition from a predominance of aerobic organisms to anaerobic organisms. Broad-spectrum coverage results in resolution within approximately 72 hours in most cases. It is a frequent complication of cesarean delivery.

62. (E) This patient has chronic lymphocytic leukemia (CLL). In many cases, review of the peripheral smear in the appropriate setting may be enough to make the diagnosis. Flow cytometry can be performed on peripheral blood to confirm monoclonality and CD5 positivity, making a bone marrow biopsy unnecessary. This patient is at low risk (Rai stage 0 or Binet stage A) for developing progressive disease, with a 5-year survival of 88% and 10-year survival of 71%. This early stage of disease also makes it unlikely that he

will require treatment of the CLL in the next year. An unusual but well-described complication of CLL is Richter syndrome, or the development of a large cell lymphoma. It occurs in about 3% of patients.

63. (D) Progressive anemia without evidence of progression of the CLL is often secondary to the development of an autoimmune hemolytic anemia (AIHA). AIHA occurs in 10 to 25% of patients sometime during the course of their disease, while as many as 35% of asymptomatic patients with CLL have a positive direct Coombs' test. An elevated reticulocyte count is diagnostic of a hemolytic anemia in this patient population.

64. (B) Benign duct papillomas account for the majority of bloody nipple discharges, while malignancy is the cause in only 10 to 30%. Prolactinomas can cause galactorrhea. Yellow, green, or brown drainage is consistent with fibrocystic changes.

65. (B) During an asthma attack, residual volume increases, as does airway hyperreactivity and mediastinal air. Lung volumes decrease along with expiratory flow rates. It is this combination that produces the symptoms of asthma and that also makes it amenable to treatment.

66. (C) Fibromas are the most common benign solid tumors of the vulva. Lipomas are also quite common lesions of the vulva but do not occur as frequently as fibromas. Hidradenomas, syringomas, and endometrioma are rare and cystic tumors of the vulva. Sebaceous cysts, blockages of the sebaceous gland ducts, are very common. The assessment of nevi is very important as 3 to 4% of melanomas in women involve the vulva.

67. (B) The manifestations of an acute overdose with propoxyphene are those of narcotic overdose. The patient is usually somnolent but may be stuporous or comatose and convulsing. Respiratory depression is characteristic, giving a respiratory acidosis. Blood pressure and heart rate are usually normal initially, but blood pressure falls and cardiac performance deteriorates, which ultimately results in pulmonary edema and circulatory collapse.

68. **(B)** Attention should be directed first to establishing a patent airway and to restoring ventilation. The narcotic antagonist naloxone will markedly reduce the degree of respiratory depression. General supportive measures, in addition to oxygen, include, when necessary, intravenous fluids, vasopressor–inotropic compounds, and, when infection is likely, antibiotics.

69. **(A)** Raynaud's phenomenon is a common occupational illness in individuals whose jobs involve exposure to extreme vibration. Jackhammer operators are a classic example of workers at risk. Carpal tunnel syndrome (which leads to pain and numbness in the affected fingers, but not particularly in association with cold) is the occupational hand injury common in keyboard specialists and others whose work involves typing. A freezer-room technician, subject to regular cold exposure, would have frequent symptoms if he had Raynaud's phenomenon, but he would not be at increased risk for developing that condition. Raynaud's is also not associated with anesthetic gas exposures, the main occupational risk factor for anesthetists, or with the many physical, biological, and chemical factors a dairy farmer may encounter.

70. **(C)** Workers exposed to loud noises on the job are at high risk for hearing loss unless they wear adequate protective equipment (ie, soundproof earphones). Repetitive motion injury is seen in a wide variety of occupations, including carpal tunnel syndrome in keyboard operators, as discussed in the answer to question 69. The other conditions listed are all common in occupational settings, but not especially among jackhammer operators.

71. **(E)** Fifty percent of all vesicoenteric fistulas are secondary to sigmoid diverticulitis. Col-

orectal tumors account for an additional 15 to 20%. Crohn's disease is associated with 10 to 15% of these fistulas, and primary bladder malignancy is the cause of about 5% of all vesicoenteric fistulas.

72. **(C)** The presence of a colovesical fistula is generally not a surgical emergency. Sometimes, the fistula can be small and seal on its own. Small fistulas can also be difficult to detect and may require different diagnostic modalities for diagnosis. Up to 50% of patients with diverticulitis may have the fistula close spontaneously. Generally, the surgical intervention is that of separating the colon from the bladder and resecting the bowel involved. Large bladder defects should undergo primary repair. Patients may present with refractory urinary tract infection, pneumaturia, or fecaluria.

73. **(C)** Aches and stiffness simulating fibrositis may appear early in hypothyroidism; untreated, this may progress to proximal myopathy, with elevated creatinine kinase levels. Serum cholesterol and triglycerides, creatinine phosphokinase, aldolase, lactic dehydrogenase, and SGOT may all be elevated in the patient with moderate to severe hypothyroidism. All of the other signs and symptoms are commonly seen in hypothyroidism as it remains untreated.

74. **(D)** Hashimoto's thyroiditis (an autoimmune process) accounts for the majority of cases of primary hypothyroidism. Idiopathic myxedema (probably a variant of Hashimoto's thyroiditis) and thyroid destruction resulting from radioactive iodine therapy or surgery for hyperthyroidism account for additional cases. The long-term survival of patients treated with radiation for Hodgkin's and other malignancies of the neck and thorax are starting to account for a large number of patients with hypothyroidism as well.

75. **(E)** Renal dysfunction is not a complication of hypothyroidism. An elevated TSH is indicative of thyroid gland failure. Anemia is a common complication of hypothyroidism,

usually being normocytic in nature. However, iron deficiency with a microcytic anemia is frequent secondary to menorrhagia. Macrocytosis is also not unusual, as about 50% of patients with pernicious anemia have antithyroid antibodies, which would give a low B_{12} level but does not affect the folate.

76. **(A)** Gynecomastia occurs at midpuberty in about 50% of boys and may involve only one breast. Gynecomastia is usually of great concern to the male adolescent, and counseling may be necessary to stress the transient nature of the phenomenon. Steroids or other medications are not recommended.

77. **(C)** Sexual maturation in a female begins with thelarche. This occurs at Tanner 3 or 4 (ages 8 to 13), while the growth spurt occurs at Tanner 2 or 3.

78. **(A)** The appearance of pubic hair growth usually follows the increase in size of the testes, which coincides with the onset of the adolescent growth (height) spurt. Facial, body, and axillary hair usually appear approximately 2 years after the growth of pubic hair.

79. **(D)** This patient's diagnosis is severe preeclampsia. The history does not support an alternative. New-onset hypertension and proteinuria in pregnancy is preeclampsia until proven otherwise. The presence of significant complications such as blood pressure greater than 170/110, proteinuria greater than 5 g/24 h or +3 or +4, pulmonary edema, oliguria, DIC, and so on increase it from mild to severe.

80. **(A)** The only cure for preeclampsia is delivery, and only real concern about the consequences of severe prematurity will cause a prudent physician to temporize on this plan. Management then dictates that a decision be made about the route of delivery. Obviously, if the cervix is effaced and dilated with the fetus vertex in the pelvis, prompt induction of labor is the optimal approach. In cases in which the cervix remains undilated and unef-

faced, additional steps in evaluation may be undertaken while "ripening" the cervix. However, these efforts at evaluation should be limited to tests that will affect management. For example, low or rapidly falling platelets may affect the decision about route of delivery if an extended induction is required. Conversely, no value on the 24-hour urine will change the management at this stage.

81. **(E)** Delivery and the removal of the placenta is the only cure for preeclampsia; all other measures treat symptoms. Magnesium sulfate is used to prevent or stop eclamptic seizures. The anticonvulsive effect is due to direct action on the cerebral cortex and not to peripheral effects at the neuromuscular junction, as some have erroneously claimed. The initial intravenous bolus may have a transient effect of lowering maternal blood pressure, but blood pressure returns to basal levels in a short period of time. Control of blood pressure must be maintained through the use of other medications such as hydralazine or labetolol. Similarly, a small increase in uterine blood flow may result temporarily from administration of magnesium. Serum levels greater than 7 mg/dL are associated with loss of patellar reflexes, somnolence, respiratory difficulty, and cardiac arrest.

82. **(A)** This patient is exhibiting many of the signs of major depressive disorder: subjective, depressed mood; inability to sleep; loss of appetite; diminished concentration; feelings of self-worthlessness; and guilt. This is the patient's first known depressive episode. She is not exhibiting a manic symptomatology, and a diagnosis of bipolar disorder would be inappropriate without such a history. Similarly, while she is potentially abusing benzodiazepines (an issue that should be discussed during the session), DSM-IV allows the diagnosis of benzodiazepine dependence only in the absence of another mental disorder that could better explain the symptoms.

83. (A) Fluoxetine, a selective serotonin reuptake inhibitor (SSRI) antidepressant, is the most appropriate therapy. Carbamazepine is an antiepilepsy medication used for manic depression, symptoms of which this patient does not have. Similarly, in a patient without psychotic symptoms, neither fluphenazine (a typical antipsychotic) nor risperidone (a newer generation antipsychotic) is appropriate. Diphenhydramine is an anticholinergic medication sometimes used in managing extrapyramidal side effects of antipsychotic medications.

84. (D) Sexual dysfunction and anorgasmia have been reported in men and women taking SSRIs for depression.

85. (A) There is evidence that the sexual dysfunction associated with SSRI usage is dose-related.

86. (A) Intubation can injure the tissues of the mouth and pharynx, causing pain that inhibits breast feeding. A postdates baby can be put to the mother's breast in the delivery room before delivery of the placenta. Most babies will root for the nipple and maintain an alert state after delivery. Early attachment and opportunities to breast feed enhance the longevity of the experience.

87. (E) Serum glucose levels decline after birth in the first 3 hours. Early feeding reduces the incidence. Postdates infants are not one of the four groups of infants at highest risk, although the presence of meconium staining should alert medical providers of the potential of reduced glycogen stores. Standard approaches to the treatment of a stable infant with a low Dextrostix test include obtaining a quantitative measure of glucose by the glucose oxidase method, placing the infant to breast, observing for symptoms, and repeating a Dextrostix test. If the serum glucose returns with a value of 45 mg/dL or less, the infant may need a feeding of 5% glucose water. For the breast-feeding infant, the water can be administered by the finger-feeding technique.

88. (C) Metronidazole should be avoided in breast-feeding women. The other medications are probably safe but should be given only when needed.

89. (A) Clinicians are required to report all cases of suspected abuse of children they see in all jurisdictions in the United States. The law does not leave the issue to a clinician's discretion.

90. (B) Calcification within the prostate is not a feature of BPH; the condition is known as prostatic calculi.

91. (E) In BPH, an enlarged prostate alone is not an indication for surgery. Even though enlarged, it may be asymptomatic.

92. (B) Removal of a diverticulum requires open operation.

93. (D) Operant conditioning is a form of learning in which behavior is directly punished or rewarded. In continual reinforcement, every response is reinforced, producing the most rapid acquisition of behavior. In positive reinforcement, a desired behavior is rewarded. In negative reinforcement, a desired behavior removes an unwanted stimulus. In partial reinforcement, a desired behavior is intermittently rewarded. In classical or Pavlovian conditioning, a stimulus that once had no ability to bring on a specific response becomes able to do so.

94. (C) According to the American Association on Mental Deficiency's classification, the degree of mental retardation depicted in options A through D correspond to a classification of profound, severe, moderate, and mild, respectively.

95. (A) The patient's painless ulceration was most likely primary syphilis. The serologic tests become positive 4 to 6 weeks after the primary infection. The treponemal-specific fluorescent treponemal antibody-absorption test (FTA-ABS) will become positive before the VDRL. The patient later presents with

secondary syphilis and may also have condy-loma lata of the vulva.

96. **(C)** Typical deformity in a displaced fracture of the femoral neck is shortening and external rotation of the limb. The internal rotator muscles are no longer able to act because of the fracture, and the limb falls laterally by its weight and the unopposed action of the external rotators.

97. **(E)** Dysuria and frequency in the absence of significant bacteriuria (presence of significant numbers of bacteria in the urine to denote active infection rather than contamination) are common problems among young men and women. This entity has been called the acute urethral syndrome, and in 35 to 50% of patients is caused by *Chlamydia trachomatis.*

98. **(D)** Gonococcal urethritis in males is characterized by a yellowish, purulent urethral discharge and dysuria. On Gram stain, it is a gram-negative diplococcus.

99. **(C)** Because of the prevalence of penicillin-resistant gonococcus, amoxicillin is not recommended. Ceftriaxone, cefixime, and spectinomycin are used, but as single doses; repeating them for 2 to 10 days is not necessary. In addition to the single dose of antibiotic for the treatment of gonococcal urethritis or cervicitis, treatment for coexisting chlamydial infection is recommended (doxycycline, 100 mg bid for 7 days, or a single dose of azithromycin, 1 g PO).

100. **(E)** The history is classic for hypertrophic pyloric stenosis. Gastroesophageal reflux is the primary differential diagnosis. Duodenal stenosis, adrenogenital syndrome, and amino-aciduria are rare.

101. **(D)** The hypertrophied pylorus is palpable in the epigastrium of a quiet infant with an empty stomach. Gastric contractions may be visible in the upper abdomen. No abdominal distention or tenderness is present, and bowel sounds are normal.

102. **(C)** In the rare case in which the "olive" is nonpalpable, a hypertrophic pylorus can usually be identified by ultrasound examination (see Figure 5.9), which shows longitudinal and cross-section images of an elongated pyloric channel with thickened musculature. This finding is called a "target" sign. If ultrasound is not diagnostic, and the infant continues to vomit, an upper GI series is obtained.

103. **(C)** Many antenatally diagnosed IUGR babies are actually constitutionally small and not at increased risk for adverse outcome. Maternal vascular disease is the most common cause of growth restriction, especially asymmetric. Symmetric growth restriction has multiple etiologies, including congenital infections, cytogenetic abnormality, congenital malformation, maternal drug ingestion, maternal smoking, and maternal alcohol abuse.

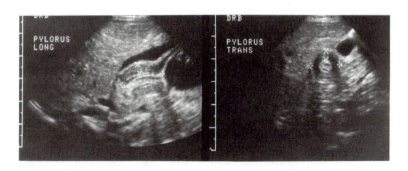

Figure 5.9

104. (B) Polycythemia rubra vera is a myelo-proliferative disorder characterized by the malignant (ie, monocolonal) expansion of erythroid, myeloid, and megakaryocytic elements within the bone marrow. This results in an increased red blood cell (RBC) mass and frequently elevated peripheral granulocyte and platelet counts. When iron deficiency anemia develops, as evidenced by the decreased mean corpuscular volume (MCV) in the patient described, the hematocrit may be within normal range.

105. (C) The most useful physical finding in terms of differential diagnosis is splenomegaly, which is present in about 75% of patients, and reflects principally the development of extramedullary hematopoiesis.

106. (D) The bone marrow in polycythemia rubra vera is typically hyperplastic and reveals a panmyelosis (expansion of all the cell lines). Red cell morphology usually reveals hypochromic microcytic cells, with a reduced MCV, suggestive of iron-deficient erythropoiesis. This suggestion is frequently confirmed by a low serum iron and absence of bone marrow stores. The leukocyte alkaline phosphatase is generally elevated, unlike chronic myelogenous leukemia, in which it is extremely low. Elevation of urine and serum uric acid is seen as a result of rapid cell turnover and ineffective erythropoiesis. A normal arterial blood gas, specifically the PO_2 is required for the diagnosis of polycythemia rubra vera.

107. (D) While HELLP syndrome may result in platelet counts similar to that seen in this case, hypofibrinogenemia is generally not a component of this disorder. In view of the significant bleeding and no previa on ultrasound, a diagnosis of placental abruption must be made, even if it is not apparent on the scan. Once DIC has developed as a result of abruption, the only acceptable course is elimination of the cause (ie, delivery). Medical management may be required postpartum, but such attempts at correction of the

lab tests should not delay elimination of the etiology of the problem.

108. (D) Significant hypertension, either essential or pregnancy induced, is the most common condition associated with abruptio placentae. Cigarette smoking may cause up to 40% of cases. Both placenta previa and abruptions increase with both increasing maternal age and increasing parity. Cocaine was recently identified as a common cause of abruption.

109. (A) The U.S. infant mortality rate has dropped more than tenfold since 1900 and continues to decline. African-American infants are roughly twice as likely to die during infancy as Caucasian infants. Despite unsurpassed capabilities in caring for high-risk newborns, the United States has one of the highest infant mortality rates in the industrialized world, related to our extremely high incidence of preterm delivery and low birth weight. There is significant geographic variation in infant mortality rates among states within this country, and even among neighborhoods within a single city; the variation is related more to rates of poverty and prematurity than to specialty health care access. Roughly 70% of infant deaths occur in the first four weeks of life—the neonatal period.

110. (D) A recent Institute of Medicine report estimated that 60% of pregnancies are unintended at the time of conception, leading to significant health risks and socioeconomic problems for mothers, infants, and their families. Poor access to family planning services is a major contributing factor. Because most parts of the United States have systems of regionalized perinatal care, high-risk mothers and infants have good access to appropriate levels of care. This country's high-risk orientation in addressing the problem of infant mortality—through neonatal intensive care and prenatal and preconceptional testing—is an expensive, and ultimately not very effective, means of preventing infant deaths.

111. (C) Neural tube defects (NTDs), including anencephaly and meningomyelocele, can be prevented through dietary supplementation with folic acid. The U.S. government recently added folic acid to some dietary staples to reduce the risk of NTDs. In order to be effective, adequate folate must be consumed very early in pregnancy, so all women of childbearing age, not just those who know they are pregnant, should eat folate-rich foods such as fresh vegetables, fruits, and fortified grain products. The other birth defects listed are not as susceptible to population-based primary prevention efforts. At the individual level, some can be detected prenatally through ultrasound and/or genetic testing (eg, tetralogy of Fallot, renal agenesis, dwarfism). Many once life-threatening malformations (eg, pyloric stenosis) are now very treatable through advances in medical and surgical techniques.

112. **(D)** The Apgar score is of limited utility in modern obstetrics. Forty-five years ago, the Apgar score was a quick way to evaluate the condition of the newborn and a guide to resuscitative efforts. Currently, resuscitation should be started before the neonate is 1 minute of age. The 5-minute Apgar score may be used to evaluate the effectiveness of resuscitation and has a *very* modest correlation with long-term sequelae. The umbilical artery pH and base excess is prognostically more significant. A pH greater than 7.2 indicates that the labor events did not result in neonatal depression. Only acidosis with at least a metabolic component and of long duration will result in serious injury to the fetus. Studies have indicated that such damage is rare if the pH is above 7.0.

113. **(E)** For a child with only a moderately elevated blood level, it is unlikely that a major single point of exposure will be found. Instead, he probably has low-level exposure to lead from a variety of sources, including all of the ones listed. Lead is ubiquitous and persistent in the environment. The use of lead in household paint and gasoline was banned over two decades ago, but it is still present in high levels, particularly in urban environments. Much of the housing stock in U.S.

cities predates the ban, and many children live in houses with lead paint that chips, peels, and/or deteriorates into dust. Lead released in car exhaust many years ago may still linger in the dirt and dust outside. Many municipal and household water supplies run through pipes containing lead or lead solder that leaches into the water.

114. **(B)** Handwashing to remove lead dust before eating is a simple and important means of reducing lead exposure. Small children get their hands dirty while playing and then ingest the dirt (and lead) when they handle their food or suck their thumbs. Sanding and sweeping should be avoided because they make the lead dust airborne; careful scraping and damp-mopping are preferable. Increasing *iron* and *calcium* in the diet can reduce lead absorption in the gut. Chelation therapy is not indicated at this level of lead poisoning, particularly not before environmental approaches are tried.

115. **(A)** Children with even low-level lead poisoning can show long-term behavioral and intellectual problems. Saturnine gout is a manifestation of acute, high-level lead exposure. None of the other conditions are related to lead.

116. **(D)** Repeat cesarean section is responsible for approximately 35% of all cesarean deliveries. That indication also was associated with the greatest increase between 1980 and 1988. Dystocia or failure to progress is diagnosed in approximately 30% of cesarean sections. Breech presentation is present in approximately 10% of cesarean deliveries. Fetal distress or nonreassuring fetal monitoring is present in 9%. The recommendation of the American College of Obstetricians and Gynecologists is that a woman with one or two prior transverse cesarean section should be counseled to undergo a trial of labor with her subsequent pregnancy. Multifetal gestations are successfully delivered vaginally. Oxytocin induction and augmentation as well as epidural anesthesia can be given to women who have had prior cesarean sections.

117. (B) This woman is strongly addicted to nicotine and has never quit long enough to get past acute withdrawal. Trying nicotine replacement therapy may help her quit permanently. The fact that she has tried to quit so many times suggests that she is highly motivated and does not need persuasion. She has a potential source of support in her husband, but he needs to be counseled about how to help rather than undermine her efforts. Research indicates that the more times a person tries to quit smoking—or make other significant behavioral change—the more likely he or she is to eventually succeed.

118. (C) Restricting smoking in public places encourages current smokers to quit by increasing the social stigma of smoking and making it inconvenient to smoke. Cigarette tax increases, prevention of illegal cigarette sales, and prohibitions on advertising and vending machine sales have the greatest impact on smoking by discouraging individuals (primarily adolescents) from *starting* to smoke. (See Figure 5.10.)

119. (B) Cervical cancer is significantly more common in women who smoke than in nonsmokers, even after controlling for potential confounding variables, such as sexual history. The other female cancers are less affected by smoking. Vaginal clear cell carcinoma is closely associated with another chemical exposure: diethylstilbestrol (DES) exposure in utero.

120. (B) Phenothiazines, especially chlorpromazine and thioridazine, can result in pigmentation of the lens. Pigmentary retinopathy is most likely to occur during treatment with high doses of medication. Lithium, maprotiline HCL, haloperidol, and amitriptyline do not cause pigmentary retinopathy.

121. (E) Malpractice is the term referring to professional negligence. An expert must establish the four D's of malpractice: "A Dereliction of a Duty that Directly leads to Damages." In negligence: (1) a standard of care must exist; (2) the person who is answer-

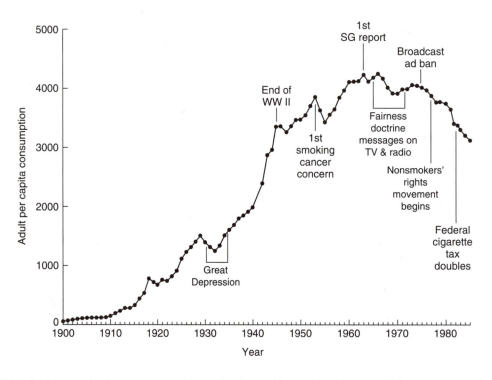

Figure 5.10. Adult per capita cigarette consumption and major smoking-and-health events. (Adapted from Warner, 1985.)

able for his or her conduct must owe a duty; (3) the plaintiff must be owed the duty; and (4) a breach of the duty is the legal cause for injury or damage.

122. **(C)** Useful laboratory findings in confirming the diagnosis of alcoholism include blood alcohol level; elevated liver enzymes, particularly GGT; macrocytosis; and folate deficiency. Radiology studies often reveal fractures, subdural hematomas, pneumonia, and other pulmonary problems.

123. **(A)** Anxiety disorders had the highest prevalence rates: 8.9% for 6 months and 14.6% for lifetime. Six-month and lifetime prevalence rates for affective (mood) disorders were 5.8% and 8.3%, respectively, compared to 0.8% and 1.3% for schizophrenia. Men were more likely to have alcohol dependence than women. Depression rates among women were twice as high as for men. Substance abuse was more common among individuals under 30 years of age than in older adults.

124. **(D)** The infant may be infected at any time contact with body fluids occurs. The variable period from exposure to the virus to the onset of symptoms has not yet been explained, but may well be related to genetic host factors.

125. **(E)** Factors associated with subsequent suicide in those who attempt suicide include: age above 45 years, male sex, unemployed or retired, living alone, poor physical health, medical treatment within the last 6 months, having a psychiatric disorder, and having made previous attempts by violent methods. Eight out of 10 individuals who successfully commit suicide have given warnings of their intent.

126. **(A)** Amnestic syndrome is most often caused by a combination of alcohol abuse and thiamine deficiency, known as Korsakoff syndrome. Patients with this syndrome may be alert and oriented but unable to express any memory of events more than a few hours old.

Delusional psychoses and tactile hallucinations are not part of the amnestic syndrome.

127. **(A)** One half of suicide completers suffer from depression, compared to 30% who suffer from alcoholism, and a smaller percentage who suffer from other illnesses, such as schizophrenia, anxiety disorders, and drug dependence.

128. **(A)** At least one third of patients sustaining subarachnoid hemorrhage develop it during sleep. Note the hyperdense blood in the interhemispheric fissure, sylvian fissures, and paramesencephalic cistern. This scenario is characteristic of subarachnoid hemorrhage.

129. **(H)** Toxoplasmosis is a common disease of birds and mammals caused by *Toxoplasma gondii*, an obligate intracellular protozoan that infects over 500 million humans worldwide. The most common manifestation in patients with AIDS is central nervous system (CNS) involvement. CT scan usually shows one or more lesions that are contrast enhancing in a ring pattern. Patients can present with such varied symptoms as fever, headache, confusion progressing to coma, focal neurologic signs, and seizures.

130. **(C)** Much of the morbidity and some mortality associated with AIDS has been ascribed to CMV infections of the liver, brain, gastrointestinal tract, lungs, and eyes. Ganciclovir, foscarnet, and cidofovir are effective antiviral agents used in control of CMV infections. Therapy is lifelong.

131. **(F)** *Cryptococcus neoformans* is a yeastlike, round or oval fungus that is the most common etiologic agent of fungal meningitis. Among HIV-infected individuals, the incidence of cryptococcosis (systemic dissemination) varies from 5 to 10%. Meningitis is the most common manifestation of CNS involvement. The mortality rate approaches 30%. Treatment is with amphotericin B. Fluconazole is another effective agent.

132. **(E)** Cryptosporidiosis is a gastrointestinal infection characterized by watery diarrhea, abdominal cramps, malabsorption, and weight loss. It is usually a severe, unrelenting illness in immunocompromised patients, particularly those with AIDS. It tends to be a self-limited disease in the immunologically normal host.

133. **(A)** The most desirable approach to therapy for pneumocystis carinii pneumonia (PCP) is prevention. A number of controlled studies have shown that the attack rate can be reduced by 5 to 10 times in HIV-infected patients who are at the highest risk (those who have less than 200 CD4 lymphocytes and those who have already experienced an episode of PCP). The most widely used agent for prophylaxis is trimethoprim–sulfamethoxazole.

134. **(B)** MAC is one of a large number of opportunistic pathogens responsible for chronic diarrhea in AIDS patients. Patients who develop disseminated MAC are usually severely immunocompromised from the standpoint of cellular immune function. Therefore, in patients with AIDS, the CD4 count is usually quite low. Diagnosis is most commonly made by biopsy and culture of liver, bone marrow, lymph nodes, or blood.

135. **(J)** Kaposi's sarcoma is the most frequent neoplasm of HIV patients. It forms one of the CDC's criteria that define an individual as having AIDS. Although classically an indolent neoplasm in HIV-negative individuals, in AIDS lymphatic involvement is not unusual and visceral involvement may occur. Unlike "classic" Kaposi's sarcoma, which is usually confined to the lower extremities, cutaneous Kaposi's sarcoma in AIDS can form large, confluent plaques anywhere on the body.

136–139. **(136-E, 137-C, 138-A, 139-B)** Speech and language development is important to assess at every encounter with a young child. Knowing some basic milestones, such as those presented, enables you to sort out those who need further evaluation. Brain damage, mental retardation, autism, and deprivation, as well as hearing difficulties, may contribute to an impaired development in this important area.

140. **(E)** Myoclonic seizures are sudden, brief, single, or repetitive muscle contractions involving one body part or the entire body. Loss of consciousness does not occur unless other types of seizures coexist. These seizures can be idiopathic or associated with Creutzfeldt–Jakob disease, uremia, hepatic failure, subacute leukoencephalopathies, and some hereditary disorders. Recent evidence has linked a variant form of Creutzfeldt–Jakob disease with bovine spongiform encephalopathy, a prior disease of cattle. This variant form usually presents with ataxia and behavior changes prior to myoclonus and dementia.

141. **(B)** Complex partial seizures were once classified as temporal lobe epilepsy. Although the temporal lobe (especially the hippocampus or amygdala) is the most common site of origin, some seizures have been shown to originate from mesial parasagittal or orbital frontal regions.

142. **(D)** Pure absence seizures consist of the sudden cessation of ongoing conscious activity without convulsive muscular activity or loss of postural control. They can be so brief as to be unapparent, but can last several minutes. There is usually no period of postictal confusion.

143. **(A)** Simple partial seizures can occur with motor, sensory, autonomic, or psychic symptoms. When a partial motor seizure spreads to adjacent neurons, a "Jacksonian march" can occur (eg, right thumb to right hand and right arm to the right side of the face). Face and hand movements are frequently linked because their cortical regions are adjacent.

144. **(D)** Absence seizures almost always begin in young children (ages 6 to 14). They may first

present as learning difficulties in school. The EEG is diagnostic, revealing brief, 3-Hz spikes and wave discharges occurring synchronously throughout all leads.

145–150. (145-D, 146-E, 147-C, 148-A, 149-B, 150-E) The diagnosis of intussusception is confirmed by barium enema. This procedure can be curative and is indicated if perforation has not occurred. Bloody stool is common. There is a high incidence of duodenal atresia in Down syndrome. Chalasia is not considered a surgical problem. Pyloric stenosis is seen more commonly in males. Esophageal atresia can be diagnosed by the passage of a radiopaque catheter.

Practice Test 6
Questions

DIRECTIONS (Questions 1 through 28): Each group of items in this section consists of lettered headings followed by a set of numbered words or phrases. For each numbered word or phrase, select the ONE lettered heading that is most closely associated with it. Each lettered heading may be selected once, more than once, or not at all.

Questions 1 Through 5

There is a wide variety of common epidemiologic study designs. Selection of the appropriate design for a given study depends on a variety of factors: time and resources available, as well as characteristics of the condition under investigation. Identify which type of study is described in each of the following examples.

    (A) case–control
    (B) prospective cohort
    (C) cross-sectional
    (D) randomized controlled trial
    (E) time series

1. Five hundred women with breast cancer and 500 age-matched women without breast cancer are interviewed about their dietary history to study the connection between breast cancer and diet.

2. Patients with urinary tract infections (UTIs) are given either standard or single-dose antibiotic therapy to evaluate the effectiveness of single-dose therapy in the treatment of UTI.

3. The incidence of fatal motor vehicle accidents from 1975 to 1998 is studied to assess the effect of changes in the interstate speed limit on mortality due to motor vehicle accidents.

4. Forty patients with angina (20 stable and 20 unstable) are followed for 2 years to compare the incidence of myocardial infarction and death in the two groups.

5. Textile industry workers are surveyed regarding their health status and medical problems to determine the prevalence of occupational illnesses in various job groups.

Questions 6 Through 10

Match the appropriate approximate age in children with the correct milestone of visual–motor development.

    (A) 1 to 2 months
    (B) 3 to 5 months
    (C) 6 to 8 months
    (D) 9 to 11 months
    (E) 12 months
    (F) 18 months
    (G) 24 months
    (H) 3 years

6. Can throw a ball

7. Grasps and brings objects to mouth

8. Sits alone briefly

9. Follows objects through visual field

10. Imitates patty cake

Questions 11 Through 16

Match the following clinical situations with the immunologic defect.

(A) B-cell deficiency/dysfunction
(B) mixed T- and B-cell deficiency/dysfunction
(C) T-lymphocyte deficiency/dysfunction
(D) neutropenia
(E) chemotaxis
(F) C3 deficiency (complement 3)

11. A 73-year-old man has an immunoglobulin G (IgG) spike.

12. A 22-year-old woman has Hodgkin's disease.

13. A 73-year-old man has 30,000 mature lymphocytes on his blood film.

14. A 24-year-old woman has a malar rash, thrombocytopenia, and arthralgias.

15. A 69-year-old man is receiving chemotherapy for acute leukemia.

16. A young woman has ataxia–telangiectasia.

Questions 17 Through 19

For each of the statements below, identify which of the following health care programs it describes.

(A) independent practice association or open-model health maintenance organization (HMO)
(B) closed panel or staff-model health maintenance organization
(C) preferred provider organization (PPO)

17. The plan contracts with or directly hires providers who care exclusively for enrollees.

18. The plan contracts with community-based providers who are not exclusively bound to enrollees.

19. The plan negotiates with community-based providers to obtain discounted fees.

Questions 20 Through 22

The U.S. government is a major payer for health care services. For each of the statements below, identify which of the following government insurance programs it describes.

(A) Medicaid
(B) Medicare
(C) Veterans Administration
(D) Indian Health Service
(E) CHAMPUS

20. Major source of health care coverage for individuals 65 years old and over

21. Could be considered among the largest "closed panel" managed care systems in the United States

22. Largest single source of payment for long-term care

Question 23 Through 25

Match the clinical situations of blood in the stools with the following diagnoses.

(A) inflammatory bowel disease
(B) milk allergy
(C) Giardia infections
(D) hookworm infections
(E) hemolytic uremic syndrome (HUS)
(F) pinworms
(G) fecal impaction
(H) cutanea larva migrans

23. Bloody diarrhea, Escherichia coli infections, and purpura

24. Cough, eosinophilia, intermittent diarrhea, and positive stool guaiac

25. Abdominal pain, blood in stools, lymphoid hyperplasia, narrowing of intestinal lumen

Questions 26 Through 28

For the following questions, select the virus most strongly implicated as a cause for the cancer listed.

(A) hepatitis B virus (HBV)
(B) human immunodeficiency virus (HIV)
(C) human papillomavirus (HPV)
(D) herpes simplex virus-2 (HSV-2)
(E) Epstein–Barr virus (EBV)

26. Cervical cancer

27. Hepatocellular carcinoma

28. Non-Hodgkin's lymphoma

DIRECTIONS (Questions 29 through 150): Each of the numbered items or incomplete statements in this section is followed by answers or by completions of the statement. Select the ONE lettered answer or completion that is BEST in each case.

29. Which of the following is the MOST appropriate position for a pelvic examination in a 5-year-old girl?

(A) dorsal lithotomy position
(B) knee/chest position
(C) in her mother's lap
(D) lateral position with leg adducted
(E) any examination is inappropriate

30. The MOST common etiology for ambiguous genitalia is

(A) androgen insensitivity syndrome
(B) androgen-secreting tumor
(C) excess androgen by mother
(D) congenital adrenal hyperplasia
(E) placental aromatase deficiency

31. In a neonate born with ambiguous genitalia, the MOST important laboratory test to order immediately is

(A) karyotype
(B) serum testosterone

(C) electrolytes
(D) 17-hydroxyprogesterone
(E) 11-deoxycorticosterone

32. A 4-month-old baby boy is evaluated in your office. The examination reveals no abnormalities. The baby's weight is 14 lb, 10 oz. His parents report that there is obesity in the family and that the baby's birth weight was 7 lb, 5 oz. The parents are concerned if the baby is gaining weight at the correct rate. You tell the parents that the expected time for a baby to double its birth weight is

(A) 4 to 6 months
(B) 9 months
(C) 12 months
(D) 15 months
(E) 2 years

Questions 33 Through 37

One of your patients calls the office to say she found a lump in her breast. She is 54 years old, had her last menstrual period at age 48 when she had a total hysterectomy for fibroids, and has been taking hormone replacement (HRT) since that time. She comes to the office for your assessment and you also feel a 2-cm firm mass in the upper outer quadrant of the right breast. You send her for a mammogram, which is reported as normal.

33. You call her to give her the results of the mammogram. You also tell her:

(A) "Don't worry because the mammogram was normal. Make a follow-up appointment in three months to see what's happening."
(B) "Let's check it again after your next cycle of the HRT."
(C) "You will need an ultrasound-guided biopsy of the mass."
(D) "You should see a surgeon for further evaluation."
(E) "Stop the HRT and let's see what it's like in 3 months."

34. A biopsy reveals a 1.5-cm infiltrating ductal carcinoma, which is estrogen- and progesterone-receptor positive. The Ki67 is 18% (unfavorable), and the tumor is aneuploid. Her surgeon has given her the choice of either a modified radical mastectomy or lumpectomy followed by radiation. Which of the following is true concerning her choices?

    (A) The survival is better for patients who have a mastectomy.
    (B) The survival is the same in either case.
    (C) The local recurrence rate is lower in the patients who have a lumpectomy and radiation.
    (D) With mastectomy, she will have to wait 6 to 12 months before reconstruction.
    (E) She will not need adjuvant hormonal or chemotherapy after mastectomy.

35. She elects to have a lumpectomy, which shows no residual tumor in the excised tissue, but 3 out of 15 lymph nodes are involved with metastatic disease. Her medical oncologist has now given her several choices. The standard therapy is considered

    (A) close follow-up with physical examination and mammogram
    (B) tamoxifen for 5 years
    (C) chemotherapy for 6 months
    (D) chemotherapy followed by tamoxifen
    (E) high-dose chemotherapy followed by autologous stem cell infusion

36. She elects to take the tamoxifen and starts on 20 mg daily. She calls to say that although she had some hot flashes when she came off the HRT, she is now having drenching sweats several times a day. You review the side effects and benefits of tamoxifen with her, which include

    (A) a decreased risk of endometrial cancer
    (B) no effect on bone density
    (C) a decreased risk of recurrence of her breast cancer
    (D) an increased risk of developing a new breast cancer
    (E) a decreased risk of venous thrombosis

37. Her last question as she is leaving your office is what should her three daughters do now that she has had breast cancer. You tell her:

    (A) "They should start getting mammograms every year, starting now."
    (B) "They should start taking tamoxifen."
    (C) "They should see their own physicians to review their individual risk profile before any recommendations can be made."
    (D) You suggest prophylactic mastectomies.
    (E) You recommend early and frequent pregnancies.

Questions 38 and 39

A 62-year-old man sustained an electrical injury by contact with a high-voltage power line. He has full-thickness skin loss on his thumb, as shown in Figure 6.1.

38. Initial management should be

    (A) conservative debridement and immediate skin grafting
    (B) amputation of the thumb to avoid systemic complications
    (C) fluid resuscitation and monitoring urine output/pH

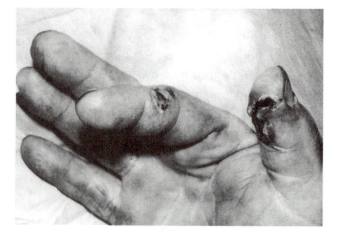

Figure 6.1

(D) imediate debridement and flap coverage

(E) urgent fasciotomies of the hand and forearm compartments

39. Common complications associated with an electrical burn injury include

(A) cardiac rhythm abnormalities

(B) fractures

(C) limb loss

(D) renal failure

(E) all of the above

Questions 40 Through 42

A 33-year-old multigravid woman presents at the office with the chief complaint of painful menstrual cramps which start 3 days prior to her menses and last 2 more days after the flow has begun. They have been progressively severe over the last 3 years. She has had one sexual partner for the past 13 years. She denies a history of sexually transmitted diseases (STDs). She has used no contraception for the past 5 years. She denies entrance dyspareunia but does have deep thrust dyspareunia.

40. Her chief complaint is BEST characterized as

(A) primary dysmenorrhea

(B) secondary dysmenorrhea

(C) primary infertility

(D) primary dyspareunia

(E) secondary dyspareunia

41. Her MOST likely diagnosis is

(A) acute salpingitis

(B) adenomyosis

(C) leiomyomata uteri

(D) endometriosis

(E) pelvic congestion syndrome

42. Optimal treatment would be

(A) total abdominal hysterectomy and bilateral salpingo-oophorectomy (TAH BSO)

(B) laser ablation of endometriosis

(C) gonadotropin-releasing hormone (GnRH) agonists

(D) continuous oral contraceptives

(E) endometrial ablation

43. When can children safely graduate from specially designed car seats to adult lap/shoulder belts with a booster seat?

(A) at 1 year of age

(B) at 25 lb

(C) at 40 lb

(D) at 3 years of age

(E) at 55 lb

Questions 44 and 45

A 42-year-old woman took an intentional massive dose of acetaminophen.

44. Which of the following is the MOST likely organ to be severely affected in this patient?

(A) heart

(B) lungs

(C) liver

(D) kidney

(E) brain

45. Which of the following is the MOST effective antidote for the patient above?

(A) acetylcysteine

(B) sodium bicarbonate

(C) phenobarbital

(D) sodium nitroprusside

(E) British anti-Lewisite (BAL)

46. The MOST common reason for a postdate pregnancy is

(A) inaccurate gestational age

(B) fetal anencephaly

(C) oligohydramnios

(D) intrauterine growth retardation

(E) advanced maternal age

47. In fetal anencephaly, absence of the pituitary, or adrenal insufficiency, prolonged pregnancy is associated with

   (A) low levels of dehydroisoandrosterone, resulting in low estrogen levels
   (B) low levels of dehydroisoandrosterone, resulting in elevated estrogen levels
   (C) increased progesterone level
   (D) decreased production of oxytocin
   (E) increased estrogen and progesterone levels

48. Postterm pregnancy is associated with which of the following complications?

   (A) preeclampsia, oligohydramnios, meconium aspiration
   (B) intrauterine growth retardation, oligohydramnios, diabetes
   (C) meconium aspiration, macrosomia, diabetes
   (D) oligohydramnios, meconium aspiration, macrosomia
   (E) preeclampsia, intrauterine growth retardation, diabetes

49. You are called to see a 6-hour-old full-term male who developed rapid breathing at a rate of 100/min. There are mild substernal retractions and grunting during expiration but no cyanosis. There are clear breath sounds, and no rales or rhonchi. Chest x-ray shows prominent pulmonary vascular markings, mild hyperaeration, and flattening of the diaphragm. The heart is normal. The MOST likely diagnosis is

   (A) myaline membrane disease
   (B) transient tachypnea of the newborn
   (C) meconium aspiration
   (D) viral pneumonia
   (E) congestive heart failure

50. A 64-year-old woman has multiple complaints, including malaise, severe unilateral headache, and pain and stiffness in her neck, shoulders, and back. Her appetite is poor and she has recently lost weight. Her examining physician finds that she has an oral temperature of 100.5°F, her hematocrit is 11.8%, and the sedimentation rate is 104 mm/hr. Which of the following is the MOST likely diagnosis?

   (A) multiple sclerosis
   (B) polymyalgia rheumatica
   (C) rheumatoid arthritis
   (D) polyarteritis nodosa
   (E) gastric carcinoma

51. The MOST feared complication of giant cell arteritis (temporal arteritis) is

   (A) thrombosis of the cranial artery
   (B) exquisite hyperesthesia
   (C) substantial fever
   (D) blindness
   (E) tongue pain

52. An asymptomatic patient presents for a routine visit and has a reactive Venereal Disease Research Laboratory (VDRL) test with a titer of 1:8, and a fluorescent treponemal antibody-absorption test (FTA-ABS) was also reactive. A VDRL test performed 10 months ago was nonreactive. An HIV antibody test was also done during her current first prenatal visit and was nonreactive. This patient should be treated with which antibiotic regimen?

   (A) benzathine penicillin G, 2.4 million units IM
   (B) benzathine penicillin G, 2.4 million units IM given weekly for 3 consecutive weeks
   (C) aqueous procaine penicillin G, 4.8 million units IM, and probenecid, 1 g orally just before the injection, plus doxycycline, 100 mg orally bid for 7 days
   (D) cefixime, 400 mg orally, plus doxycycline, 100 mg orally bid for 7 days
   (E) amoxicillin, 500 mg orally tid for 7 to 10 days

53. Which of the following would be BEST treated by Mohs' chemosurgery?

   (A) 2-cm diameter melanoma of the back
   (B) subungual acral lentiginous melanoma

(C) nodular basal cell carcinoma of the malar area

(D) morphemic basal cell carcinoma of the medial canthus

(E) squamous cell carcinoma of the lower lip

Questions 54 Through 57

A 30-year-old man presents with a history of recurrent pneumonias and a chronic cough productive of foul-smelling, purulent sputum, occasionally blood-tinged, which is worse in the morning and on lying down. On physical examination, the patient appears chronically ill with clubbing of the fingers. Wet inspiratory rales are heard at the lung bases posteriorly.

54. The MOST likely diagnosis is

(A) bronchiectasis

(B) chronic bronchitis

(C) disseminated pulmonary tuberculosis

(D) pulmonary neoplasm

(E) chronic obstructive emphysema

55. This syndrome is MOST likely to be associated with

(A) lung cancer

(B) dextrocardia

(C) fungal infection

(D) carcinoid syndrome

(E) Hodgkin's disease

56. The MOST important procedure necessary to define the extent of the disease would be

(A) computed tomography (CT)

(B) bronchoscopy

(C) bronchography

(D) open thoracotomy

(E) bronchoalveolar lavage

57. Therapy for this disease might include

(A) antibiotics and postural drainage

(B) steroids

(C) radiotherapy

(D) aerosols

(E) isoniazid

58. A 19-year-old man arrives at the emergency department after a motorcycle accident, complaining of severe thigh pain. He has swelling and tenderness of the thigh, but distal neurovascular examination is intact. Radiographs disclose a comminuted and displaced fracture of the femur. Optimal treatment of this injury would be

(A) application of a traction boot and immobilization until the swelling subsides

(B) immediate internal fixation of the fracture

(C) application of a cylinder cast for 6 weeks

(D) insertion of a tibial traction pin with balanced traction to produce anatomic reduction and continued nonoperative management in this manner

(E) immediate placement of external fixator

59. A continuing-care retirement community that receives payment from residents on a capitated, prepaid basis is interested in minimizing its exposure to major financial losses. You have been hired to advise them on preventive interventions in which they should invest. Which of the following immunizations should be offered annually to each resident?

(A) HBV

(B) pneumococcal vaccine

(C) influenza vaccine

(D) tetanus booster

(E) bacillus Calmette–Guérin (BCG) immunization

60. Which feature BEST describes cerebral palsy?

(A) mental retardation

(B) basal ganglion sclerosis

(C) generalized spasticity

(D) choreiform movements

(E) nonprogressive motor defects

Questions 61 Through 63

A 24-year-old, previously healthy Latina woman presented to the community health center with fever and persistent cough. Her condition did not improve with antibiotic treatment for presumed mycoplasma pneumonia. Testing showed that she is suffering from pneumocystis carinii pneumonia (PCP), secondary to HIV infection.

61. If the woman's HIV infection had been detected a year ago during its asymptomatic phase, what intervention could have prevented this case of pneumonia?

   (A) trimethoprim–sulfamethoxazole
   (B) penicillin
   (C) rifampin
   (D) zidovudine (AZT)
   (E) flu vaccine

62. If PCP prophylaxis were provided to a larger number of asymptomatic HIV-positive people in the community, what would be the direct effect on the local epidemiology of HIV/AIDS?

   (A) would increase prevalence of HIV infection by increasing incidence of HIV
   (B) would increase prevalence of HIV infection by increasing duration of infection
   (C) would not change HIV or AIDS prevalence significantly
   (D) would increase incidence of AIDS
   (E) would reduce the positive predictive value of western blot testing for HIV

63. Each time the CDC broadens the case definition for AIDS, adding new AIDS-defining conditions, which of the following happens (assuming no real change in patterns of disease)?

   (A) The incidence of AIDS increases, but the prevalence remains unchanged.
   (B) The incidence of AIDS increases acutely, then falls to prechange level.
   (C) The prevalence of AIDS rises after a hiatus, coinciding with the incubation period.

   (D) The incidence of AIDS decreases, because individuals are diagnosed earlier in the course of their illness.
   (E) The life expectancy of individuals with AIDS falls because of greater disease burden.

64. You are called to evaluate the electrocardiogram (ECG) of a 9-year-old child who sustained blunt chest trauma. Which of the following statements is true concerning children's ECGs in comparison with adults?

   (A) The rate is relatively slower.
   (B) Variations in the normal are less diverse.
   (C) The P-R interval is relatively normal.
   (D) The Q-R-S interval is relatively longer.
   (E) Sinus arrhythmia is more frequent.

65. Which of the following statements is true regarding ovarian steroid feedback on gonadotropin secretion?

   (A) Estradiol stimulates follicle-stimulating hormone (FSH) and luteinizing hormone (LH).
   (B) Estradiol inhibits FSH and LH secretion, but rising estradiol levels after exceeding a certain threshold cause a positive feedback on LH secretion.
   (C) Progesterone has no effect on FSH secretion.
   (D) The pituitary response to estradiol is elicited only by endogenous (ovarian) and not exogenous estradiol.
   (E) The positive feedback of ovarian steroids on gonadotropin secretion operates at a low set point before initiation of puberty (ie, even low levels of sex steroids lead to significant secretion of gonadotropins).

66. The normal pH of the vagina in women of reproductive age is

   (A) 2.5 to 3.5
   (B) 3.5 to 4.5
   (C) 4.5 to 5.5
   (D) 5.5 to 6.5
   (E) 6.5 to 7.5

Questions 67 Through 71

A 22-year-old intoxicated man is brought into the emergency department after being an unrestrained passenger in an automobile accident. His blood pressure is 80/60 mm Hg; pulse 160 beats/min; and respiratory rate, 40 breaths/min, labored. He has an obvious open left femur fracture and is complaining vigorously of left chest pain and inability to get his breath. He refuses to lie flat.

67. Which of the following tests would NOT be included in the initial assessment?

   (A) auscultation of both lung fields
   (B) palpation of the position of the trachea
   (C) sending the patient for chest x-ray
   (D) looking to see if neck veins are distended
   (E) cardiac auscultation

68. His neck veins are found to be distended, the trachea is shifted to the right, and breath sounds are absent on the left. Crepitance is present on the left side of the chest. He is becoming more agitated and is demanding that someone help him breathe. The MOST appropriate intervention would be to

   (A) order a stat chest x-ray
   (B) paralyze and intubate the patient
   (C) perform a left chest tube thoracostomy
   (D) perform a nasotracheal intubation
   (E) order abdominal x-rays

69. Appropriate treatment was performed, and the patient is breathing easier now. His blood pressure is 80/60; pulse, 140; and respiratory rate, 35. His breath sounds are equal bilaterally, and his neck veins are flat. The initial treatment of his shock would include all of the following EXCEPT

   (A) transfusion of uncrossmatched blood
   (B) starting two large-bore intravenous lines
   (C) infusing 2 L of Ringer's lactate as rapidly as possible

   (D) controlling any external hemorrhage
   (E) placing him on high-flow oxygen

70. His hypotension continues; your NEXT intervention would be to

   (A) order a CT scan of his abdomen
   (B) continue transfusion of crystalloid and order O-negative or type-specific blood for immediate transfusion
   (C) continue transfusion of crystalloid only
   (D) start dopamine infusion
   (E) order blood transfusion as soon as fully typed and crossmatched blood is available

71. Appropriate initial treatment of his hypotension has been carried out. His blood pressure is now 130/90; pulse, 100; and respiration, 25. External hemorrhage is controlled and the neck veins are flat. Chest x-ray shows no evidence of hemorrhage, and chest tube drainage is minimal. He is beginning to complain of left upper quadrant pain and is requiring an intravenous rate of 300 mL/hr to prevent hypotension from recurring. Which of the following would NOT be appropriate?

   (A) diagnostic peritoneal lavage
   (B) x-ray of the pelvis
   (C) monitoring of urine output
   (D) placement of a central venous line for monitoring
   (E) pericardiocentesis

Questions 72 Through 75

A 34-year-old woman has been complaining of a 2-year history of increasing dyspnea and fatigue. Physical examination reveals increased jugular venous pressure and a reduced carotid pulse. Precordial examination reveals a left parasternal lift, loud P2, and right-sided S3 and S4. There are no audible murmurs. Chest x-ray reveals clear lung fields, and an ECG shows evidence of right ventricular hypertrophy. Pulmonary function tests show a slight restrictive pattern.

72. The MOST likely diagnosis is

    (A) asthma (without wheezing)
    (B) primary pulmonary hypertension
    (C) pulmonary veno-occlusive disease
    (D) pulmonary leiomyomatosis
    (E) "silent" tricuspid valve disease

73. Confirmation of the diagnosis usually requires

    (A) open lung biopsy
    (B) pulmonary angiography
    (C) cardiac catheterization
    (D) noninvasive exercise testing
    (E) electrophysiologic testing

74. The MOST common form of treatment is

    (A) anticoagulants
    (B) nitrates
    (C) alpha-adrenergic blockers
    (D) calcium channel blockers
    (E) angiotensin-converting enzyme (ACE) inhibitors

75. The MOST likely cause of death is

    (A) intractable left ventricular failure
    (B) intractable respiratory failure
    (C) massive pulmonary embolism
    (D) sudden death
    (E) myocardial infarction

76. The development of the female external genitalia is dependent upon

    (A) the Y chromosome
    (B) müllerian inhibiting factor
    (C) reaggression of the müllerian duct system
    (D) estrogen secretion by the ovary
    (E) the absence of a functioning testis

Questions 77 and 78

A 21-year-old mother complains that her son has started to scream and cry when she leaves him with a babysitter. She says that in the past he did not object to being left with a babysitter and asks you why he becomes so upset now.

77. You tell her that

    (A) she must not be spending enough time with her son
    (B) stranger anxiety is normal at her son's age
    (C) stranger anxiety suggests that her son is autistic
    (D) stranger anxiety will improve when the child can move away from the stranger effectively

78. Stranger anxiety is characteristic of what age?

    (A) 2 to 4 weeks
    (B) 2 to 3 months
    (C) 7 to 8 months
    (D) 12 to 18 months
    (E) 2 years

79. A 22-year-old patient is 34 weeks pregnant and presents because in the last month she has noted the bumps on her vulva have rapidly grown in size and number. They are nontender and fleshy, involving the perineum and the labia minora. The MOST likely diagnosis is

    (A) bacterial vaginosis
    (B) *Treponema pallidum*
    (C) *Chlamydia trachomatis*

(D) human papillomavirus 6 or 11

(E) human papillomavirus 16, 18, 31, or 45

Questions 80 Through 82

You have been asked to advise a friend who is planning to buy a house about what precautions she should take to be sure there are no environmental hazards. The house she is interested in was built in 1908. It was professionally renovated 2 years ago, including new wiring, plumbing, and heating systems, as well as repapering, painting, and new energy-efficient windows.

80. Which of the following should your friend be MOST concerned about?

(A) radon in the basement

(B) lead in the underlying layers of old paint

(C) asbestos insulation in the walls

(D) volatile organic compounds used as solvents during the renovation work

81. What illness would the woman be at increased risk for if that hazard were present?

(A) bladder cancer

(B) lung cancer

(C) peripheral neuropathy

(D) subcortical dementia

(E) asthma

82. Which of the house renovations could have compounded this problem?

(A) replacing heating system

(B) repainting

(C) installing new windows

(D) replacing old wiring

(E) new plumbing system

83. A 65-year-old woman presents with a chief complaint of a breast mass. On physical examination, she has a 3-cm mass in the upper outer quadrant of the left breast and no axillary lymphadenopathy. No discrete lesion is seen on mammogram. Fine-needle aspiration is positive for malignant cells. Which of the following would be an appropriate treatment option?

(A) follow-up examination in 6 weeks

(B) excision of this fibroadenoma

(C) follow-up mammogram in 3 months to determine if a lesion becomes apparent

(D) lumpectomy, axillary dissection, irradiation

(E) radiation and chemotherapy

Questions 84 Through 86

You are called to the emergency department to evaluate a 50-year-old man who complains of shortness of breath for 3 weeks and swelling of his face. On physical examination, you note distention of the veins of the neck and chest wall in addition to facial edema.

84. Which of the following is a correct statement concerning his condition?

(A) The most likely cause is lymphoma.

(B) He will improve with diuretics alone.

(C) He needs emergency radiation therapy.

(D) Squamous cell cancer is the second most common cause.

(E) This is an oncologic emergency and treatment should begin immediately.

85. A CT-guided biopsy is obtained and, while awaiting the reading on the tissue, you receive a call from the laboratory saying that the patient's calcium is 13.2 mg/dL. The MOST likely malignancy to be associated with hypercalcemia in a patient with this process is

(A) small cell carcinoma

(B) metastatic parathyroid carcinoma

(C) squamous cell carcinoma

(D) lymphoma

(E) germ cell tumor of the mediastinum

86. You do a neurologic examination and find that he is lethargic but otherwise has no deficits. Management of his hypercalcemia MUST include

    (A) mithramycin
    (B) hydrochlorothiazide
    (C) intravenous saline
    (D) insulin
    (E) gallium nitrate

87. The MOST common cardiac cause of cyanosis in the newborn is

    (A) tetralogy of Fallot
    (B) patent ductus arteriosus
    (C) hypoplastic left heart syndrome
    (D) pulmonary hypertension
    (E) transposition of the great vessels

Questions 88 and 89

A 52-year-old man presents to the emergency department with a 2-month history of mid-epigastric pain and a 1-hour history of vomiting bright red blood. On physical examination, he is confused about the day and date but is oriented to person and place. He is unsteady walking from the parking lot to the waiting room. His abdominal examination is positive for diffuse tenderness in the midepigastric area, but there is no rebound or rigidity. Rectal exam shows no masses, but the stool in the vault is tarry-black and positive for occult blood. His blood alcohol level is elevated.

88. His complete blood count (CBC) is MOST likely to show

    (A) a macrocytic anemia
    (B) a microcytic anemia
    (C) a normocytic anemia
    (D) leukopenia
    (E) thrombocytosis

89. Alcohol is toxic to platelets and megakaryocytes. The thrombocytopenia secondary to acute alcohol use usually lasts

    (A) 1 to 2 hours
    (B) 3 to 7 days

(C) 1 to 2 weeks
(D) 3 to 4 weeks
(E) none of the above; alcohol affects platelet function and not numbers

90. A morbidly obese woman underwent a total abdominal hysterectomy for fibroids 4 days ago. She now is febrile, with a temperature of 38.6°C. Her physical exam is significant for lung fields that are clear to auscultation, no costovertebral tenderness, and an abdomen that has normal bowel sounds and is non-tender. Her incision is erythematous, indurated, warm to the touch, and tender. The next step in this patient's management would be to

    (A) begin parenteral antibiotics for superficial wound infection
    (B) remove every other staple to allow any fluid in the wound to drain
    (C) remove the staples and probe the wound to allow any fluid to drain as well as probe the fascia for any defects
    (D) begin using a warm heating pad over the incision
    (E) check urine analysis for evidence of a lower urinary tract infection

Questions 91 and 92

A 34-year-old man complains of right upper quadrant discomfort. On physical evaluation, he has enlargement of the liver and spleen. A bone marrow biopsy is done while awaiting blood studies. The bone marrow biopsy shows large reticulate cells containing glucocerebrosides.

91. The MOST likely diagnosis is

    (A) large cell lymphoma
    (B) Gaucher's disease
    (C) glycogen storage disease
    (D) sarcoidosis
    (E) persistent parvovirus infection

92. Treatment options for this patient include

    (A) chemotherapy using cyclophosphamide hydroxydaunorubicin vincristine prednisone (CHOP)

(B) intravenous administration of al-glucerase (glucocerebrosidase-beta-glucosidase)

(C) avoidance of phenylketones

(D) prednisone

(E) antiretrovirals

Questions 93 and 94

93. A 30-year-old Caucasian woman presents with a 1.5-cm diameter nevus on her left leg. She noted that it was increasing in size over the past few months. The appropriate method for diagnosis of the lesion is

(A) lymphoscintigraphy

(B) shave biopsy

(C) magnetic resonance imaging (MRI) scan

(D) excisional biopsy

(E) fine-needle aspiration

94. The patient's diagnosis is superficial spreading malignant melanoma with 0.55-mm thickness. An appropriate treatment plan would be

(A) chemotherapy with radiation therapy

(B) wide local excision

(C) wide local excision with groin dissection

(D) radiation therapy

(E) chemotherapy

Questions 95 and 96

A 54-year-old female is found to have small cell carcinoma after being evaluated for hoarseness.

95. Which of the following statements is true about her disease?

(A) The hoarseness is probably from involvement of the recurrent laryngeal nerve.

(B) Weight loss is an atypical presenting sign, and a bowel primary should be sought.

(C) No further staging evaluation is necessary.

(D) Metastasis to the brain is unusual in small cell carcinoma.

(E) The lung is the sole site of development of small cell carcinoma.

96. Which of the following hormones can be secreted by small cell carcinomas?

(A) insulin

(B) antidiuretic hormone (ADH)

(C) erythropoietin

(D) osteoclast-activating factor (OAF)

(E) growth hormone–releasing hormone (GHRH)

97. A male has mental retardation; high, prominent forehead; prominent supraorbital ridges; long, narrow face; large ears; prominent mandible; and interstitial fibrosis of the testes. His behavior includes hyperactivity, hand flapping, gaze avoidance, and repetitive behavior. What diagnosis is suggested?

(A) autism

(B) William syndrome

(C) Burte Sloan syndrome

(D) fragile X syndrome

(E) XXY syndrome

Questions 98 Through 101

A 73-year-old nulliparous woman presents to your office for the first time for a general physical exam. She has recently moved to your community, and her last pelvic exam was 5 years ago. She complains of incontinence while trying to open her front door on arriving home from her daily errands. As part of your physical exam, you do a Papanicolaou (Pap) smear that is reported as atypical glandular cells of uncertain significance.

98. Which of the following statements represents the current use of Pap smears in the care of women?

(A) They are no longer necessary after age 65.

(B) They should be done annually as a screening technique for cervical and endometrial pathology.

(C) They need to be performed only on sexually active women.

(D) They are a screening technique to pick up preinvasive cervical pathology.

(E) They have a false-negative rate of less than 5%.

99. Cervical dysplasia and the progression to cervical cancer have been associated with which of the following viruses 95% of the time?

    (A) cytomegalovirus (CMV)
    (B) HSV-2
    (C) HIV
    (D) HPV
    (E) Squamous dysplasia virus (SDV)

100. Based on this Pap smear report, you ask her to

    (A) return for a repeat smear in 3 months
    (B) use vaginal estrogen cream
    (C) undergo colposcopy
    (D) undergo colposcopy and endocervical curettage
    (E) undergo colposcopy, endocervical curettage, and endometrial biopsy

101. The initial evaluation does not reveal the source of the abnormal cytology. You

    (A) believe the report was a laboratory error but ask her to return for another Pap smear as soon as possible
    (B) recommend that she use vaginal estrogen cream and return for a repeat smear in 3 months
    (C) recommend that she undergo colposcopy in 6 months
    (D) recommend a cold-knife cone biopsy
    (E) recommend a vaginal hysterectomy and anterior repair to take care of both the abnormal Pap smear and stress incontinence at once

102. Which of the following terms describes the thought pattern marked by speech that is indirect and tedious in detail but eventually arrives at a coherent goal?

    (A) tangentiality
    (B) word salad
    (C) circumstantiality
    (D) derailment
    (E) Klang associations

103. Which of the following patients would be a more appropriate candidate for a CT scan than for MRI?

    (A) a young woman with multiple sclerosis
    (B) a child with a suspected abnormality in the size of his ventricles
    (C) a man with an implanted cardiac pacemaker
    (D) a woman with suspected temporal lobe disease
    (E) a child with autism

104. X-rays of a normal newborn would reveal ossification centers in which of the following?

    (A) clavicle
    (B) proximal femur
    (C) talus
    (D) distal tibia
    (E) none of the above

105. Allegations of malpractice are common in obstetrical practice. To prove that malpractice has occurred, which of the following must have occurred?

    (A) There must have been an injury to the plaintiff.
    (B) The defendant must have deliberately injured the plaintiff.
    (C) There must be a violation of a standard of care by the defendant that resulted in an injury to the plaintiff.
    (D) There must be a violation of a standard of care and an injury, but causation may be assumed.
    (E) Causation must be established beyond a reasonable doubt.

106. The best approach to minimizing the risk of your being named in a malpractice suit is to

    (A) communicate frequently with the risk management department at the hospital
    (B) refer all complicated cases to the teaching service
    (C) communicate effectively with the patient and order all tests and consults requested

(D) communicate effectively with the patient and document compliance with the standard of care

(E) obtain frequent consultation with a variety of specialists

Questions 107 and 108

Mrs. Jones has come to your office many times for a variety of complaints. In spite of multiple examinations and laboratory tests, you have not been able to find an organic basis for any of her symptoms. She responds to your favorable report of her tests with a new list of symptoms.

107. At this point, it would be most useful to say:

(A) "Mrs. Jones, there is absolutely nothing wrong with you."

(B) "I think you should see a psychiatrist."

(C) "I have another medicine that I would like you to try."

(D) "I'm puzzled, Mrs. Jones, about your response to the good news. Do you have any ideas about that?"

(E) "I think your problem is emotional, Mrs. Jones. I can't find anything wrong with you."

108. Of the following diagnoses, the most likely cause of Mrs. Jones' chronic complaints is

(A) cancer

(B) a viral infection

(C) domestic violence

(D) mental retardation

(E) a bacterial infection

109. A 70-year-old married man, father of two, has been hospitalized for a course of treatment for prostatic cancer. According to Elizabeth Kübler-Ross, the stages of response that this patient may experience upon being told that he has metastatic disease include

(A) denial, anxiety, depression, acceptance

(B) anger, intellectualization, bargaining, acceptance

(C) isolation of affect, bargaining, depression, acceptance

(D) fear, denial, depression, acceptance

(E) anger, bargaining, depression, acceptance

Questions 110 and 111

A 64-year-old man has a complaint of anorexia and weight loss (20 lb). On physical examination, he is a cachectic man. His abdominal examination shows no abnormalities. On rectal examination, he is heme positive. His hemoglobin is 8.5 mg/dL. On upper endoscopy, an ulcer is noted in the antrum. Multiple biopsies were taken. The pathology report was positive for adenocarcinoma.

110. All of the following statements regarding prognosis for gastric cancer are correct EXCEPT

(A) tumor located in the pyloric antrum has a better outcome than tumor located in the proximal two thirds of the stomach

(B) metastasis with four or fewer lymph nodes is associated with a better outcome

(C) CT scan is accurate for predicting the operability of a lesion

(D) a lesion limited to the mucosa and submucosa has a better chance for cure

(E) positive physical findings such as an enlarged supraclavicular lymph node, jaundice, ascites, or pelvic mass suggest advanced disease and a worse prognosis

111. All of the following conditions are associated with gastric cancer EXCEPT

(A) higher socioeconomic groups

(B) pernicious anemia

(C) chronic atrophic gastritis

(D) adenomatous polyps

(E) a high intake of dietary nitrates

112. A 60-year-old man with schizophrenia had been taking large doses of a phenothiazine for several years. On examination, his muscles are rigid, and he is tremulous. He walks with a shuffling gait. On occasion, drooling is noted. The patient MOST likely is displaying

    (A) echopraxia
    (B) catatonia
    (C) a pyramidal system disorder
    (D) an extrapyramidal system disorder
    (E) an irreversible side effect of his medication

113. Which of the following is associated with a particularly poor prognosis of schizophrenia?

    (A) acute onset
    (B) affective symptoms
    (C) clouded sensorium
    (D) positive family history of schizophrenia
    (E) marriage

114. When a terminal illness occurs in an individual, which of the following is often observed in the family members?

    (A) remission of any preexisting psychopathology
    (B) intensification of family conflicts
    (C) solidification of roles
    (D) transient psychotic episodes
    (E) stable patterns of maintaining discipline

115. Which of the following conditions BEST describes the growth chart in Figure 6.2?

    (A) growth hormone deficiency
    (B) genetic short stature
    (C) constitutional growth delay
    (D) chronic illness
    (E) normal variation

Questions 116 Through 118

A 37-year-old man is brought to the emergency department by the police. As you interview him, you note that he is drowsy and unable to focus his at-

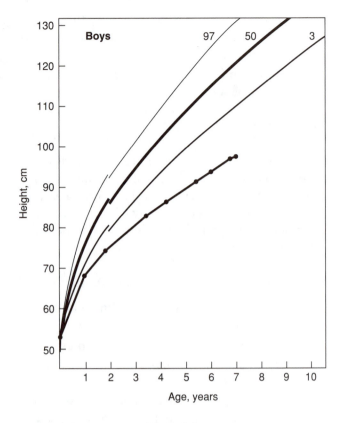

Figure 6.2.

tention on your questions. Also, his speech is slurred. On physical exam, his pupils are 1 mm in diameter.

116. This man is MOST likely experiencing

    (A) opiate intoxication
    (B) cocaine intoxication
    (C) alcohol intoxication
    (D) amphetamine intoxication
    (E) cannabis intoxication

117. In order to acutely reverse the effect of the drug, you could administer

    (A) methadone
    (B) cocaine
    (C) alcohol
    (D) naloxone
    (E) clonidine

118. After this patient recovers, a treatment program that includes which of the following medications would be most effective in preventing relapse?

    (A) methadone
    (B) disulfiram
    (C) olanzapine
    (D) naloxone
    (E) clonidine

119. A premature baby is MOST likely to be deficient to a clinically significant degree in which of the following compounds or cells?

    (A) alpha-1-antitrypsin
    (B) surfactant
    (C) eosinophils
    (D) elastin
    (E) mast cells

Questions 120 and 121

A 30-year-old man presents with a several-month history of epigastric pain relieved by foods and antacids. Earlier this evening, his pain became much worse. On physical examination, he has a diffusely tender abdomen and is positive for rebound tenderness. He is initially hypotensive and requires volume resuscitation. His upright abdominal x-ray is shown for Figure 6.3.

120. The MOST important aspect of his treatment is

    (A) hydration alone
    (B) emergency exploratory laparotomy
    (C) antibiotics alone
    (D) upper endoscopy
    (E) a CT scan of the abdomen

121. The pathologic process that caused his abdominal pain is duodenal ulcer disease. Which of the following statements about duodenal ulcer disease is correct?

    (A) The majority of duodenal ulcers are located in the duodenal bulb.
    (B) Cigarette smoking has not been implicated.

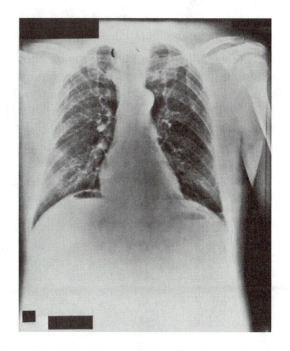

Figure 6.3. Abdominal x-ray showing dilated loops of small and large bowel without air-fluid levels, typical of diffuse peritonitis.

    (C) NSAIDs do not increase the risk of peptic ulcer disease.
    (D) *Helicobacter pylori* has been implicated in gastric but not duodenal ulcers.
    (E) Duodenal ulcer disease is more common in women than in men.

122. A 7-year-old girl is evaluated in your office and found to have an enlarged spleen. A large spleen is associated with all of the following EXCEPT

    (A) Gaucher disease
    (B) Epstein–Barr virus infection
    (C) alpha-1-antitrypsin deficiency
    (D) chronic myelogenous leukemia
    (E) metastatic Wilms' tumor

Questions 123 and 124

On entering middle school, a 12-year-old boy is tested and found to be of above-average intelligence, but his school work does not reflect this. He is often inattentive during class, but not restless. He does not act out and is described by his teachers as "daydreaming" frequently in class. An electroencephalogram (EEG) shows brief 3-Hz spike-and-wave discharges occurring synchronously throughout all leads.

123. The medicine MOST likely to be helpful is

    (A) phenytoin
    (B) carbamazepine
    (C) phenobarbital
    (D) clonazepam
    (E) valproic acid

124. Which of the following is true of the medication?

    (A) can be used to treat typical and atypical seizures
    (B) causes sedation
    (C) impairs cognitive ability
    (D) CBCs need not be monitored
    (E) renal function should be monitored

125. You are asked to see a 15-month-old boy who had a seizure for the first time. The parents report that the seizure took place several hours after the onset of a fever. On physical examination, you discover that the child has an otitis media. The remainder of the examination is normal, including a neurologic examination performed by yourself. Which of the following is the MOST likely diagnosis?

    (A) meningitis
    (B) septicemia
    (C) pneumococcus
    (D) epilepsy
    (E) febrile seizure

Questions 126 and 127

A 34-year-old woman with alcohol dependence had previously undergone psychodynamic psy-chotherapy unsuccessfully in an attempt to discontinue alcohol abuse. She then went to a behavioral therapist who, after counseling, allowed her to drink but gave her disulfiram to take each morning.

126. A patient who is taking disulfiram daily and who begins to drink alcohol is most likely to experience which of the following symptoms?

    (A) constipation
    (B) diaphoresis
    (C) bradycardia
    (D) dry mouth
    (E) somnolence

127. Which of the following types of therapy was being used?

    (A) abreaction
    (B) confrontation
    (C) psychoanalytic
    (D) aversion
    (E) masochism

128. A 16-year-old boy presents to your clinic with the complaint of discharge from his penis. You perform a Gram stain on the urethral exudate (see Figure 6.4). The MOST likely diagnosis is

    (A) syphilis
    (B) gonorrhea
    (C) Reiter syndrome
    (D) herpes
    (E) chanchroid

Questions 129 and 130

A 26-year-old woman took an overdose of aspirin.

129. Which of the following would be considered a mild manifestation of aspirin toxicity?

    (A) renal failure
    (B) bradycardia

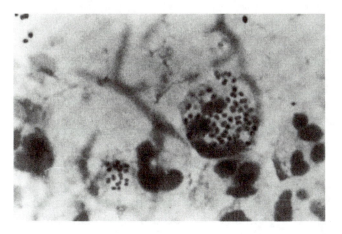

Figure 6.4

(C) convulsions

(D) respiratory acidosis

(E) respiratory alkalosis

130. Which of the following is appropriate treatment of this patient in the emergency department?

(A) dialysis

(B) subcutaneous injection of vitamin K

(C) oral rehydration

(D) intravenous methylene blue

(E) protection of the airway and oxygen administration

131. You have just completed your evaluation of an infant in the emergency department. The parents report that the infant has had diarrhea for 2 days. On examination, you noted the infant to be irritable without tears. His mouth was dry. His skin was dry but did not tent up when pinched. His diaper was minimally wet. Your estimate of the degree of dehydration was

(A) 2%

(B) 3 to 5%

(C) 5 to 7%

(D) 8 to 12%

(E) cannot estimate from this information

Questions 132 and 133

A 70-year-old woman with multiple medical conditions comes in for a routine gynecologic exam. She has a 2-week history of loss of urine with coughing and sneezing associated with some urgency. On exam, she is found to have a small first-degree cystocele and her cervix comes halfway down her vagina.

132. The next step in the investigation of this patient that is MOST likely to be beneficial is

(A) urinalysis

(B) cystometry

(C) voiding cystourethrogram

(D) blood glucose

(E) neurologic exam

133. The MOST appropriate treatment of her cystocele would be

(A) Kegel exercises to reverse the pelvic relaxation

(B) fitting her with a pessary

(C) a colpocliesis (Lefort type)

(D) a uterine suspension

(E) observation

134. You examine a newborn in the nursery and discover that the child exhibits a flat midface, narrow palpebral fissures, and low nasal bridge. He also has a short, upturned nose and a narrow vermilion border of his upper lip. These children may be small for gestational age and show poor growth. Others may have cleft lip, atrial and ventricular septal defects, and microphthalmia. The findings BEST describe

(A) cocaine exposure in utero

(B) HIV infection

(C) fetal alcohol syndrome

(D) heroin exposure

(E) toxoplasmosis

135. Hypoparathyroidism in adults is MOST commonly a result of

    (A) development of antiparathyroid antibodies (Schmidt syndrome)
    (B) prior neck surgery
    (C) ^{131}I therapy
    (D) lack of parathyroid-stimulating factor (PSF) from the pituitary
    (E) congenital absence of parathyroid glands (DiGeorge syndrome)

136. A newborn failed the state screening program, with thyroxine (T_4) values of 5.4 and thyroid-stimulating hormone (TSH) of 448. He is breast fed and looks well at age 8 days. He is active. He cries with hunger. The physical examination is normal. The repeat findings are T_4, 2; TSH, 476; and thyroxine-binding globulin (TBG, 3.1. Your assessment of these results is

    (A) thyroiditis
    (B) transient hypothyroidism
    (C) immune hypothyroidism
    (D) congenital hypothyroidism
    (E) normal

Questions 137 and 138

A 30-year-old woman has experienced loss of appetite, anhedonia, early morning awakening, depressed mood, and a pervasive feeling of hopelessness for the past 8 months.

137. If she were studied in the sleep laboratory, the results would MOST likely show
    (A) increased time of sleep before the first rapid eye movement (REM) period
    (B) decreased time of sleep until the first REM period
    (C) no REM sleep
    (D) no non-REM sleep
    (E) no true sleep at all

138. Prior to the testing in the sleep laboratory, the physician considers obtaining informed consent. Which of the following statements is true with regard to informed consent?

    (A) To perform any procedure or any touching of a patient in a medical center without consent constitutes battery.
    (B) Detailed and specific consent forms may substitute for a physician–patient dialogue.
    (C) If a patient is over 90 years old, consent should be obtained from a family member rather than from the patient.
    (D) If a patient is fearful of a procedure, the physician does not need to explain the risks of the procedure when obtaining consent.
    (E) The consent process contains two elements: information and voluntariness.

139. The fetus is in a left occiput transverse position, full dilatation at a +3 station. A posterior asynclitism is noted. From the following choices, select the proper instrument and technique for delivery.

    (A) Tucker–McLean forceps with the Scanzoni maneuver
    (B) Simpson's forceps with the Scanzoni maneuver
    (C) Kielland forceps with a Scanzoni rotation
    (D) Kielland forceps with axial rotation around the shaft
    (E) Tucker forceps with a shaft axial rotation

Questions 140 Through 142

A 72-year-old man who has been coming to you for a number of years for mild hypertension comes in for a regular check-up complaining of the recent onset of low back pain. He cannot pinpoint a specific time of onset. He has not had any kind of chronic pain prior to this. A routine CBC at his last office visit 3 months ago showed normal WBC and platelet counts, but the hemoglobin was 12 g/dL with a mean corpuscular volume (MCV) of 92. His creatine at that time was 1.2 mg/dL.

140. What should you do next?

    (A) Reassure him that this is likely just arthritis and prescribe an NSAID.
    (B) Repeat the CBC.

(C) Repeat the CBC and also check serum iron, B$_{12}$, and folate levels.

(D) Repeat the CBC and a serum protein electrophoresis.

(E) Order a bone scan to evaluate his back pain.

141. What proportion of patients with this diagnosis have a normal SPEP?

(A) none
(B) 20%
(C) 50%
(D) 75%
(E) 100%

142. Therapy for this problem should include

(A) chiropractic manipulation of the spine
(B) strontium
(C) methotrexate
(D) calcium supplementation and exercise
(E) pamidronate

143. The scarf sign in the newborn is

(A) a reddening of the neck area from having the umbilical cord wrapped around the neck
(B) enlargement of the lymphatics in the neck region—cystic hygroma
(C) cyanosis from pulmonary hypertension
(D) accumulation of skin in the chest wall seen in postmature babies
(E) a test to help identify the gestational age of a premature baby

144. Which of the following types of injury leads to the greatest amount of preventable morbidity among the elderly?

(A) falls
(B) burns
(C) poisoning
(D) attempted suicide
(E) motor vehicle accidents, including pedestrian injuries

145. A middle-aged man comes to you because he fears his wife will leave him. He tells you that his wife has moved out of the house and that he is impotent and cannot satisfy her. He drinks some wine before dinner and three or four gin and tonics afterward. He states that for the past several weeks he has had trouble sleeping, awakening early. He is not able to concentrate on his work and finds pleasure in nothing, saying, "Things just don't look good." He sighs deeply and pauses. At this point, it would be most helpful to say, "Tell me more about

(A) your drinking problem"
(B) what's wrong at work"
(C) your wife's moving out"
(D) your sexual problems"
(E) things not looking good"

146. The first step in the management of shoulder dystocia is

(A) Zavenelli maneuver
(B) Woods' screw
(C) McRoberts maneuver
(D) to call for help, drain bladder, and ensure an adequate perineal opening
(E) suprapubic pressure

Questions 147 and 148

A 40-year-old woman with schizophrenia is being treated with haloperidol. On physical examination, she is noted to be fidgeting with her hands and rocking at the waist, and she appears to be generally restless.

147. Which of the following is she MOST likely to have?

(A) automatism
(B) akinesia
(C) akathisia
(D) agitated depression
(E) apraxia

148. Which of the following is a positive symptom of schizophrenia?

    (A) flattened affect
    (B) poverty of speech
    (C) apathy
    (D) impaired hygiene
    (E) auditory hallucinations

149. In order to differentiate functional from organic impotence, which of the following techniques is most useful?

    (A) MMPI-2
    (B) Rorschach
    (C) nocturnal penile tumescence recording
    (D) WAIS-R
    (E) skull x-rays

150. Test results reveal metastatic disease to the bone, brain, and liver in a 70-year-old man. Which of the following is the MOST appropriate behavior for the patient's physician in conveying the bad news? The physician should

    (A) discuss the test results individually with the patient on morning rounds
    (B) make arrangements to sit down with the patient, his spouse, and other family members to discuss the findings and treatment
    (C) set aside time for a lengthy detailed discussion initially, in order to avoid the need for ongoing discussions
    (D) discuss the findings with the patient's spouse and other family members alone, since recent studies show that most patients prefer not to be informed of a diagnosis of advanced malignancy
    (E) request that a psychiatric consultant convey the bad news to the patient

Answers and Explanations

1. **(A)** Case-control studies involve investigation of past exposures in two groups of individuals: one with the condition under investigation and the other free of that condition. It is most useful in studying the causes of rare conditions.

2. **(D)** When studying the effectiveness of a particular intervention, the best study design is generally the randomized controlled trial, in which patients are assigned randomly to receive either the treatment under investigation or an alternative. When there is a well-established treatment for the condition, the alternative should be the standard treatment. When there is no known treatment for the condition, the alternative is a placebo—a pharmacologically inactive preparation that appears as much as possible like the actual treatment.

3. **(E)** Time series studies are most useful in studying the effect of major changes, as in this example, where it would be difficult or impossible to find an appropriate, concurrent control group.

4. **(B)** Cohort studies are used to investigate to what degree a particular exposure or condition is a risk factor for the outcome(s) of interest. It can be used only if the outcome is expected to be fairly common in the population being studied.

5. **(C)** Cross-sectional studies are useful in assessing the prevalence of health conditions in a population and in developing hypotheses that should be investigated further. Because they look at only one point in time, they cannot be used to draw firm conclusions about cause.

6-10. **(6-F, 7-B, 8-C, 9-A, 10-D)** Knowing the approximate age in children for significant developmental milestones is critical for the USMLE examination and for real medical practice as well.

11. **(A)** Multiple myeloma is associated with B-cell deficiency/dysfunction because of the proliferation of the malignant clone.

12. **(C)** Hodgkin's disease, acquired immune deficiency syndrome (AIDS), sarcoidosis, and thymic aplasia or hypoplasia result in T-cell deficiency/dysfunction.

13. **(A)** Chronic lymphocytic leukemia, like myeloma, results in B-cell deficiency/dysfunction because of the proliferation of the malignant clone.

14. **(F)** Systemic lupus erythematosus (SLE) has been associated with C3 deficiency, but most severe complement deficiencies result from inherited disorders.

15. **(D)** While the malignancy itself can result in a variety of immunologic dysfunctions, the most common problem associated with the treatment of hematologic malignancy is neutropenia.

16. **(B)** Ataxia–telangiectasia, common variable hypogammaglobulinemia, severe combined immunodeficiency, and Wiskott–Aldrich

syndrome have mixed T- and B-cell deficiencies.

17–19. **(17-B, 18-A, 19-C)** In the staff model HMO, the plan contracts with or directly hires providers who care exclusively for enrollees in the plan. The independent practice association (or open-model or foundation HMO) contract with community-based providers who are not exclusively bound to the enrollees in the plan and who care for other patients as well. In a PPO, the plan negotiates with the community-based providers to obtain discounted fees.

20. **(B)** Medicare provides universal health insurance for people over age 65 and for a variety of other individuals, such as those with end-stage renal disease.

21. **(C)** The Veterans Administration provides outpatient and inpatient care (including long-term care) to veterans of the armed forces through a system of Veterans Administration Medical Centers around the country. It does not cover care provided in other settings.

22. **(A)** The Medicaid program was established to provide health care coverage to low-income individuals and families. While roughly three quarters of Medicaid *beneficiaries* are poor women and children, roughly three quarters of Medicaid *spending* goes to long-term care. Medicare covers long-term care only for a transitional period following an acute hospitalization, but Medicaid covers it indefinitely for those who qualify. Because long-term care is very expensive, many middle-income individuals qualify for Medicaid coverage when they move into a nursing home by "spending down" their assets and having health care expenses that exceed their income.

23. **(E)** HUS, characterized by hemolytic anemia, thrombocytopenia, and renal insufficiency, usually starts with a mild illness with cough, vomiting, and mild diarrhea. When the child becomes markedly ill, with hemolysis, bleeding, and decreased platelets, three systems are involved; the kidney, the gastrointestinal (GI) tract, and brain. The symptoms include anemia, purpura, and bleeding in the kidneys, intestines, and brain. The peripheral smear shows burr and helmit cells, along with schistocytes. The urine will show red cells, protein, and red cell casts. The patient may be anuric for several days to many weeks. Usually, the anuria lasts about 2 weeks. Many cases are associated with an *E. coli* infection. Some cases will be confused with ulcerative colitis.

24. **(D)** Hookworm infection is caused by either *Necator americanus* or *Ancylostoma duodenale*, which are found most commonly in the Southern United States. The initial infection is characterized by a skin rash, followed by a cough, low-grade fever, acute abdominal disturbance, intermittent diarrhea, and eosinophilia. Symptoms depend on the nutritional status of the patient and the number of reinfections. The diagnosis is made by finding ova in the stool. Most infections are not significant clinically unless the number of ova is high when the patient develops anemia. Cutanea larva migrans is also termed "creeping eruption" and is a skin disorder caused by migrating nematode larvae in the skin (see Figure 6.5).

25. **(A)** Inflammatory bowel disease includes both Crohn's disease and ulcerative colitis. Crohn's disease frequently involves the ileocecal area. It typically presents with diarrhea and weight loss. Patients may have periumbilical pain, which is increased with meals. They may also have abscesses or bowel perforation (see Figure 6.6). Ulcerative colitis usually presents with rectal bleeding and a change in bowel consistency. Abdominal pain, fever, weight loss, and anemia are other symptoms or signs. Many clinical and laboratory features are similar in the two conditions. Endoscopy and radiologic studies help differentiate the two problems.

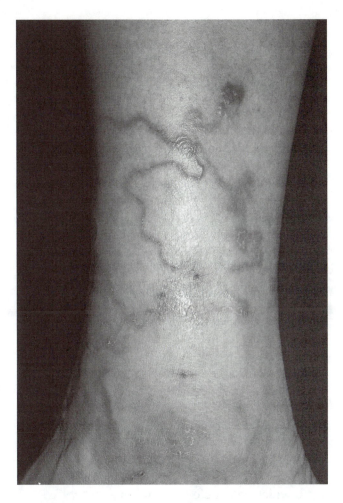

Figure 6.5. Cutanea larva migrans. Serpentine, erythematous, threadlike, vesicular, raised lesions on the lower leg.

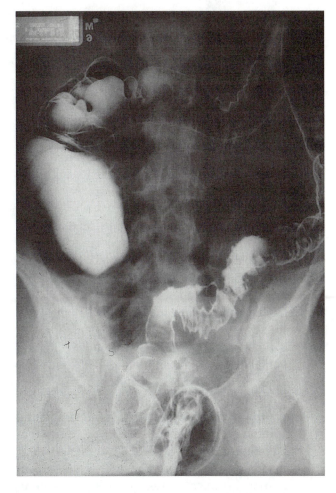

Figure 6.6. Crohn's disease. Barium radiograph. Changes seen are characteristic of Crohn's disease. There is segmented intestinal involvement where the walls are rigid and there is lumenal stenosis.

26. (C) There is strong epidemiologic *and* genetic evidence of HPV involvement in the etiology of cervical cancer. Serologic associations have also been identified between cervical cancer and herpes simplex-2 virus, but those appear to be more coincidental than causal. HSV-2 seems at most to be a cofactor. Invasive cervical cancer in an individual with HIV infection is considered an AIDS-defining condition, as of the Centers for Disease Control and Prevention (CDC's) 1993 revision of the AIDS case definition. As with HSV-2, HIV appears to be a cofactor, facilitating the unrestrained growth of cervical cancer, but it has not been implicated as a causative agent in the cancer.

27. (A) Hepatocellular carcinoma is a well-recognized late complication of chronic infection with the hepatitis B virus. Periodic screening of HBV-infected individuals, via ultrasound or alpha-fetoprotein titers, can detect the cancer at an early, treatable stage. Hepatitis C virus also appears to be a risk factor for hepatocellular carcinoma and may be a more common risk factor than HBV in some parts of the world (eg, Japan).

28. (E) One of the earliest identified associations between viral infection and neoplastic disease was the association between EBV virus infection and a form of non-Hodgkin's B-cell lymphoma known as Burkitt's lymphoma.

As was noted above with invasive cervical cancer, there is a strong association between non-Hodgkin's lymphomas and HIV infection; B-cell lymphoma was one of the original AIDS-defining conditions. But also as with cervical cancer, HIV infection seems to be a promoter of tumor growth, rather than an initiator. In some parts of the world, over 90% of lymphomas contain EBV genetic material in all tumor cells, in patients with and without associated HIV infection.

29. **(C)** It is not a routine part of the pediatric examination, but may be necessary if symptoms are present. The best approach is to examine the patient while she is sitting on her mother's lap. If the cervix needs to be visualized, it can be performed in a knee/chest position by gently spreading the labia apart. It is not necessary to place a young child in a dorsal lithotomy position.

30. **(D)** Of all infants with ambiguous genitalia, approximately 40 to 45% have congenital adrenal hyperplasia (CAH). Androgen-secreting tumors, placental aromatase deficiency, and excessive maternal androgen ingestion are also causes of ambiguous genitalia. In androgen insensitivity syndrome, the external genitalia are normally female in appearance.

31. **(C)** Neonates born with ambiguous genitalia are at risk for a salt-wasting CAH. The electrolyte imbalance can be life-threatening and is significant immediately after birth. Notification of the sex assignment should be delayed until the proper evaluation has been expeditiously completed.

32. **(A)** The weight gain of infants averages 20 g/day for the first 6 months and 15 g/day until 1 year old. They double their birth weight by 4 to 6 months and triple the birth weight in a year. They quadruple their weight by 2 years.

33. **(D)** Neither a mammogram nor a physical examination is 100% sensitive in detecting breast cancer. Many palpable lesions are not seen on mammogram. Therefore, any suspicious mass—and one that has recently developed is suspicious—should be evaluated by a surgeon. Many radiology units will automatically do an ultrasound on a palpable lesion to rule out a cyst, but if the lesion is palpable, ultrasound is not necessary for biopsy and only adds to the expense. For nonpalpable lesions picked up on mammogram, needle localization can be done using the mammogram to assist the surgeon in biopsying the correct area.

34. **(B)** Several studies now show that the overall survival for women is equivalent whether they choose mastectomy or lumpectomy with radiation. The local recurrence rate is higher, on the order of 6 to 10% for those who chose the lumpectomy with radiation, but many are salvaged with mastectomy at that point. Reconstruction can be performed immediately or delayed, depending on the wishes of the patient and the requirements for adjuvant radiation. The surgical options deal only with the breast and do not address the possibility of systemic disease; therefore, adjuvant therapy of some type may still be necessary whichever choice she makes.

35. **(B)** With positive lymph nodes, most oncologists would strongly urge the patients to receive some type of adjuvant therapy. The 5-year recurrence rate for a 1.5-cm tumor with positive nodes is about 35%. This can be reduced to about 24% with tamoxifen in patients over the age of 50. Although there is a tendency to add chemotherapy to patients with bad prognostic signs, there has yet to be a trial conclusively demonstrating the advantage of this. High-dose chemotherapy should be considered experimental.

36. **(C)** Tamoxifen increases the risk of endometrial cancer from about 1 per 2000 in the general population to 2 per 2000. Of course, this woman has had a hysterectomy so it is not an issue. It will reduce her risk of recurrence by 30% and developing a new cancer by at least the same amount. The results of the Breast Cancer Prevention Trial have yet to be pub-

lished in a peer-reviewed journal but are likely to confirm an even greater advantage in prevention than the 30 to 40% seen in other studies. There is an increased risk of thrombosis, which is more pronounced in women with other risk factors such as obesity and tobacco use. The Prevention Trial will also show an increase in bone density, which has been suggested by previous studies.

37. **(C)** Making recommendations to patients you have never seen is risky business, although patients will often ask you to do so. Mammograms are not perfect tests, and a recent study confirmed the high incidence of false positives. Mammograms show the greatest benefit for women between the ages of 50 and 75, where the incidence of the disease is greatest. It would be best for the daughters to sit down with a physician and review their risk profile, which would include onset of menstruation, age at first term pregnancy, age at menopause, number of first-degree relatives with breast cancer, and tobacco use, as well as some less certain ones such as percentage of body fat, exercise, and breast feeding. Early and frequent pregnancies do seem to be associated with a smaller incidence of breast cancer but can hardly be routinely recommended. Prophylactic mastectomies are sometimes performed but only under very extreme circumstances.

38. **(C)** Electrical injuries can be deceptively extensive. Aside from the obvious local injury, often extensive distant injury (neurologic, vascular, and muscular) is present. The zone of obvious injury frequently enlarges to a sigificantly greater area over the first 7 to 14 days following the injury. Early debridement is important; however, tissue that appears graftable (and may well support a graft initially) frequently progresses to necrosis. It is the knowledge of this natural history of electrical injuries that makes most surgeons cautious about early coverage of wounds. While occasionally necessary to avoid compressive injury to deep tissues, fasciotomies should not be done routinely, but the need for them must be constantly kept in mind. Likewise, amputations should not be a routine procedure but may need to be done as the tissue necrosis or functional loss dictates. The extensive injury frequently causes myonecrosis, and urine should be checked routinely for myoglobin. If myoglobinuria is present, fluid resuscitation should be aggressive to maintain a good urine output and the urine alkalinized to minimize the precipitation in the kidney and resultant renal insufficiency.

39. **(E)** All the listed problems can be complications in electrical burn patients. Fractures occur secondary to falling at the time of the electrical injury.

40. **(B)** Secondary dysmenorrhea is associated with a variety of organic causes such as endometriosis, adenomyosis, and leiomyomata, and tends to occur later in reproductive life. Primary dysmenorrhea, a condition associated with ovulatory cycles, is due to myometrial contractions induced by prostaglandins originating in secretory endometrium, and begins with regular menses. With an increased production of prostaglandins, associated symptoms may include headache, nausea, vomiting, backache, and diarrhea. Nonsteroidal anti-inflammatory drugs (NSAIDs) are usually very effective treatment, particularly if started prior to the onset of symptoms. She also has infertility, with a 5-year history of no contraceptive use. However, as she is multigravid, it would be characterized as secondary infertility.

41. **(D)** Endometriosis is a term indicating ectopic endometrial glands and stroma. Its incidence is 3 to 10% of reproductive-age women. It should be suspected in all women complaining of infertility. Other common symptoms include dysmenorrhea (especially following a period of pain-free menses), deep thrust dyspareunia, and dyschezia. Most patients with leiomyomata are asymptomatic. Adenomyosis is not usually associated with infertility. Salpingitis is not usually a cause of dysmenorrhea.

42. **(B)** The definitive treatment for endometriosis is TAH BSO. Surgical ablation using the cautery or CO_2 laser is used as a conservative therapy to remove as much of the endometriotic tissue as possible, return the pelvic anatomy to normal, and hopefully restore fertility. Hormonal therapy of endometriosis, aimed at pain relief, has been successfully accomplished using GnRH agonists, progestational agents, combined oral contraceptives, and danazol. Endometrial ablation of the uterine cavity would not be effective in treating ectopic inflammation of endometriosis.

43. **(C)** The general guidelines depend mainly on weight. At 20 pounds, children may sit facing the front of a car. Above 60 pounds, they may use an adult lap/shoulder belt alone. At 60 pounds and a height of over 48 inches, they use a lap/shoulder belt on the normal seat of the car.

44. **(C)** This readily available analgesic and antipyretic is a classic example of an intrinsic, dose-dependent hepatotoxin, causing zonal necrosis and acute liver failure, often associated with renal failure. Significant liver injury usually occurs with doses in excess of 10 to 15 g, most frequently taken in a suicide attempt. Within a few hours, the patient develops nausea, vomiting, and diarrhea; a relatively asymptomatic period ensues. Clinical and laboratory signs of liver damage become evident within 10 hours of acetaminophen ingestion.

45. **(A)** The initial treatment of acetaminophen overdose consists of supportive measures and gastric lavage. Acetylcysteine should be administered to high-risk patients, in whom it may significantly reduce the severity of liver necrosis and its attendant mortality. This agent appears to act mainly by providing cysteine for glutathione synthesis and is most effective when given within 10 hours of acetaminophen ingestion.

46. **(A)** As is the case with premature labor, an accurate estimate of gestational age is extremely important in providing optimal care. The majority of pregnancies believed to be beyond 42 menstrual weeks are actually less far advanced.

47. **(A)** These fetal conditions result in low levels of dehydroisoandrosterone production by the fetal adrenals. Low levels of this precursor result in decreased estrogen production.

48. **(D)** Amniotic fluid volume normally falls after 38 weeks of gestation and oligohydramnios is recognized as an indicator of an increased risk of fetal distress. Meconium-stained amniotic fluid is also more common in postdate pregnancy and presents a poor prognosis for vaginal delivery. An increase in fetal macrosomia and the resulting increase in shoulder dystocia are well-established complications of postdate pregnancy.

49. **(B)** This description of a newborn with rapid respirations and no other major findings suggests transient tachypnea of the newborn (TTN) or persistent postnatal pulmonary edema. Not all infants have tachypnea, and some may have the fluid enter the lungs postnatally. There may be cyanosis, which clears with supplemental oxygen. TTN usually resolves by day 3 or 4. Abnormal breath sounds and radiographs will help diagnose the other conditions.

50. **(B)** Polymyalgia rheumatica (PMR), the most likely diagnosis in this patient, is characterized by aching and morning stiffness in the shoulder and hip girdles, the proximal extremities, the neck, and the torso. Fatigue, sense of weakness, loss of weight, and a low-grade fever may be present. A moderate normochromic normocytic anemia is typical. Usually, the erythrocyte sedimentation rate is elevated.

51. **(D)** This disease affects large and medium-sized arteries, especially those branching from the proximal aorta that supply the neck and the extracranial structure of the head. Temporal artery biopsy shows a granuloma-

tous inflammatory infiltrate. Visual symptoms are present in about one third of patients. Permanent visual loss may be partial or complete and may occur without warning.

52. **(A)** HIV is an important part of the evaluation of any patient being seen for STDs. Persons with a documented seroconversion to syphilis using a nontreponemal test (such as VDRL) of less than one year's duration; a fourfold or greater increase in titer of a nontreponemal test; history of symptoms of primary or secondary syphilis; or a sex partner with primary, secondary, or latent syphilis (documented independently as duration of less than 1 year) are classified as having *early latent syphilis.* They should be treated with a single dose of benzathine penicillin G, 2.4 million units IM. Late latent syphilis is treated with three doses of benzathine penicillin G, 2.4 million units IM, each a week apart.

53. **(D)** Mohs' chemosurgery was developed to allow the ablative surgeon to assess the margins of excision as the lesion is being excised. Its best uses are for difficult lesions situated in critical areas (eg, eyelids, canthal areas, nose, etc.), where the least amount of excision that will provide adequate margin is needed. Morphemic basal cell carcinomata are notorious for their treacherously infiltrative spread and high recurrence rate. A morphemic basal cell carcinoma in the medial canthal region is an excellent situation in which to use the Mohs' technique. All the other lesions described can be handled well with standard surgical excision with frozen section, permanent pathologic control, or both.

54. **(A)** Bronchiectasis is defined as a permanent abnormal dilatation of large bronchi due to destruction of the wall. It is a consequence of inflammation, usually an infection. Other causes include toxins or immune response. Persistent cough and purulent sputum production are the hallmark symptoms.

55. **(B)** Kartagener syndrome consists of situs inversus (with dextrocardia), bronchiectasis, and nasal polyps. The bronchiectasis results from impaired ciliary function.

56. **(A)** Bronchography has been superseded by CT scan in defining the extent of bronchiectasis. Occasionally, advanced cases of saccular bronchiectasis can be diagnosed by routine chest x-ray. The use of high-resolution CT scanning, in which images are 1.5 mm thick, has resulted in excellent diagnostic accuracy.

57. **(A)** Antibiotics and postural drainage might be included in therapy. The choise of antimicrobial agents is guided by the sputum culture, but ampicillin and tetracycline are used if normal flora are found. The general principles of therapy include eliminating underlying problems, improved clearance of secretions, control of infections, and reversal of airflow obstruction.

58. **(B)** Immediate internal fixation provides the best opportunity for rapid recovery and avoidance of complications due to long enforced bedrest, necessary for the other treatments.

59. **(C)** A new influenza vaccine is issued annually by the CDC, incorporating influenza strains that are predicted, via epidemiologic forecasting, to be important pathogens in the coming flu season. In order to be maximally protected from the flu each year, annual vaccination is recommended for the elderly, others at risk of serious influenza complications, and individuals who work in long-term care facilities and other settings where they are in close contact with individuals at risk. Hepatitis B vaccine is administered in three sequential doses and confers life-long immunity. Pneumococcal vaccine is multivalent and provides long-term protection against the most common strains of pneumococcus; annual boosters are not needed. Inoculation with tetanus toxoid is recommended every 10 years, in combination with a diphtheria booster. BCG immunization is a questionably effective vaccine for preventing tuberculosis

and it is not generally used in this country (see Figure 6.7).

60. **(E)** The definition of cerebral palsy (CP) concentrates on the nonprogressive motor defects, not intelligence. While many children have no known cause, some will have a history notable for events such as meningitis, maternal drug use, head trauma, and asphyxia. Two main groups, spastic and nonspastic CP, correlate somewhat with the location of the brain defects: Spastic CP involves the motor cortex, nonspastic in the other areas. Associated disabilities include strabismus, feeding and speech disorders, motor disabilities, constipation, orthopedic deformities, and behavior difficulties.

61. **(A)** Trimethoprim–sulfamethoxazole is an effective means of preventing PCP in persons with HIV infection. AZT is an antiretroviral drug that could slow the general progression of HIV disease, thereby decreasing the risk of PCP, but it is not a specific prophylaxis against PCP. The other treatments listed each have specific prophylactic indications other than in HIV disease, including the following examples: penicillin to prevent bacterial endocarditis in individuals with valvular heart disease, and rifampin to prevent meningococcal disease in close contacts of individuals with meningococcal meningitis or meningococcemia.

62. **(B)** Because PCP is a common opportunistic infection in individuals with HIV and it has a high case-fatality rate, prophylaxis to prevent PCP can significantly prolong the life of HIV-infected individuals. Prevalence is a product of both the incidence and duration of illness, so increasing the life expectancy of infected people will increase the prevalence. By itself, a change in life expectancy will not affect *incidence* of the disease (ie, the rate at which individuals become infected). Without prophylaxis, PCP is often the first opportunistic infection a person with HIV experiences, marking their transition to AIDS. Preventing PCP will generally postpone the first AIDS-defining condition, and will therefore *decrease* the incidence of AIDS.

63. **(B)** When the AIDS case definition (or that of any chronic, progressive disease) is broadened, individuals will be counted as having the condition earlier in the course of their illness. The number of cases of the disease will rise acutely just after the definition changes, but it will soon return to previous levels, because the change in definition has no actual effect on the rate at which individuals become infected; it just changes the point at which they are counted. Unless something happens to change the course of the illness, the prevalence of the disease will parallel the incidence, rising abruptly just after the change in case definition and then returning

Age	Vaccine/Toxoid						
	Influenza	Pneumococcal	Measles	Mumps	Rubella	Varicella	Td[1]
18–24			X	X	X	X	X
25–64			X[2]	X	X[3]	X	X
65	X	X				X	X

[1]Td = Tetanus and diphtheria toxoids, adsorbed (for adult use), which is a combined preparation containing < 2 flocculation units of diphtheria toxoid.

[2]One dose for all persons born in 1957 or later, two doses for health care workers, college students, travelers born in 1957 or later.

[3]Those born after 1956.

Figure 6.7. Vaccines and toxoids recommended for adults, by age groups, United States.

to its baseline rate of growth. Even without any advances in treatment, an expansion of the case definition will lead to an apparent increase in the life expectancy of infected individuals: The individual will carry the diagnosis of AIDS for a longer time, by picking it up earlier, rather than by living longer. Because changes in case definitions and advances in treatment often take place at the same time, the effects on incidence and prevalence are rarely as clear-cut as this example, but it is important to remember the artifactual changes produced by different ways of counting cases. Otherwise, treatment effects may be perceived as being more or less significant than they really are.

64. **(E)** Sinus arrhythmia is often related to respiratory phases, with speeding of the heart during inspiration and slowing during expiration. Both phasic and nonphasic forms of sinus arrhythmia are especially common in children and require no treatment.

65. **(B)** Both estradiol and progesterone inhibit gonadotropin (FSH and LH) secretion, except during the preovulatory phase of the cycle. During this phase, rising estradiol levels reaching a certain threshold (typically over 300 pg/mL) lead to a positive feedback on LH secretion. This positive feedback in turn results in a rapid rise in LH, leading to ovulation.

66. **(B)** The normal pH of the vagina is 3.5 to 4.2 in women of reproductive age. Exposure to semen, menstrual blood, and vaginal infections typically raises the pH of the vagina.

67. **(C)** The patient is in severe respiratory distress. Sending him for any study is not indicated until his condition can be stabilized.

68. **(C)** All findings presented are consistent with the presence of a left-sided tension pneumothorax. The emergent treatment this patient requires is chest tube insertion.

69. **(A)** The patient has received no prior fluid resuscitation. Whereas uncrossmatched blood

may eventually be indicated, vigorous crystalloid fluid infusion is appropriate at this point.

70. **(B)** Uncrossmatched blood is now indicated, but crystalloid infusion should be continued, pending the availability of blood.

71. **(E)** Low probability exists for tamponade. Pericardiocentesis is not indicated in this situation.

72. **(B)** This presentation is characteristic of primary pulmonary hypertension. Pulmonary veno-occlusive disease is much less common. The predominant pathology, plexogenic arteriopathy, is characterized by medial hypertrophy associated with laminar intimal fibrosis and plexiform lesions. The thrombotic arteriopathy is characterized by eccentric intimal fibrosis with medial hypertrophy, fibroelastic intimal pads in the arteries and arterioles, and evidence of old recanalized thrombi. There is a female predominance, and the third or fourth decade is the most common age at presentation. By the time of diagnosis, the pulmonary hypertension is usually severe.

73. **(C)** Open lung biopsy is not required. Pulmonary angiography is usually performed if a lung scan suggests thromboembolic disease. Cardiac catheterization is useful to exclude an underlying cardiac shunt as the cause of the pulmonary hypertension. The pulmonary capillary wedge pressure is normal but can be difficult to obtain.

74. **(D)** Patients frequently are subjected to test doses of a short-acting vasodilator such as intravenous prostacyclin or adenosine, or inhaled nitric oxide. About half of these responders will then respond to high oral doses of nifedipine or diltiazem. Prostacyclin is also available as a treatment, but its applicability is limited by the necessity to administer it as a continuous intravenous infusion.

75. **(D)** The natural history of the disease is unclear because it is asymptomatic for a long

period. Survival from diagnosis is dependent on the functional class of the patient. Functional class IV dyspnea suggests a mean survival of only 6 months. Death is usually the result of either right heart failure or sudden death.

76. **(E)** In the absence of a functioning testis, the sexually indifferent fetus will undergo female differentiation irrespective of the genetic sex of the fetus. The male phenotype occurs because the functioning testis secretes müllerian inhibiting factor and testosterone.

77. **(D)** Stranger anxiety occurs as part of normal child development and appears when the child has some capacity for mental representation. The development of stranger anxiety is not related to the amount of time a mother spends with her child and is not related to the child's ability to run away from strangers. Typically, stranger anxiety is stronger toward totally unknown persons than toward more familiar ones. Autistic children lack this developmental marker.

78. **(C)** Stranger anxiety is evidence of the development of a strong attachment bond and usually appears by 7 to 8 months of age.

79. **(D)** Human papillomavirus is the most common viral STD. It clinically presents with vaginal and vulvar warts. Serotypes 6 and 11 are usually associated with vulvovaginal warts. Serotypes HPV-16, -18, -31, and -45 are associated with an increased incidence of cervical neoplasia. The koilocyte is histologically characteristic. They are occasionally confused with condyloma lata.

80. **(A)** Radon is a colorless, odorless, radioactive gas that is found in high concentrations in many homes throughout the United States. It enters the house through the basement slab as a result of radioactive decay in the underlying soil. Radon levels are impossible to predict based on knowledge of average local levels. Levels vary widely even between neighboring houses because of specific geo-

logic configurations. Lead paint is a major problem only if it is old, chipped, or peeling; encasing peeling lead paint (eg, with other paint or drywall) is an adequate means of preventing health effects. Similarly, asbestos is not a problem if it is enclosed within the walls. Volatile organic compounds involved in renovation could have posed a health threat to the workers dealing with them, but because they are volatile, they would not linger long enough in the house to affect the residents' health.

81. **(B)** Second to tobacco smoke, radon is the most significant risk factor for lung cancer in this country. After being inhaled, some of the radon decomposes into particles (referred to as "radon daughters") that remain in the lung, leading to chronic low-level radiation exposure within the lung. Bladder cancer, peripheral neuropathy, and asthma are all associated with environmental exposures: analine dyes, organic peticides, and various irritants and allergens, respectively. There is no known environmental risk factor for subcortical dementia.

82. **(C)** Installation of energy-efficient windows reduces the exchange of air between indoors and outdoors, trapping in the house indoor pollutants, including radon. The other renovations would not have affected the radon hazard but might alter other risks in the indoor environment. If done carelessly, replacing the heating, wiring, and plumbing systems could have led to increased asbestos exposure if the renovation involved disrupting asbestos insulation. Repainting and installing new plumbing would have reduced the likelihood of lead poisoning by covering deteriorating lead-based paint with an intact layer of new paint and by eliminating lead pipes and lead solder.

83. **(D)** For carcinoma of the breast, the appropriate treatment plan is either modified radical mastectomy or lumpectomy, axillary dissection, and irradiation. With the diagnosis of malignancy, it would be inappropriate to

follow this lesion with serial examinations or mammograms. Fine-needle aspiration is accurate if it is interpreted by an experienced cytopathologist. A palpable lesion does not need to be visualized on mammogram to be considered a risk for malignancy. A fibroadenoma is a benign breast mass.

84. **(D)** The most common cause of superior vena cava syndrome is lung cancer, of which 38% are small cell carcinomas. Squamous cell accounts for 20% and lymphomas for about 9%. Other causes include mediastinal fibrosis, thrombosis usually secondary to instrumentation and other malignancies. Diuretics may help ease some of the pressure initially but the patient will require chemotherapy or radiation. Superior vena cava syndrome is an oncologic emergency, but time should still be taken to obtain tissue before instituting any kind of therapy. This is, however, a time for getting radiation and pathology in on a weekend.

85. **(C)** Hypercalcemia is most commonly seen with squamous cell carcinoma. Previously, cancer-related hypercalcemia was divided into "humorally related" and secondary to bone metastasis. It is clear now that hypercalcemia is caused by factors released by the malignant cells that cause bone resorption. A parathyroid-related hormone has been identified. Tumors that secrete this hormone are more resistant to antihypercalcemic drugs.

86. **(C)** Patients with long-standing hypercalcemia can have very few signs or symptoms and agressive intervention is not necessary. Treatment with fluids and furosemide (not hydrochlorothiazide) is often adequate while beginning therapy for the underlying problem. In more resistant cases, especially those associated with parathyroid hormone–releasing hormone (PTHRH), pamidronate can be very useful and some clinicians give it as a routine. Gallium nitrate can be useful in resistant cases. Mithramycin is almost never used because it causes neutropenia and thrombocytopenia, which can interfere with the administration of more active chemotherapeutic agents and because other effective agents are available. There is no role for insulin in these patients.

87. **(E)** Though tetralogy of Fallot is the most common cyanotic heart lesion in patients with congenital heart disease who survive beyond infancy, transposition of the great arteries is the most common cause of cyanosis in the neonate. In this lesion, the aortic root arises from the right ventricle, and the main pulmonary artery arises form the left ventricle. Patent ductus arteriosus is considered a left-to-right shunt, and blood flows from the aorta to the pulmonary artery. It is not a cyanotic heart lesion. Hypoplastic left heart syndrome is incorrect because there is underdevelopment of the entire left heart. Affected patients present with varying degrees of cyanosis and heart failure. Pulmonary hypertension of the newborn describes the persistence of fetal circulation and is characterized by cyanosis and respiratory distress. It is often associated with infection, central nervous system abnormalities, polycythemia, and pulmonary parenchymal disorders.

88. **(B)** Patients with acute gastrointestinal (GI) bleeds may have a normocytic anemia. The red cells are being produced normally until the point at which they are rapidly being lost. Patients who have chronic blood loss via the GI tract usually have a microcytic anemia secondary to iron deficiency. The melena and history of pain suggest a possible longer-term process in addition to the acute one. Thrombocytosis can be seen in patients who are iron deficient but would be unlikely in the face of the consumption process accompanying an acute GI bleed. Leukopenia is not expected in a typical GI bleed.

89. **(B)** Although alcohol has some beneficial effects on platelet function when used in moderation, it is still a very toxic substance to the hematopoietic system. It is directly toxic to both platelets and megakaryocytes. It affects folate and iron metabolism and therefore he-

moglobin production in the red blood cell. Acute alcohol use can cause a decrease in both the number and the function of platelets. If megakaryocyte function is still adequate—usually more an indicator of chronic alcohol intake—the thrombocytopenia will resolve in 3 to 7 days. Chronic heavy use can result in thrombocytopenia lasting many weeks. As heavy alcohol use continues, hepatic dysfunction can cause hypersplenism and thrombocytopenia of a different etiology.

90. **(C)** Five to ten percent of abdominal hysterectomies will develop a wound infection. For wounds that are indurated, tender, or have exudate in a patient who is febrile, the wound should be inspected and, if felt to be infected, the wound should be opened. Wound infections usually occur on the fourth to fifth postoperative days and may be the result of a seroma or a hematoma within the subcutaneous tissue. Any wound that is opened should be explored to ascertain whether the fascia is intact.

91. **(B)** This is a classic presentation for Gaucher's disease. Glucocerebrosides are breakdown products of lipids from the membranes of senescent leukocytes and erythrocytes. The diagnosis can be made on bone marrow biopsy, but there is also now available a beta-glucocerebrosidase level from commercial laboratories. The juvenile form may have neurologic symptoms, including mental retardation, muscle spasticity, and ataxia. This disorder is most commonly seen in Ashkenazi Jews.

92. **(B)** The treatment for Gaucher's used to be supportive. Splenectomy was performed for symptoms. Blood and platelets were transfused as needed. Bone pain was managed with anti-inflammatories and narcotics. When large quantities of alglucerase became available, it altered the approach from watching the patient's gradual decline to intervening and preventing the accumulation of glucocerebrosides and their end-organ damage. Initially, the cost of the therapy exceeded $300,000 per year. Fortunately, newer dosing

recommendations have cut the cost to $100,000 per year, but obviously the cost is still staggering.

93. **(D)** Excisional biopsy is the correct method for diagnosis of this lesion. A shave biopsy is not a good method because the true depth of the lesion cannot be measured accurately. It is the depth of the lesion that affects treatment plan and prognosis. Fine-needle aspiration is not a good method of diagnosing this type of lesion. Lymphoscintigraphy and MRI are imaging studies and will not provide a diagnosis.

94. **(B)** This melanoma is considered a superficial lesion (< 0.76-mm thickness) with a high likelihood of cure. The correct management of this lesion is wide local excision. In this case, a 1-cm margin would be adequate. Regional lymph node dissection is used in situations of more advanced disease, that is, intermediate-thickness lesions (controversial), thick lesions (> 4 mm), limited lymphatic drainage area involved, or clinically positive lymph nodes with no unresectable distant metastases. Melanoma can be radioresistant, and standard radiation therapy is generally used for palliative measures. Chemotherapy is reserved for more advanced lesions.

95. **(A)** Hoarseness secondary to involvement of the recurrent laryngeal nerve is the most common reason for hoarseness in patients with mediastinal tumors. Weight loss in small cell carcinoma is very common, and, although small cell carcinomas can occur in almost any part of the body, it is not necessary in this patient to look further than the lung for a primary site. Further evaluation is indicated as 19 to 38% have bone involvement, 17 to 23% have marrow involvement, up to 14% have brain involvement, and 3 to 11% have soft-tissue involvement at the time of presentation.

96. **(B)** Adrenocorticotropic hormone (ACTH) and ADH are commonly produced by small cell carcinomas, giving typical paraneoplastic syndromes. Small cell carcinomas can also

produce calcitonin and chromogranin A, but no paraneoplastic syndrome has been described for these. GHRH production has been reported in pancreatic and bronchial carcinoids but has not been documented in small cell carcinoma. Insulin can be produced by endocrine tumors of the pancreas, erythropoietin by renal cell tumors, and OAF by myelomas.

97. **(D)** This form of mental retardation accounts for 40% of X-linked mental retardation involving 4 to 5 per 10,000 males. About one third of female carriers are reported as slow. These patients may exhibit signs of autism. Reports state that a significant percentage of males with autism have fragile X syndrome. Patients with William syndrome have growth delay, mental retardation, stellate iris, hypoplastic nails, supravalvular aortic stenosis, and characteristic facies. XXY syndrome, or Klinefelter syndrome (seminiferous tubule dysgenesis), is associated with mental retardation in some cases. These patients are tall males with small, firm testes and poorly developed secondary sexual characteristics.

98. **(D)** Cervical cytopathology is a screening technique, which, when done on a regular basis, may detect cervical disease at a preinvasive stage to allow treatment of premalignant disease. It has a reported false-negative rate of 10 to 20%. It should be performed at age 18 or when a woman becomes sexually active and continued throughout life.

99. **(D)** HPV genotypes have been found in up to 95% of high-grade dysplasias or cervical cancers. HIV may decrease the time interval of progression due to changes in immunocompetence. HSV-2 is associated with dysplasia but not as strongly as HPV.

100. **(E)** Glandular abnormalities tend to be more aggressive than squamous abnormalities and should be evaluated without delay. Glandular cells could arise from either the endometrium or the endocervix; thus, endometrial biopsy should be added to the evaluation unless there is an obvious lesion at colposcopy.

101. **(D)** Repeat Pap smears done earlier than 3 months tend to have a high false-negative rate and cannot be relied on. Indications for cervical conization include neoplasia on biopsy with unsatisfactory colposcopy (entire lesion or transition zone not seen); neoplasia on endocervical curettage; significant discrepancy between Pap smear and colposcopically directed biopsy (apparent diagnosis on Pap smear more than one step worse than biopsy); and microinvasive squamous cell cancer on biopsy. Her incontinence symptoms are of the "urge" rather than the "stress" variety and are unlikely to be improved by surgery.

102. **(C)** Circumstantiality is marked by long-windedness that is goal directed. Tangentiality is a type of speech reflecting thoughts that may be related to the question in an oblique way, but in which the goal of speech is never reached. Word salad is a pattern of speech that is incomprehensible. Derailment consists of a thought pattern resulting in speech in which ideas slip off the track onto a completely different track. Klang associations are groupings of similar sounding or rhyming words.

103. **(C)** MRIs generally provide better resolution than CTs but are more expensive. The risk of CT scans is of radiation exposure, whereas that of MRI scans is of exposure to a strong electromagnetic field. Because of the strength of the electromagnetic field, MRI scans are contraindicated in patients with implanted cardiac pacemakers.

104. **(E)** The correct answer is the distal femur and proximal tibial epiphyses, cuboid, and proximal humeral epiphysis.

105. **(C)** The concept of a tort is generally not well understood among physicians beyond its ability to cause sleepless nights. In general, a tort requires that an obligation or duty exists, that the duty was abrogated, that an injury occurred, and that the injury resulted from the abrogation of that duty. This need not be shown "beyond a reasonable doubt," the

standard for criminal cases, but the conclusion must be supported by the preponderance of the evidence; that is, it is "more likely than not." While the legal definition is relatively straightforward, its application in reality is rarely that clear. Physicians must keep in mind that attorneys are trained to act as advocates for their clients, and they may in turn be judged guilty of legal malpractice if they do not assume this role. The circumstances of any given case are not always clear, and therefore an effective advocate will always attempt to shade those events in a manner that benefits his or her client. Furthermore, there is nothing unique to medicine about this issue—an explosion of litigation has affected all aspects of American life, from the corporate boardroom to the Little League field. Physicians must learn to treat these issues objectively, rather than taking all cases personally, if they hope to survive in the current climate and hopefully alter the process for the future.

106. **(D)** Sadly, being named in a malpractice suit is a fate that awaits most clinicians. Open and honest communication with the patient, competent practice, and meticulous documentation will minimize the practitioner's risk, but nothing can eliminate it altogether. The strategies mentioned will also enhance the ability of the physician to aid in his or her defense should a case be brought. Excessive ordering of tests and consults may well work against the practitioner. Higher costs will bring these practices to the attention of third-party payers, and generally reflect negatively on the individual physician and medicine in general.

107. **(D)** The patient should feel that you are concerned and interested in her, not her symptoms. While she may well be depressed or have a somatization disorder or hypochondriasis, it is much too abrupt to tell her she should see a psychiatrist. She will likely feel discounted and think that you are telling her that "nothing is wrong" with her or that "it is all in her head" when she knows she is suffering.

108. **(C)** Domestic violence, including physical, sexual, and/or emotional abuse, is common and physicians should routinely ask all female patients specifically about abuse. Domestic violence impacts significantly upon the victim's physical and mental health. Many complaints, nonspecific complaints, and repeated injuries should alert the physician to the possibility that an individual is being mistreated at home. Cancer or an infection would most likely be identified on the physical examination or in the laboratory tests. The presence of chronic medical complaints is not typical of mental retardation.

109. **(E)** Kübler-Ross conceptualized five stages experienced by people when they receive news of a fatal illness: shock and denial, anger, bargaining, depression, and acceptance. These stages are widely encountered and may help the clinician to better understand the patient, although individuals do not necessarily experience all stages, nor do reactions necessarily follow a strict sequence.

110. **(C)** CT scan is not always accurate to predict which lesions are resectable. The operability of a gastric tumor is best determined at surgical exploration. All of the other statements are correct.

111. **(A)** Patients with achlorhydria (pernicious anemia and chronic atrophic gastritis) are at increased risk of developing gastric cancer. Adenomatous gastric polyps can be precursors of cancer, and some evidence exists implicating the formation of nitrosamines from nitrates in the cause of gastric cancer. The incidence of gastric cancer is greater in lower socioeconomic groups.

112. **(D)** The use of psychotropic medications, especially phenothiazines, may result in an extrapyramidal syndrome, manifested by parkinsonian symptoms, such as rigidity, tremor, and akinesia. Parkinsonian symptoms can be treated during continued medication use and are reversible upon discontinuation of the medication. Echopraxia is the pathological imitation of movements of one

person by another. Catatonia is defined as abnormal motor behavior associated with an abnormal mental state and is classified as excited, stuporous, rigid, or posturing. Catatonia should resolve with neuroleptic medication use. A pyramidal system disorder is not a defined disorder.

113. **(D)** Schizophrenia has a better prognosis in married patients who have had an acute onset of an illness with affective symptoms or a clouded sensorium and who have no family history of schizophrenia. Patients with a positive family history of schizophrenia, however, fall into the poor-prognosis group of schizophrenic patients.

114. **(B)** At times of great external stress, such as the impending death of a family member, family conflicts may intensify. Reevaluation and changes in family member roles, as well as changes in patterns of maintaining discipline, are commonly seen. Psychotic episodes are not common.

115. **(A)** Patients with growth hormone deficiency will have satisfactory growth in the first year of life as they react to insulin. Then the growth curve flattens as the failure of the growth hormone takes effect.

116. **(A)** Opiate intoxication causes pupillary constriction. Pupillary constriction is not seen in other intoxication states.

117. **(D)** Naloxone is an opioid antagonist and will acutely reverse opiate intoxication. Naloxone must be used with caution in order to avoid causing severe opiate withdrawal symptoms. Methadone is an opiate itself and thus will not reverse heroin intoxication. Cocaine acts on different receptors than opiates and thus will not reverse opiate intoxication. Similarly, alcohol does not reverse the effects of heroin. Clonidine suppresses the autonomic signs of opiate withdrawal and thus is used to ease the discomfort of opiate withdrawal.

118. **(A)** Methadone is an opiate with a longer half-life than heroin that does not produce the euphoria of heroin. Methadone can be taken once per day, and its dosage may be decreased gradually without an abrupt change in blood level. Methadone treatment programs can be extremely effective in allowing an individual to overcome heroin addiction and repair his or her life. Disulfiram, or Antabuse, is used to treat alcohol abuse. Olanzapine is an antipsychotic used to treat psychotic disorders, such as schizophrenia. Naloxone is an opiate antagonist used to acutely reverse opiate intoxication. Clonidine is an antiadrenergic agent used to treat symptoms of opioid, alcohol, and nicotine withdrawal.

119. **(B)** Surfactant is a mixture of phospholipids and proteins, and appears in the amniotic fluid at approximately 30 weeks' gestation. It reduces surface tension in the air spaces of the lung. When there is a deficiency, as in premature infants, surface tension is high at the interface between alveolar gas and the alveolar wall. This results in progressive atelectasis and the development of hyaline membrane disease. Alpha-1-antitrypsin deficiency is an inherited autosomal recessive condition that involves the lungs and liver of affected patients. Peripheral eosinophils are low in all newborns. Mast cells are specialized cells that play a role in atopic diseases. Elastin is a yellow, elastic, fibrous mucoprotein that is found in the connective tissue of elastic structures. It may be overproduced in patients with Hurler syndrome.

120. **(B)** Figure 6.3 demonstrates a pneumoperitoneum that indicates the patent has a perforated viscus. This is a surgical emergency, and the patient should be taken to the operating room for an exploratory laparotomy. Hydration and antibiotics are important in the management of this patient, but each alone would be inappropriate. In view of the perforated viscus, further diagnostic studies are not warranted.

121. (B) Approximately 95% of ulcers are located in the duodenal bulb. Cigarette smoking has been associated with duodenal ulcers. NSAIDs are associated with ulcer development. *Helicobacter pylori* infection is implicated in gastric and duodenal ulcers. Duodenal ulcers are more common in men than in women.

122. (E) The causes of splenomegaly include hemolytic disease (thalassemia, spherocytosis), inflammatory and infectious diseases (malaria, subacute bacterial endocarditis, tuberculosis, lupus), and malignancy (leukemia, lymphoma, Hodgkin's disease). Except for neuroblastoma, few solid malignancies metastasize to the spleen. Wilms' tumors are felt to arise from the metanephric blastema. (See Figure 6.8.)

123. (E) The boy has absence seizures, also called petit mal. They begin most commonly in children and often present as learning difficulties. There is not generalized convulsive muscular activity. The drug of choice is valproic acid.

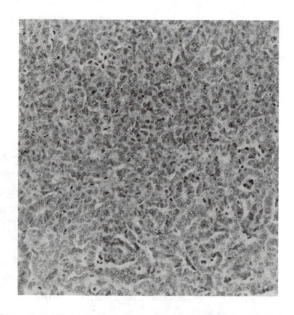

Figure 6.8. Wilms' tumor with characteristic tubular/glomerulid structures and blastema (original magnification, × 40).

124. (A) Valproic acid can be used in a variety of situations, although it is usually the first drug used in absence seizures. It causes little sedation or change in cognitive ability. Drug levels as well as CBCs and liver enzymes should be monitored intermittently during treatment, but it has no significant renal toxicity.

125. (E) Febrile seizures occur after the onset of a fever in susceptible infants. It classically lasts a few minutes, with no abnormality of the neurologic exam when the patient awakens. If the patient looks well, there is no need to investigate the cause of the seizure—this time. Observation is required to ensure that the patient remains well. Treatment and laboratory testing are dependent on the philosophy of the doctors.

126. (B) Disulfiram (Antabuse) inhibits the enzyme acetaldehyde dehydrogenase, resulting in toxic acetaldehyde accumulation 15 to 30 minutes after alcohol consumption. Common symptoms include nausea, vomiting, tachycardia, dyspnea, skin flushing, diaphoresis, headache, and anxiety. The usual dose is 250 to 500 mg/day. Patients should be aware that they may react to even small amounts of alcohol present in food, mouthwash, and over-the-counter medications.

127. (D) The patient was undergoing aversion therapy in which the subject's undesirable behavior (drinking alcohol), was being coupled with an unpleasant stimulus (an emetic agent). This is a form of behavior therapy. Antabuse is frequently used to establish an aversive reaction to alcohol by inducing nausea and other unpleasant effects when alcohol is consumed. Antabuse blocks the oxidation of alcohol at the acetaldehyde stage, causing toxic accumulation of acetaldehyde. Abreaction is the process of bringing to consciousness a painful experience or conflict and reliving the painful emotions, with the goal of providing relief and gaining insight. Confrontation is a psychotherapeutic intervention in which the therapist makes the patient aware of a feeling that the patient was denying or suppressing. Psychoanalytic psychotherapy, first developed by Sigmund Freud, involves free association of thoughts and feelings during the course of intensive treatment in order to bring to consciousness repressed fears and conflicts. Masochism is not a type or technique of psychotherapy.

128. **(B)** Typical bean-shaped gram-negative diplococci are clearly seen within polymorphonuclear leukocytes in a Gram stain of the urethral exudate. This finding is consistent with a diagnosis of gonorrhea.

129. **(E)** Manifestations of mild salicylate poisoning include vomiting, tachycardia, hyperpnea, fever, tinnitus, lethargy, confusion, respiratory alkalosis, and an alkaline urine (pH > 6). In severe poisoning, convulsions, coma, and respiratory and cardiovascular failure may occur. Vomiting, poor intake, and hyperventilation may cause severe dehydration, acute renal failure, and acidosis.

130. **(E)** Emergency and supportive measures should include, first and foremost, protection of the airway, with endotracheal intubation if necessary. Oxygen should be administered as indicated by arterial blood gas analysis. Parenteral fluids, not oral, should be given to produce a brisk urine flow, though care should be taken to avoid the development of pulmonary edema. Prolongation of the prothrombin time should be corrected with intravenous vitamin K. The subcutaneous route should not be used in this critically ill patient, given the relatively slow and possible erratic absorption time inherent for this method of administration. If bleeding is an acute problem, plasma products should be used to correct the coagulopathy. Dialysis is not a useful intervention, nor is methylene blue, for aspirin overdose.

131. **(C)** Minimal dehydration (3 to 5%) is characterized by dry mucous membranes and thirst. Moderate dehydration (5 to 7%) includes loss of fluid around the eyes and dry skin, which may tent. The patient with severe dehydration will have tachycardia, oliguria, and marked decrease in skin turgor.

132. **(A)** A patient with a recent onset of urinary incontinence, especially if it is associated with urgency, should be evaluated for a urinary tract infection. Dysuria as a symptom of urinary tract infection is often absent in elderly women. If this is negative, then proceeding with a more in-depth work-up would be appropriate.

133. **(E)** In a 70-year-old woman who is asymptomatic with mild pelvic relaxation, the most appropriate and prudent approach would be observation. Since the damage is to endopelvic fascia, exercise would not reverse the relaxation. A pessary would provide some support but does have problems such as ulceration and is therefore not without some risk.

134. **(C)** As few as two drinks a day may produce these defects. All pregnant women should avoid alcohol. These patients with fetal alcohol syndrome also may have developmental delay, mental retardation, and hyperactivity.

135. **(B)** Prior surgery on the neck, especially thyroid surgery, accounts for the greater majority of hypoparathyroidism in adults. Injury to, or removal of, the parathyroid glands is the cause.

136. **(D)** The signs of hypothyroidism in the newborn are absent or subtle. Some may have prolonged jaundice, transient hypothermia, enlarged posterior fontanel, or respiratory distress. (The normal values are $T_4 > 6$ U/dL and TSH, 20 U/mL). In this case, the high TSH indicates that the thyroid is not responding to the stimulus of TSH. The state programs select out the lower 10% of the babies for further study so that they can detect the rare case before brain damage takes place.

137. **(B)** Depressed patients typically show "reduced REM latency," a shorter time from the onset of sleep until the first REM period.

138. **(A)** Informed consent requires that the physician relate sufficient information to the patient in order to allow him or her to decide if the procedure is acceptable in light of its risks and benefits. The consent process contains three elements: information, competence, and voluntariness. Consent forms must not substitute for physician–patient dialogue, and informed consent must be freely given, not induced in a frenzied situation. The patient's age or anxiety regarding the procedure do not affect the need to obtain informed consent.

139. **(D)** The patient described is in a deep transverse arrest with asynclitism. Presuming that the prerequisites for a forceps delivery are met, this would be best handled by using the Kielland forceps first, with correction of asynclitism, taking advantage of the sliding lock, then a rotation around the axis of the shaft of the instrument. The Kielland lacks a pelvic curve; therefore, the instrument is directly rotated on its shaft. The Scanzoni maneuver requires the handles to be rotated in a wide arc so that the axis of the rotation in the vagina is made parallel to the axis of the pelvic curve. The Simpson's forceps are preferable to the Tucker–McLean forceps because the fenestrated blade of the Simpson's is less prone to slipping during rotation.

140. **(D)** New onset of back pain in an older man with a normocytic anemia is myeloma until proven otherwise. It is hard to know when to worry about someone with chronic back pain, although most end up with a serum protein electrophoresis (SPEP) at some point. Most clinicians would probably order iron, B_{12}, and folate levels, but they are not going to answer the question of his back pain. Myeloma is associated with lytic lesions, and therefore if any radiologic study is ordered, it should be a skeletal survey.

141. **(B)** Eighty percent of patients with myeloma will have a monoclonal spike on SPEP. Performing a urine protein electrophoresis will pick up an additional 10%, but about 10% of myelomas will be completely nonsecreting.

142. **(E)** Manipulation of the spine in patients with potentially lytic lesions is absolutely contraindicated. Strontium is helpful in treating refractory blastic lesions but not very helpful in lytic lesions. NSAIDs and radiation are often used to control the pain associated with the bony lesions. Dexamethasone is used alone and in combination with other chemotherapeutic agents to treat myeloma. Methotrexate is not one of the active agents in this disease. Calcium supplementation and exercise are reasonable and benign interventions but are not as useful as pamidronate. Pamidronate has been shown to decrease fractures in patients with stage II and III myeloma, resulting in an improved quality of life and possibly an improved survival time.

143. **(E)** This sign is elicited by pulling the hand across the chest wall to the opposite shoulder. In a 28-week-old newborn, the elbow can reach the other shoulder. At 32 weeks, there is some resistance. At 36 weeks, the elbow just passes the midline, and in full-term babies, the elbow does not reach the midline. The other features of the Dubowitz tests are posture, heel-to-ear maneuver, popliteal angle, dorsiflexion angle of the foot, and return to flexion of the forearm.

144. **(A)** Injuries are a major cause of morbidity and mortality in both the young and the old, but the specific distribution of injury types is very different at different stages in the life cycle. In the elderly, falls account for most injury morbidity and mortality. Factors that put older adults at risk for falls include visual impairment, osteoporosis, and medication side effects such as orthostatic hypotension. Burns are also common among the elderly, but less common than falls. Poisoning is more prevalent among small children, whose curiosity exceeds their good sense. The highest incidence of attempted suicide and motor vehicle accidents is in the adolescent and early adult years, though motor vehicle–related injuries (including pedestrian accidents) remain an important cause of death and disability throughout life.

145. **(E)** It is important to recognize when a patient is depressed and ask more about the patient's feelings of hopelessness, including directly asking him or her about suicide. There is time for investigation and treatment of premature ejaculation, alcoholism, difficulty at work, and marital conflict—but not if the patient is already dead.

146. **(D)** Obtaining help and an adequate number of personnel, including assistance, anesthesia, and a pediatrician, is the first step in managing shoulder dystocia, and the distended bladder should be drained. If there is any possibility of perineal resistance, an episiotomy should be widened. The next step should be suprapubic pressure provided by the assistant as gentle downward traction applied to the fetal head. The McRoberts maneuver is the next step. If these are unsuccessful, then the Woods' screw and delivery of the posterior arm, followed by intentional fractures of the clavicle or the Zavenelli maneuver, are appropriate.

147. **(C)** Akathisia, a pattern of involuntary movements such as fidgety hands, rocking at the waist, and shifting from foot to foot, is a common side effect of antipsychotic medications. In addition to akathisia, acute dystonic reaction, Parkinson-like syndrome, and tardive dyskinesia are the major extrapyramidal side effects of antipsychotic medications. Akathisia may be confused with agitation and often does not respond to antiparkinsonian agents used in the treatment of other extrapyramidal side effects, causing it to be a particularly troublesome side effect. Automatism is a symptom of temporal lobe epilepsy in which patients perform repetitive well-organized movements. The term *akinesia* refers to the loss of normal muscular tonicity or responsiveness, resulting in slowness and fatigue. Akinesia is a parkinsonian symptom. As mentioned, akathisia can be confused with agitation but, in this patient, the classic signs of akathisia are present and the patient is treated with a neuroleptic. The term *apraxia* refers to the inability to make skilled movements with accuracy, a result of disease in the cerebral cortex.

148. **(E)** Positive symptoms of schizophrenia include hallucinations, delusions, bizarre behavior, and marked formal thought disorder. Flat affect, poverty of speech, apathy, and impaired hygiene are negative symptoms of schizophrenia.

149. **(C)** If erections occur in a man while he is asleep, a psychological cause of impotence is likely. Other useful tests to rule out an organic cause are measuring penile blood pressure and testing pudendal nerve latency time. The Minnesota Multiphasic Personality Inventory-2 (MMPI-2) is a nonprojective personality test. The Rorschach (inkblot) test is a projective test. The Wechsler Adult Intelligence Scale–Revised (WAIS-R) is an intelligence test. Skull x-rays can identify fractures in the skull bones.

150. **(B)** Studies have shown that patients and families informed of bad news simultaneously have fewer emotional difficulties. Communicating a diagnosis is best done in private and briefly, leaving the opportunity of ongoing dialogue with the patient and family. Most studies asking whether patients wish to be told the truth about malignancy show an overwhelming desire for truth. There is no need for a psychiatric consultant. Any news is best heard from the physician whom the family knows best.

References

American Psychiatric Association. *Diagnostic and Statistical Manual of Mental Disorders*, 4th ed. Washington, DC: American Psychiatric Association; 1994

American Public Health Association; http://www.apha.org

American Journal of Public Health. Washington, DC: American Public Health Association

Andreasen NC, Black DW. *Introductory Textbook of Psychiatry.* Washington, DC: American Psychiatric Press; 1991

Beckman, Ling, et al. *Obstetrics and Gynecology.* Williams & Wilkins; 1998

Behrman RE, Kliegman RM. *Nelson Essentials of Pediatrics,* 3rd ed. Philadelphia: WB Saunders, 1998

Benenson AS, ed. *Control of Communicable Diseases in Man,* 15th ed. Washington, DC: American Public Health Association; 1990

Benenson AS, ed. *Control of Communicable Diseases Manual,* 16th ed. Washington, DC: American Public Health Association; 1995

Bennett JC, Plum F, eds. *Cecil Textbook of Medicine,* 20th ed. Philadelphia: WB Saunders; 1996

Berek, ed. *Novak's Gynecology,* 11th ed. Williams & Wilkins; 1998

Brunwald E, Isselbacher KJ, Wilson JV. *Harrison's Principles of Internal Medicine,* 13th ed. New York: McGraw-Hill; 1994

Cunningham FG, McDonald PC, Gant NF, eds. *Williams Obstetrics,* 20th ed. Appleton & Lange; 1997

David TJ, ed. *Recent Advances in Pediatrics.* New York: Churchill Livingstone; 1998

DeVita VT Jr, Hellman S, Rosenberg SA. *Cancer Principles & Practice of Oncology,* 5th ed. Philadelphia: Lippincott-Raven; 1997

Evans AS, Kaslow RA, eds. *Viral Infections of Humans: Epidemiology and Control,* 4th ed. New York: Plenum Publishing Corporation; 1997

Gant NF, Cunningham FG, eds. *Basic Obstetrics and Gynecology.* Appleton & Lange; 1993

Goldman HH. *Review of General Psychiatry,* 3rd ed. Norwalk, CT: Appleton & Lange; 1992.

Greenberg RS, et al. *Medical Epidemiology.* Norwalk CT: Appleton & Lange; 1993

Greenfield LJ, Mulholland MW, Oldham KT, Zelenock GB, eds. *Surgery: Scientific Principles and Practice.* Philadelphia: JB Lippincott; 1993

Hatcher RA, et al. *Contraceptive Technology.* New York: Irvington Publishers; 1994

Henretig FM, King C, eds. *Textbook of Pediatric Emergency Procedures.* Baltimore: Williams & Wilkins; 1997

Herbst, Mishell, Stenchever, Droegemueller, eds. *Comprehensive Gynecology,* 2nd ed. St. Louis: CV Mosby, 1992

Institute of Medicine. *America's Vital Interest in Global Health.* Washington, DC: National Academy Press; 1997

Institute of Medicine. *The Hidden Epidemic: Confronting Sexually Transmitted Diseases.* Washington, DC: National Academy Press; 1996

Kaplan HI, Sadock BJ, eds. *Comprehensive Textbook of Psychiatry,* 6th ed. Baltimore: Williams & Wilkins; 1995

Kaplan HI, Sadock BJ. *Kaplan and Sadock's Synopsis of Psychiatry: Behavioral Science/Clinical Psychiatry,* 8th ed. Baltimore: Williams & Wilkins; 1998

Kuzma J. *Basic Statistics for the Health Sciences.* Mountain View, CA: Mayfield Publishing Co; 1984

Last JM, Wallace RB, eds. *Maxcy-Rosenau-Last Public Health and Preventive Medicine,* 3rd ed. Norwalk, CT: Appleton & Lange; 1992

McGinnis JM, Foege WH. Actual causes of death in the United States. *Journal of the American Medical Association,* 270(18):2207–2212; 1993

McKenzie JF, Pinger RR. *An Introduction to Community Health.* Sudbury, MA: Jones & Bartlett Publishers; 1997

Morbidity and Mortality Weekly Report. Atlanta: Centers for Disease Control and Prevention

Morgan JW. *Concise Epidemiology,* 3rd ed. Bryn Mawr, CA: MDM Consulting; 1994

Nyhus LM, Baker RJ, Fischer JE, eds. *Mastery of Surgery,* 3rd ed. Boston: Little, Brown and Co; 1997

Polk HC, Gardner B, Stone HE, eds. *Basic Surgery,* 4th ed. St Louis: Quality Medical Publishing; 1993

Sabiston DC, ed. *Textbook of Surgery: The Biologic Basis of Modern Surgical Practice,* 15th ed. Philadelphia: WB Saunders; 1997

Schwartz SI, Shires GT, Spencer FC, eds. *Principles of Surgery,* 5th ed. New York: McGraw-Hill; 1994

Scientific American Medicine, updated to 1998, Scientific American, Inc., New York

Speroff L, Glass RH, Kase NG, eds. *Clinical Gynecologic Endocrinology and Infertility,* 5th ed. Baltimore: Williams & Wilkins; 1994

Stobo JD, Hellmann DB, Ladenson PW, Petty BG, Traill TA. *The Principles and Practice of Medicine,* 23rd ed. Stamford, CT: Appleton & Lange; 1996

Stoudemire A. *Clinical Psychiatry for Medical Students,* 2nd ed. Philadelphia: JB Lippincott; 1994

Thomas R, Harvey D. *Pediatrics Color Guide,* 2nd ed. New York: Churchill Livingstone; 1997

Tierney LM Jr, McPhee SJ, Papadakis MA. *Current Medical Diagnosis & Treatment,* 37th ed. Stamford, CT: Appleton & Lange; 1998

United States Department of Health and Human Services, Centers for Disease Control and Prevention; http://www.cdc.gov

U.S. Preventive Services Task Force. *Guide to Clinical Preventive Services: Report of the U.S. Preventive Services Task Force,* 2nd ed. Washington, DC: Williams & Wilkins; 1996

Way LW, ed. *Current Surgical Diagnosis and Treatment,* 10th ed. Norwalk, CT: Appleton & Lange, 1994

Wilmore DW, Cheung LY, Harken AH, Holcroft JW, Meakens JL, eds. *American College of Surgeons: Care of the Surgical Patient.* New York: Scientific American; 1998

Credits

Baue AE, Geha AS, Hammond GL, Naunheim KS: *Glenn's Thoracic and Cardiovascular Surgery*, 6th ed. Stamford, CT: Appleton & Lange, 1996. (Figure 4.7)

Feliciano DV, Moore EE, Mattox KL (eds): *Trauma*, 3rd ed. Stamford, CT: Appleton & Lange, 1996. (Figure 3.4)

Goldlist BJ: *Appleton & Lange's Review of Internal Medicine*, 2nd ed. Stamford, CT: Appleton & Lange, 1998. (Figures 3.2, 5.3)

Hansbarger LC: *MEPC: Pediatrics, A USMLE Step 2 Review*, 9th ed., Stamford, CT: Appleton & Lange, 1995. (Figure 4.4)

Hurwitz RM, Hood AF: *Pathology of the Skin: Atlas of Clinical–Pathological Correlation*. Stamford, CT: Appleton & Lange, 1998. (Figures 2.1, 2.6, 2.7, 2.9, 2.10, 2.13, 4.5, 5.6, 6.5, 6.6)

Jacobs SL: *MEPC: Review for the USMLE Step 2*. Stamford, CT: Appleton & Lange, 1996. (Figures 1.2, 1.4, 2.11, 2.12, 3.3, 4.8, 5.4, 6.2, 6.4)

Jenson HB, Baltimore RS: *Pediatric Infectious Diseases: Principles and Practice*. Stamford, CT: Appleton & Lange, 1995. (Figure 3.1)

Metzler MH: *MEPC: Surgery, A USMLE Step 2 Review*, 11th ed. Stamford, CT: Appleton & Lange, 1995. (Figures 5.9, 6.1)

Ross RD: *MEPC: Obstetrics & Gynecology—USMLE Step 2 Review*. Stamford, CT: Appleton & Lange, 1997. (Figure 5.1)

Saunders CE, Ho MT: *Current Emergency Diagnosis & Treatment*, 4th ed. Stamford, CT: Appleton & Lange, 1992. (Figure 6.3)

Skinner HB: *Current Diagnosis & Treatment in Orthopedics*. Stamford, CT: Appleton & Lange, 1995. (Figures 1.3, 3.5)

Stobo JD, Traill TA, Hellmann DB, et al: *The Principles and Practice of Medicine*, 23rd ed. Stamford, CT: Appleton & Lange, 1996. (Figures 2.8, 4.3, 4.6)

Tanagho EA, McAninch JW: *Smith's General Urology*, 14th ed. Stamford, CT: Appleton & Lange, 1995. (Figure 6.8)

Way LW: *Current Surgical Diagnosis & Treatment*, 10th ed. Stamford, CT: Appleton & Lange, 1994. (Figure 5.2)

Zinner MJ: *Maingot's Abdominal Operations*, 10th ed., vols. I and II. Stamford, CT: Appleton & Lange, 1997. (Figures 4.1, 4.2)